Atlas of Pediatric Ultrasound

Atlas of Pediatric Ultrasound

Edited by
Reinhard D. Schulz and Ulrich V. Willi

Contributions by
C.-L. Fawer, I. Forster, I. Gassner, S. Jequier, R. D. Schulz, K. Seitz,
K. Vergesslich and U. V. Willi

1532 illustrations

1992
Georg Thieme Verlag Stuttgart · New York
Thieme Medical Publishers, Inc., New York

Library of Congress Cataloging-in-Publication Data

Atlas der Ultraschalldiagnostik beim Kind.   English.
    Atlas of pediatric ultrasound / edited by Reinhard D.
Schulz and Ulrich V. Willi ; contributions by C.-L.
Fawer ... et al. ; translated by Terry C. Telger.
        p.   cm.
    Translation of: Atlas der Ultraschalldiagnostik
beim Kind.
    Includes bibliographical references and index.
ISBN 3-13-774201-3 (GTV, Stuttgart).--
    ISBN 0-86577-417-X (TMP, New York)
    1. Children--Diseases--Diagnosis--Atlases.
2. Diagnosis, Ultrasonic--Atlases.   I. Schulz,
Reinhard D.
II. Willi, Ulrich V.   III. Title.
    [DNLM: 1. Ultrasonography--in infancy & childhood--
atlases.   WB 17 A8805]
RJ51.U45A75 1991
618.92'007543--dc20
DNLM/DLC
for Library of Congress
                                            91-849
                                            CIP

Translated by Terry C. Telger

This book is an authorized translation of the German edition, published and copyrighted 1990 by Georg Thieme Verlag, Stuttgart, Germany
Title of the German edition:
Atlas der Ultraschalldiagnostik beim Kind

Cover illustration: Paul Klee (1879–1940)
"Büste eines Kindes" ("Bust of a child").
1930 (380), watercolor, 51 × 51 cm.
Paul-Klee-Stiftung in the Kunstmuseum Bern,
© 1989 COSMOPRESS Geneva

© 1992 Georg Thieme Verlag, Rüdigerstrasse 14,
D-7000 Stuttgart 30
Thieme Medical Publishers, Inc., 381 Park Avenue South,
New York, N.Y. 10016
Typesetting by Druckhaus Götz GmbH, D-7140 Ludwigsburg
Printed in Germany by K. Grammlich, D-7401 Pliezhausen

ISBN 3-13-774201-3   (GTV, Stuttgart)
ISBN 0-86577-417-X   (TMP, New York)

Important Note: Medicine is an ever-changing science undergoing continual development. Research and clinical experience are continually expanding our knowledge, in particular our knowledge of proper treatment and drug therapy. Insofar as this book mentions any dosage or application, readers may rest assured that the authors, editors and publishers have made every effort to ensure that such references are in accordance with the state of knowledge at the time of production of the book.

Nevertheless this does not involve, imply, or express any guarantee or responsibility on the part of the publishers in respect of any dosage instructions and forms of application stated in the book. Every user is requested to examine carefully the manufacturers' leaflets accompanying each drug and to check, if necessary in consultation with a physician or specialist, whether the dosage schedules mentioned therein or the contraindications stated by the manufacturers differ from the statements made in the present book. Such examination is particularly important with drugs that are either rarely used or have been newly released on the market. Every dosage schedule or every form of application used is entirely at the user's own risk and responsibility. The authors and publishers request every user to report to the publishers any discrepancies or inaccuracies noticed.

To our families and our teachers

Addresses

Claire-Lise Fawer, M. D.
Division de Neonatologie, Service de Pédiatrie
CHUV
1011 Lausanne
Switzerland

Ishilde Forster, M. D.
Radiologie – Kinderspital
Steinwiesstr. 75
8032 Zürich
Switzerland

I. Gaßner, M. D.
Univ.-Klinik für Kinderheilkunde
Anichstr. 35
6020 Innsbruck
Austria

Sigrid Jequier, M. D.
Department of Radiology, Montreal Children's
Hospital
2300 Tupper Street
Montreal, Quebec H3H 1P3
Canada

R. D. Schulz, M. D.
Leitender Arzt der Abteilung für Ultraschall-
diagnostik und spezielle Radiologie
Olgahospital – Pädiatrisches Zentrum
Bismarckstr. 8
7000 Stuttgart 1
Germany

K. Seitz, M. D.
Kreiskrankenhaus Böblingen, Innere Abteilung
Bunsenstr. 120
7030 Böblingen
Germany

Klara Vergesslich, M. D.
Univ.-Kinderklinik
Währinger Gürtel 18–20
1090 Wien
Austria

U. V. Willi, M. D.
Radiologie – Kinderspital
Steinwiesstr. 75
8032 Zürich
Switzerland

Preface

The concept of this book is that of a "comparative atlas". The morphologic phenomena and criteria presented herein are necessarily limited in their quantity.

We designed this book for colleagues who have a special interest in pediatric ultrasound, our intent being to make available our own case material for scrutiny and comparison. The similarity or dissimilarity of cases in this book to cases that present as "acute" problems may furnish an important diagnostic criterion. A particular case may expand the differential diagnostic spectrum in a given evaluation or may even lead to a diagnosis.

We organized our atlas on the basis of frequently encountered symptoms and typical clinical investigations. By design, then, the case arrangement is not "encyclopedic" and is somewhat arbitrary. It is a result of situations in which the indication for sonography is based not on a defined set of symptoms but on a more complex inquiry (cranial sonography in neonates), of situations that require a differential diagnosis (abnormality on a chest radiograph; hydronephrosis/hydroureter), or of cases requiring a physiologic and pathologic overview (the neonatal and infant hip). Some cases could be placed in various chapters because of their diverse symptoms; generally we took the major or cardinal symptom as our criterion. Where the same cases are illustrated in two or more chapters, a cross-reference is provided in the legend.

Cases that have the same diagnosis but a different morphologic presentation are shown side-by-side. That some legends are quite long reflects our intention to present cases in the context of their history, clinical manifestations, differential diagnosis, and treatment, with occasional references made to discrepancies between the preliminary diagnosis and the condition that was actually found.

The relatively small size of some pictures reflects our intention to use only the informative part of an image. Some images could be reduced without loss of pertinent information. At the same time, a large percentage of the illustrations are full 1:1 reproductions of the original document. In many cases we attempt to present pathologic findings in their anatomic context so that the reader can interpret the image more easily.

Some of the illustrated cases or case groups serve to present a diagnostic concept, A few cases illustrate novel diagnostic criteria.

Because symbols and analogies are helpful in conveying diagnostic insight (the "aha!" experience), and imagination is essential for intuition, we attempted to stimulate the reader's imagination by using the "punk-hairstyle" and "tiger-face" analogies in the first chapter. We do not do this to encourage idle reveries. Often we recognize only what we are looking for, and we tend to look for that which we presume or already know.

In closing, we would like to offer two seemingly contradictory observations: While the more costly technologies of computed tomography and magnetic resonance imaging are desirable and at times indispensable, the more universally available modalities of sonography combined with conventional radiography offer diagnostic capabilities that are adequate in many cases. And although the boundaries of sonography are expanding more and more, the examiner should nevertheless always strive to recognize them for the good of the patient. Especially when functional criteria are essential for a complete diagnosis (urinary system, intestinal tract, biliary tract, cardiovascular system), the diagnostician should not waste time with unrewarding sonographic follow-ups but should make the decision to proceed with the appropriate (functional) examination.

We hope that this book will enrich and invigorate the daily practice of the pediatric diagnostician, providing him or her with occasional help on the path from symptom to diagnosis.

We thank Thieme for their patience and cooperation, and we thank our patients for the illustrative case material.

Stuttgart and Zürich, Summer, 1991   R. D. Schulz
U. V. Willi

Table of Contents

1 Examination of the Brain through the Fontanelle

C.-L. Fawer

The examination of the central nervous system of the newborn infant has changed dramatically over the past 15 years. In the early 1970s, the diagnostic approach to the brain was indirect and relied on clinical examination and special studies such as transillumination, lumbar puncture, and electroencephalography. The introduction of computed tomography (CT) around 1978 and of cerebral sonography around 1980 permitted the direct visualization of brain structures. Ultrasonography (US), initially a research tool, quickly became the modality of first choice for examining the neonatal central nervous system because of its numerous advantages. Today ultrasound is used routinely in the supervision and treatment of infants at increased perinatal risk.

With the introduction of high-frequency (7.5 MHz) and sector transducers, cerebral ultrasound imaging now

- provides an accurate delineation of the main brain structures;
- permits an accurate diagnosis of various lesions (frequency, location, extent, complications, course, possible resolution);
- permits the early detection of cerebral lesions;
- aids in the identification of etiologic and pathogenetic factors.

Several longitudinal studies on the neuropsychologic development of newborns have confirmed the prognostic importance of sonographically detectable brain lesions that are diagnosed in the neonatal period.

Experience gained since 1980 in both the diagnosis and follow-up of cerebral lesions in newborns has enabled us to formulate guidelines for the use of transfontanelle sonography (Table 1.1). The indications for this procedure are diverse. Ultrasound should be used routinely in preterm infants of 34 weeks' gestation or less during the 1st, 2nd, and 3rd weeks of life, because neurologic signs are nonspecific or even absent in this age group. The examination should be performed at bedside in the neonatal unit, proceeding systematically to ensure an accurate evaluation. Small to moderate cerebral hemorrhages generally carry a good prognosis. Intraparenchymal hemorrhages are often associated with dead, and infants who survive are profoundly handicapped. Periventricular leukomalacia (PVL) should be accurately described (extent; frontal, parietal, or occipital location) due to the major prognostic significance of this lesion. A striking correlation has been found between PVL and the type and severity of a subsequent neurodevelopmental handicap. By contrast, it can be quite difficult to interpret the cranial sonogram of a full-term infant with perinatal asphyxia! Some time elapses between anoxia and the appearance of cerebral lesions, and even a normal sonogram does not necessarily confirm the integrity of brain structures.

Cerebral ultrasound also provides the clinician with a very useful diagnostic tool for the detection of lesions associated with antenatal and postnatal infections, of cerebral malformations, and of brain tumors. Like any special investigation of the central nervous system, cerebral sonography should be an integral part of the overall clinical, neurologic, and electroencephalographic workup.

References

Couture, A., L. Cadier: Echographie cérébrale par voie transfontanellaire. Vigot 1983

Fawer, C. L., P. Diebold, A. Calame: Periventricular leucomalacia and neurodevelopmental outcome in preterm infants. Arch. Dis. Childh. 62 (1987) 30–36

Naidich, T. P., R. M. Quencer: Clinical neurosonography. Neuroradiology 28 (1986) 379–641

Peters, H., K.-H. Deeg, D. Weitzel: Die Ultraschall-Untersuchung des Kindes. Springer, Berlin 1987

Acknowledgements

I thank Prof. A. Calame and Prof. E. Gautier for their support, which enabled me to complete this work. Prof. A. Anderegg, Dr. U. Willi, Dr. Milheiro Casimiro, and Dr. A. Goulao kindly provided illustrations form their personal cases files for inclusion in this chapter, helping to make it more complete. Their assistance is gratefully acknowledged. Finally, I would like to express my sincere thanks to M. Marion for typing the manuscript.

Table 1.1 Guidelines for transfontanelle sonography

Indication	Timing	Pathologic findings
Preterm infants ≤ 34 weeks	5th–7th day	Intracranial hemorrhage Periventricular leukomalacia (early stage)
	2nd–3rd week	Periventricular leukomalacia (late stage)
	2nd–4th week	Posthemorrhagic hydrocephalus
Newborns > 34 weeks		
– After perinatal asphyxia	1st–3rd day 3rd–7th day 15th day 1 month	Cerebral edema Early hypoxic/ischemic lesions Late hypoxic/ischemic lesions Cerebral atrophy
– Birth trauma Fractures Cephalhematoma	1st–5th day	Extracerebral fluid collection
– Dysmorphic signs – Chromosome abnormalities		Cerebral malformations Cerebral malformations
– Embryofetopathies		Calcifications, cysts Cerebral ventricular dilatation Lissencephaly
– Intrauterine growth retardation with micro- cephaly		Calcifications, cysts (fetopathies) Vascular malformations (periven- tricular calcifications, cysts of the stratum germinativum)
– Microcephaly		Fetopathies, cerebral malformations
– Macrocephaly		– Ventricular dilatation – Megalencephaly – Dilatation of extracerebral spaces – Cerebral malformations
– Abnormal head growth		Extracerebral fluid collection – Subarachnoid – Subdural – Internal hydrocephalus – External hydrocephalus – Cerebral malformation
– Meningitis	Early stage	Ventriculitis Parenchymal damage Abscess Extracerebral fluid collection
	Late stage	Monitoring of ventricular size
– Suspected child abuse		Subdural hematoma

Intracranial Hemorrhage in Preterm Infants and Posthemorrhagic Ventricular Enlargement

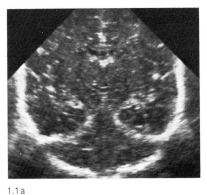 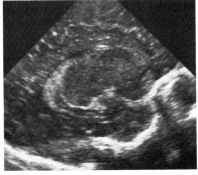 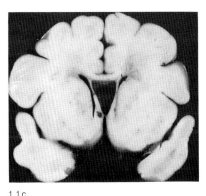

1.1a   1.1b   1.1c

1.1 Normal appearance of the brain of an immature preterm neonate: pericerebral CSF spaces enlarged, sylvian fissure shows incomplete opercularization. **a** Parietal coronal scan.

b Sagittal scan: the occipital horn is usually dilated. **c** Postmortem section.

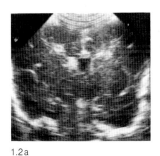 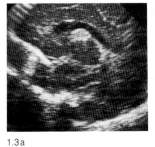 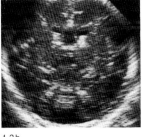

1.2a   1.2b   1.3a   1.3b

1.2 Hermorrhage in the right germinal matrix. a Parietal coronal scan. **b** Right parasagittal scan: the head of caudate nucleus is partly outlined by the hemorrhage.

1.3 Bilateral intraventricular and germinal matrix hemorrhage. a Right parasagittal scan. **b** Parieto-occipital coronal scan.

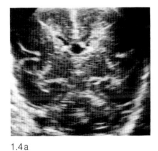 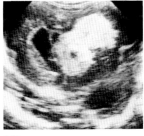 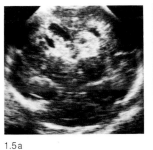 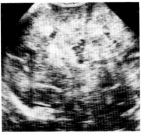

1.4a   1.4b   1.5a   1.5b

1.4 Development of an intracranial hemorrhage. Preterm neonate of 26 weeks' gestation. **a** Coronal scan 1 hour after birth: possible left-sided hemorrhage; ventricular lumen is partly obscured. **b** Coronal scan at 30 hours: massive left-sided intraventricular and intraparenchymal hemorrhage.

1.5 Massive intraventricular hemorrhage and periventricular leukomalacia (often coexist in immature preterms). **a** Parietal coronal scan: acute, severe hemorrhagic ventriculomegaly with bilateral echogenic periventricular areas. **b** Parieto-occipital coronal scan: intraventricular hemorrhage obstructs both ventricular lumina. Diffuse increased echogenicity in white matter.

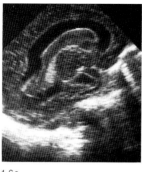
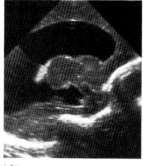
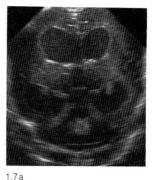
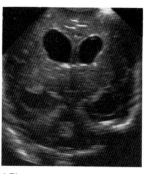

1.6a   1.6b   1.7a   1.7b

1.6 Evolution of massive intraventricular hemorrhage. a
Left parasagittal scan at the age of 3 weeks: blood adheres to the
choroid plexus and ventricular floor. Hematoma forms a "cast"
that fills the ventricular system. **b** Same view at 5 weeks: rapidly
progressive hydrocephalus, complete resolution of the
hematoma.

1.7 Development of massive intraventricular hemorrhage
in an preterm infant of 34 weeks' gestation, following severe
metabolic acidosis. At 72 hours, the hemorrhage is still confined
to the germinal matrix. **a** Coronal scan: by day 9 hemorrhage has
penetrated into the ventricular system. Massive tetraventricular
expansion. Echoes in the ventricular lumen represent fresh
blood. Treated by repeated lumbar punctures. **b** At 7 months,
hydrocephalus is nonprogressive, has been stable since the age
of 12 weeks. The child is normal at 3½ years of age.

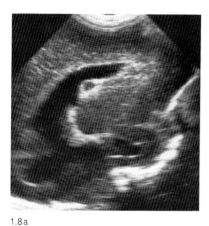
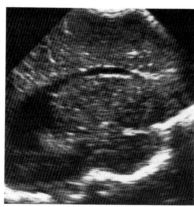
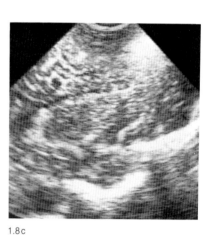

1.8a   1.8b   1.8c

1.8 Transient posthemorrhagic ventricular dilatation in a
preterm infant of 27 weeks' gestation. **a** Right parasagittal scan at
the age of 2 weeks: ventricular enlargement, cyst in the germinal
matrix. **b** At 3 months: residual dilatation of the occipital horn. **c**
At 9 months: normal findings (apparent despite very small fontanelle).

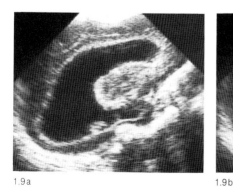
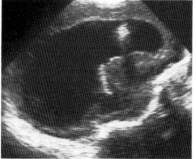
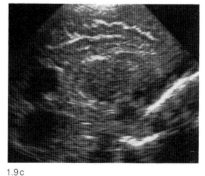

1.9a   1.9b   1.9c

**1.9 Rapidly progressive posthemorrhagic ventricular dila-
tation** in a preterm infant of 27 weeks' gestation. **a** Left parasagittal scan in the 1st month of life: massive ventricular enlargement. **b** Following insertion of a Rickham drain. **c** At 3 months,
insertion of an atrioventricular shunt, with subsequent collapse of
the ventricular system and supra- and subtentorial collection of
CSF. Complete reabsorption in a few weeks.

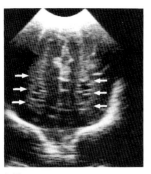
1.10a

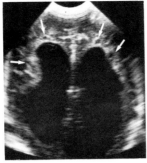
1.10b

1.10 Sequelae of a rapidly progressive posthemorrhagic internal hydrocephalus in a preterm neonate of 25 weeks gestation. **a** Frontal coronal scan: multiple periventricular cystic structures, probably a complication of hydrocephalus developing on day 10. Course: tetraparesis, visual impairment, developmental retardation, the West syndrome. **b** Parieto-occipital coronal scan: intraventricular hemorrhage on the 3rd day of life followed by very rapidly progressive hydrocephalus. *Caution:* In a very immature preterm infant, rapidly progressive hydrocephalus can lead to extensive periventricular parenchymal damage with a poor prognosis.

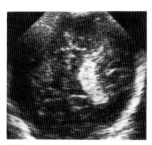
1.11a

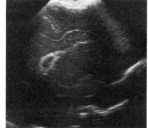
1.11b

1.11 Choroid plexus hemorrhage in a preterm infant of 33 weeks' gestation. Initial US in the first days of life was normal. Sudden apnea in week 3. The left choroid plexus is dilated, very echogenic, and completely fills the ventricular lumen. **a** Sagittal scan. **b** By 1 month, plexus echogenicity has regressed, leaving a hypoechogenic core.

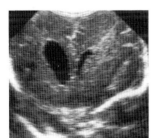
1.12a

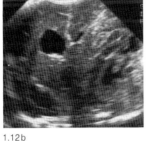
1.12b

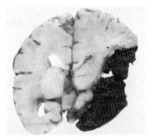
1.12c

1.12 Complex subarachnoid hemorrhage in a preterm infant of 35 weeks' gestation with intrauterine growth retardation, septic shock on day 4, a tense fontanelle, and convulsions. **a** Frontal coronal scan: mass effect with midline shift, enlargement of the right ventricular system, displacement of the left ventricle. **b** Parietal coronal scan: a heterogeneous temporal mass displacing the left ventricular system. Left subarachnoid hemorrhage confirmed by autopsy (**c**).

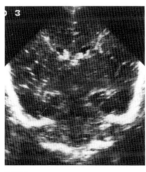
1.13a

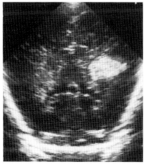
1.13b

1.13 Intraparenchymal lesion in a preterm infant of 33 weeks' gestation that had infectious complications on the 3rd day of life. **a** Parietal coronal scan: moderate bilateral interventricular and germinal matrix hemorrhages. **b** Occipital coronal scan: intraparenchymal lesion in the left occipital area. Diagnosis confirmed by MRI.

Periventricular Leukomalacia in Preterm Infants

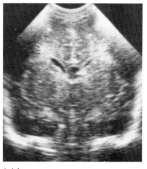

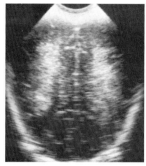

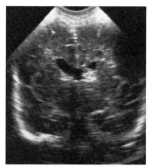

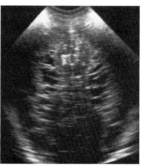

1.14a   1.14b   1.14c   1.14d

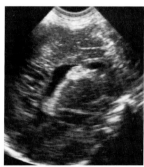

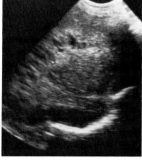

1.14e   1.14f

1.14 Hemorrhage and leukomalacia in a preterm infant of 33 weeks' gestation with group B streptococcal sepsis and severe circulatory problems. **a** Parietal and **b** occipital coronal scans at 72 hours: extensive triangular echogenicities at the external angle of the lateral ventricles. **c** Parietal and **d** occipital coronal scans at 10 days: development of multiple honeycomb-like cysts. **e** Left parasagittal scan: cysts clearly visible behind the trigone in addition to a previous germinal matrix hemorrhage. Hemorrhage and leukomalacia frequently coexist in the same infant. **f** Extent of lesions in the white matter can be accurately evaluated on far lateral parasagittal scans (here on the left side) near the sylvian fissure. Neuropsychologic prognosis depends on the extent and location of the lesions. This infant, who had frontal, parietal, and occipital lesions, later developed severe tetraparesis with visual impairment (strabismus and ambliyopia).

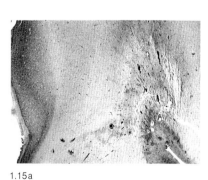

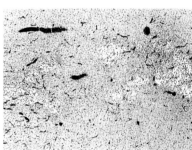

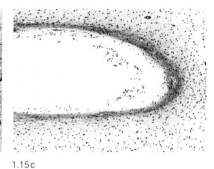

1.15a   1.15b   1.15c

1.15 Neuropathologic evolution. a Subacute necrosis of the external angle of the lateral ventricle. Vascular congestion and vacuolization. The increased echogenicity results from the presence of multiple vascular interfaces and also from the tissue changes caused by necrosis. **b** Central liquefaction, congestion, and angiogenesis. **c** Cyst well circumscribed by gliosis.

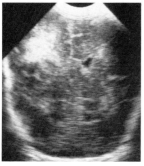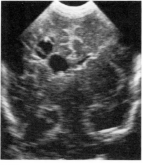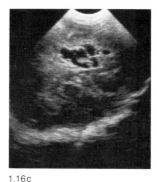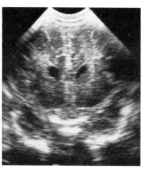

1.16a   1.16b   1.16c   1.17

1.16 Leukomalacia of the right parietal region in a preterm neonate of 29 weeks' gestation that developed left hemiplegia. **a** Parietal coronal scan (age 48 hours): triangular increased echogenicity in the right periventricular area. **b** Two weeks later: cysts in the white matter that do not communicate with the ventricular system. Ipsilateral ex vacuo ventricular enlargement. **c** Right parasagittal view: cysts clearly visible in the region of the sylvian fissure.

1.17 Gliosis and microcalcifications. Frontal coronal scan in the 3rd week of life: echogenic areas sometimes remain visible for several weeks. They are associated with a change in the size and shape of the ventricular system. Neuropathologically, they represent zones of gliosis and microcalcification. Affected infants are at an increased risk for later neuropsychologic deficits.

Hypoxic/Ischemic Lesions in Mature Neonates

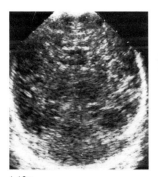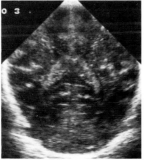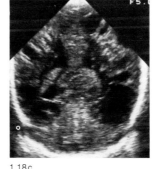

1.18a   1.18b   1.18c

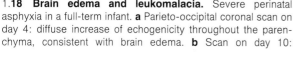

1.18 Brain edema and leukomalacia. Severe perinatal asphyxia in a full-term infant. **a** Parieto-occipital coronal scan on day 4: diffuse increase of echogenicity throughout the parenchyma, consistent with brain edema. **b** Scan on day 10:

increased subcortical echogenicity (interhemispheric fissure, sulci). **c** After 1 month, multifocal subcortical cystic lesions: subcortical leukomalacia.

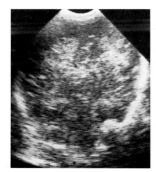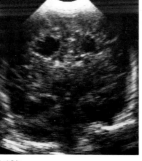

1.19 Leukomalacia. Septic shock in a mature neonate of 37 weeks' gestation. **a** Parietal coronal scan: triangular supraventricular increased echogenicity. **b** After 5 weeks, well-circumscribed cystic lesions at the same location: periventricular leukomalacia.

1.19a   1.19b

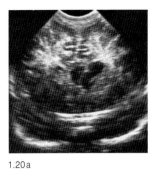 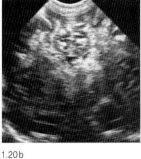 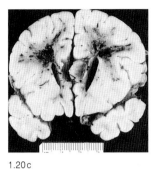 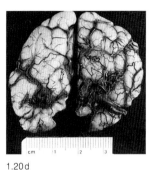

1.20a   1.20b   1.20c   1.20d

1.20 Thrombosis of the longitudinal sinus in a mature neonate with cyanotic cardiopathy; at 3 weeks, generalized seizures with a tense fontanelle. **a** Frontal and **b** parietal coronal scans: intense white matter echogenicity with a vascular (venous) pattern. **c, d** Dilatation of the ventricular system: thrombosis of the longitudinal sinus, confirmed at autopsy.

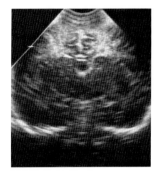 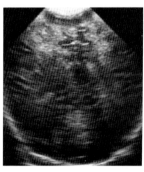 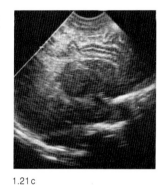

1.21a   1.21b   1.21c

1.21 Hyperechogenicity. Severe perinatal asphyxia, seizures, tense fontanelle. **a** Parietal coronal scan: diffuse increased echogenicity in white matter. **b** Parieto-occipital coronal scan and **c** left parasagittal scan: pronounced increase in white matter echogenicity, strong differentiation of gray matter. Brain edema. Hyperechogenicity regressed over 72 hours. Course: normal development at the age of 24 months.

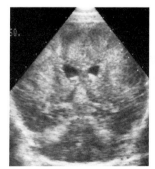 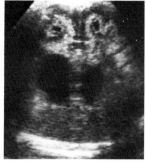

1.22a   1.22b

1.22 Hyperechogenicity. Severe perinatal asphyxia. **a** Parieto-occipital coronal scan on day 4: generally increased echogenicity of the brain parenchyma. **b** Frontal coronal scan at 1 month: subcortical cysts, widening of the interhemispheric fissure. Falx cerebri is visible. Massive asymmetric dilatation of the ventricular system.

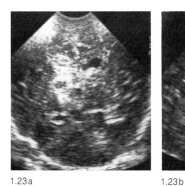 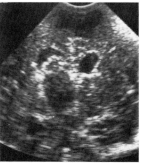 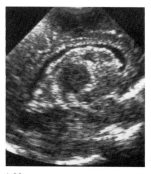

1.23a   1.23b   1.23c

1.23 Evolution of an intraventricular hemorrhage in a mature 10-day-old neonate. Unremarkable pregnancy and delivery. **a** Parietal coronal scan: massive intraventricular and intrathalamic hemorrhage on the right side. **b** Ten days later: posthemorrhagic ventricular enlargement and necrosis of the thalamus on the right side. **c** Right parasagittal scan. Course: no progression of hydrocephalus. Normal development at 5 years of age. Medically controlled epilepsy.

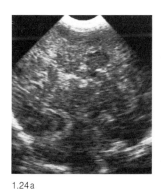 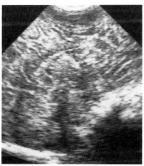 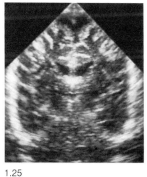 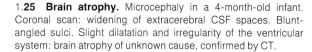

1.24a   1.24b   1.25   1.26

1.24 Brain atrophy. Recurrent, refractory seizures in a mature neonate with skin lesions. Clinical diagnosis: incontinentia pigmenti. **a** Parietal coronal scan on day 3: effacement of cerebral structures and diffuse echogenicity. **b** Sagittal scan: differentiation of cortex and white matter. Course: brain atrophy, death after 4 months.

1.25 Brain atrophy. Microcephaly in a 4-month-old infant. Coronal scan: widening of extracerebral CSF spaces. Blunt-angled sulci. Slight dilatation and irregularity of the ventricular system: brain atrophy of unknown cause, confirmed by CT.

1.26 "Normal" sonogram. Severe perinatal asphyxia in a mature neonate. Seizures. Parietal coronal scan: normal. US consistently normal. CT on day 15 was also normal. Course: severe spastic tetraparesis. *Caution:* Normal US does not always guarantee integrity of brain structures. Even severe perinatal asphyxia may be associated with normal sonographic findings.

Prenatal Infection

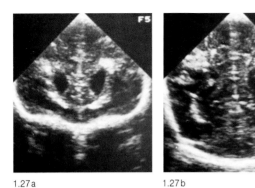
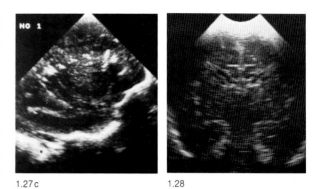

1.27a   1.27b   1.27c   1.28

1.27 Cytomegalovirus infection in a 3-month-old infant. **a** Frontal coronal scan: ventricular enlargement with periventricular areas of high echogenicity. Almost no sulci are visible. **b** Occipital coronal scan: strong dilatation of the occipital horns. Punctate sonodensities in the ventricular walls, hyperechogenic areas in the medulla. Sulci no longer visible. **c** Right parasagittal scan: prominent lesions along the ventricular wall. Classic US signs of

severe congenital CMV infection: ex vacuo ventricular enlargement (microcephaly), multiple calcifications throughout the cerebral parenchyma, lissencephaly.

1.28 Cytomegalovirus infection of moderate degree. Multiple microcysts in the germinal matrix are the only apparent abnormality.

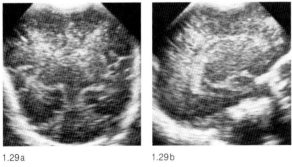
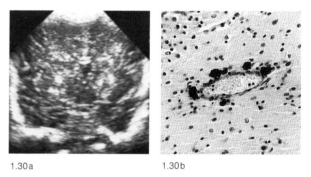

1.29a   1.29b   1.30a   1.30b

1.29 Cytomegalovirus infection. Multiple small calcifications in the periventricular region, especially in the frontal and occipital areas. **a** Parieto-occipital coronal scan. **b** Right parasagittal scan.

1.30 Congenital rubella in a neonate with microcephaly and hepatosplenomegaly. **a** Parietal coronal scan: clacifications mainly in the basal ganglia (not detectable by CT). The infant did not survive. **b** Autopsy confirmed perivascular calcifications.

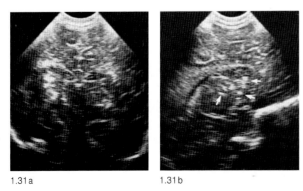

1.31a   1.31b

1.31 Congenital rubella in a neonate with cataracts. **a** Parietal coronal and **b** right parasagittal scans: multiple calcifications in the periventricular region and basal ganglia.

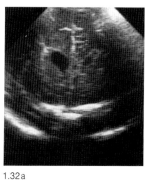 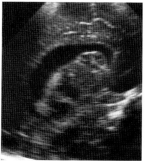 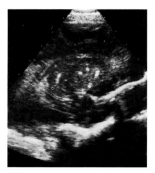

1.32a   1.32b   1.33

1.32 Congenital toxoplasmosis. Maternal infection inadequately treated during pregnancy. Apparently healthy newborn underwent routine US. **a** Frontal coronal scan: asymmetric ventricular dilatation, cysts, and small periventricular calcifications. **b** Right parasagittal scan: enlargement of the right lateral ventricle. Multiple cysts in the germinal matrix. Course: child treated for 1 year, normal at the age of 3 years.

1.33 Congenital toxoplasmosis in a growth-retarded preterm neonate of 34 weeks' gestation. Sagittal scan: multiple calcifications in the basal ganglia. Serologic analysis positive for toxoplasmosis.

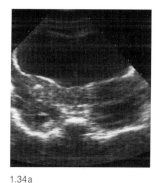 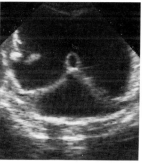 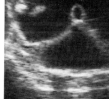

1.34a   1.34b   1.34c

1.34 Congenital toxoplasmosis. Fetal microcephaly diagnosed by US during pregnancy. Serologic analysis positive for toxoplasmosis. Term delivery. Head circumference 29.5 cm. **a** Parietal coronal, **b** occipital coronal, and **c** sagittal scans: massive enlargement of all four ventricles, very thin cortex, probable calcifications in the ventricular walls. Severe fetopathy mimics a cerebral malformation. **DD:** Dandy−Walker syndrome.

Miscellaneous Antenatal Diseases

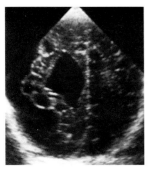 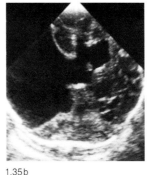

1.35a   1.35b

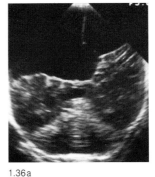 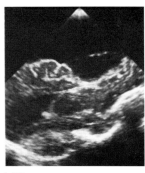

1.36a   1.36b

1.35   Suspicion of previous brain infarction in a 5-day-old infant. **a** Frontal coronal scan: dilatation of the right lateral ventricle, midline shift, fluid collection in the right frontal area. **DD:** intracerebral or extracerebral effusion? Malformation or post-ischemic condition? Malformation based on vascular occlusion? **b** Parieto-occipital coronal scan: breakthrough of effusion into the right ventricular system. Previous infarction in the anterior and middle cerebral artery territories.

1.36   Uncertain diagnosis in a 6-month-old infant with progressive macrocephaly. **a** Parieto-occipital scan: massive fluid collection in the parietotemporal region, more prominent on the right. Falx cerebri is clearly visible. **b** Right parasagittal scan: effusion displaces brain parenchyma and ventricular system downward. **DD:** extracerebral effusion? Arachnoid cyst? Post-traumatic state? Prenatal or postnatal insult? Porencephaly?

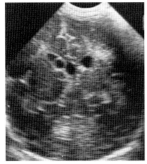 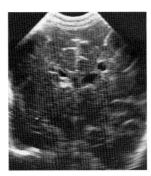

1.37   1.38

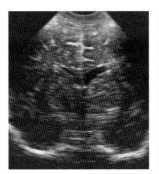 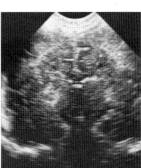

1.39   1.40

1.37   Leukomalacia in a preterm neonate of 31 weeks' gestation. First sonogram (at 48 hours): large cyst in the right germinal matrix of prenatal origin. Fresh leukomalacia, most prominent in left periventricular area. Course: moderate spastic diplegia.

1.38   Prenatal periventricular leukomalacia in a preterm neonate of 29 weeks' gestation. Initial sonogram (at 4 hours): several well-circumscribed cysts in the white matter associated with a right germinal matrix hemorrhage. Course: the child is normal at 5 years of age.

1.39   Asymmetry of the lateral ventricles. Mother suffered severe abdominal trauma in a car accident in the 27th week of pregnancy, underwent an emergency cesarean section in the 39th week due to uterine rupture. Perinatal asphyxia. Initial sonogram (at 2 hours): marked ventricular asymmetry, enlargement of the left lateral ventricle with a blunt lateral angle. No other lesions are apparent. US findings remained unchanged during the neonatal period. Course: severe tetraparesis. CT at the age of 16 months confirmed persistence of ventricular dilatation.

1.40   Sialidosis. Two mature newborn infants of healthy parents died in the neonatal period from progressive neurovisceral disease with arthrogryposis, hepatosplenomegaly, and ascites. US in both infants showed a general increase in white matter echogenicity with small, intensely echogenic foci. Autopsy revealed intracellular vacuoles and microcalcifications: storage disease in sialidosis.

Trauma

Birth Trauma

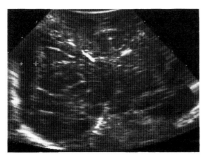 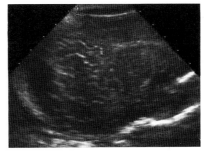

1.41a   1.41b

1.41 Extracerebral effusion in a full-term infant. Forceps delivery due to bradycardia. Huge cephalhematoma in the right parietal region. Skull film: fracture of the right parietal bone. **a** Coronal and **b** parasagittal scans: extracerebral effusion on the right side. *Caution:* Cephalhematoma may be associated with subdural effusion even without a fracture.

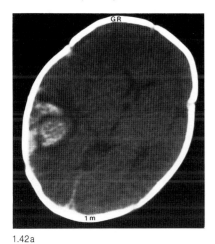 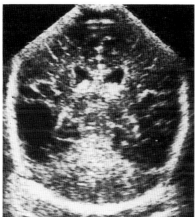 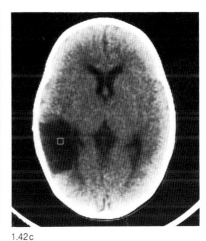

1.42a   1.42b   1.42c

1.42 Evolution of a parenchymal hemorrhage in a full-term infant. Traumatic delivery. Right-sided cephalhematoma. **a** CT at 1 month: late visualization of an intraparenchymal hemorrhage in the right parietal area, which progressed in several weeks to a hygroma. **b** Parieto-occipital coronal scan. **c** CT.

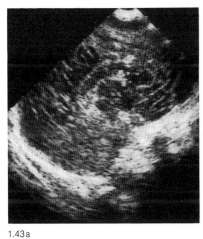 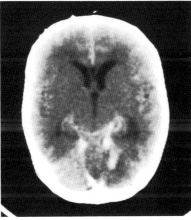

1.43a   1.43b

1.43 Hematoma in the posterior fossa of a 24-hour-old infant delivered by vacuum extractor due to bradycardia. **a** Mid-sagittal scan: Structures of the posterior fossa und tentorial region, especially the cerebellum, are poorly differentiated, im-plying a hematoma in the tentorial region. **b** CT scan 1 week later confirms hematoma in the posterior fossa.

Trauma in Abused Infants

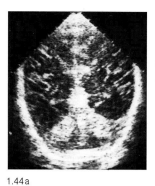
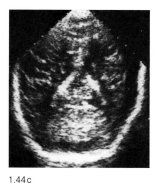
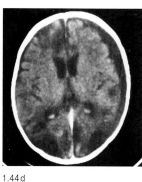

1.44a   1.44b   1.44c   1.44d

1.44 Extracerebral effusion in a 5-month-old infant with convulsions and a bloody spinal tap. **a** Parieto-occipital coronal scan. **b** CT: brain edema. Ventricles no longer visible. **c** Parieto-occipital coronal scan 1 month later: left-sided extracerebral effusion, mild ventricular dilatation. White matter lesions appear as hypoechogenic areas. **d** CT.

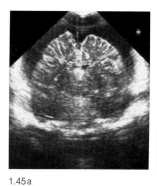
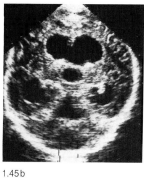
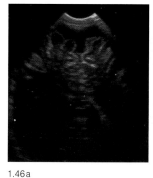
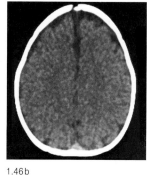

1.45a   1.45b   1.46a   1.46b

1.45 Hygroma followed by internal hydrocephalus in a 5-month-old abused infant. **a** Parietal coronal scan: massive, heterogenous, bilateral extracerebral effusions; evacuated through bur holes. **b** Three weeks later: tetraventricular hydrocephalus due to probable obstruction of the foramina of Magendie and Luschka.

1.46 Chronic subdural hematoma in a 5-month-old infant with convulsions. **a** Coronal scan: extracerebral effusion in the parietal region, blunting of the sulci, widening of the interhemispheric fissure. **b** CT. Infant did well without treatment. *Note:* chronic subdural hematoma should always arouse suspicion of child abuse.

Malformations of the Central Nervous System

Malformations of the Midline and Posterior Fossa

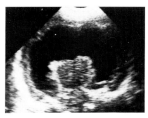 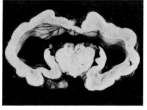

1.47a   1.47b

1.47 Alobar holoprosencephaly. Most severe form, based on dysraphic anomaly of the prosencephalon. **a** Coronal scan: failure of division of cerebral tissue into separate hemispheres; large, horseshoe-shaped single ventricle and fused thalami. Cerebral mantle very thin. Infant died shortly after birth. **b** Postmortem section.

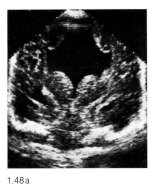 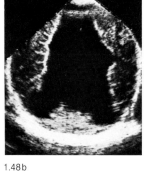

1.48a   1.48b

1.48 Labor holoprosencephaly. a Single ventricle. **b** Occipital extent of the cavity. The child is still alive at 5½ years of age.

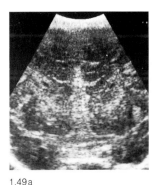 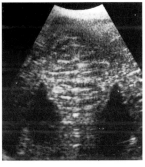

1.49a   1.49b

1.49 Agenesis of the corpus callosum in 2½-month-old infant with subtle degenerative signs. Abnormal karyotype: trisomy mosaic 8. **a** Frontoparietal coronal scan: ectasia ot the frontal horns. **b** Occipital coronal scan: ectasia and widening of

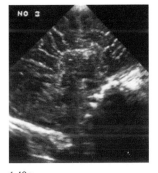

1.49c   1.49d

the occipital horn. **c** Midsagittal scan: corpus callosum not visible; on midline, striking radial arrangement of the sulci, resembling a punk hairstyle in profile (**d**).

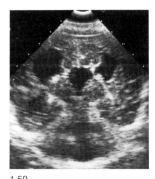

1.50

1.50 Agenesis of the corpus callosum with Dandy–Walker variant. Term neonate with too-rapid head growth and convulsions. Parieto-occipital scan: concave aspect of lateral ventricles, third ventricle elongated and displaced upward. Posterior fossa abnormal with two hypoechogenic areas: partial agenesis of the inferior cerebellar vermis and cystic expansion of the fourth ventricle. *Caution:* corpus callosum agenesis is frequently associated with a malformation of the posterior fossa.

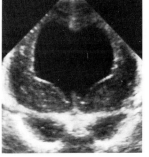

1.51a   1.51b

1.51 Chiari II malformation. Complex malformation, often associated with myelomeningocele. Small posterior fossa, elongated pons, displacement of the medulla oblongata, cerebellum, and fourth ventricle through the foramen magnum. **a** Frontal coronal scan: marked enlargement and inferior pointing of the frontal horns. **b** Midsagittal view: downward displacement of the hypoplastic cerebellum. Massive ventriculomegaly.

Arachnoid Cyst

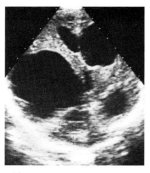 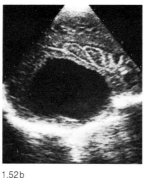 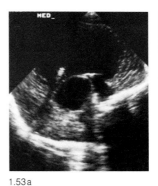 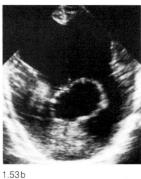

1.52a   1.52b   1.53a   1.53b

1.52 Arachnoid cyst in a 6-week-old infant. **a** Coronal scan: huge cyst in the right temporal region with displacement of the third ventricle, massive ventricular enlargement due to obstructed foramina of Monro. **b** Right parasagittal scan: cyst is in the right temporal lobe, displacing the insula toward the vertex.

1.53 Arachnoid cyst in a 5-month-old infant with cerebral compression signs and excessive head growth. **a** Midsagittal scan: cystic mass behind the third ventricle and above the cerebellum, causing aqueductal obstruction and consequent hydrocephalus. **b** Occipital coronal scan proves the severity of the hydrocephalus. **DD:** vein of Galen aneurysm. Most common sites of arachnoid cysts: temporal fossa, suprasellar region, posterior fossa, region of the quadrigeminal plate.

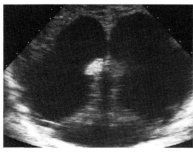 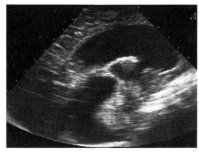

1.54a   1.54b

1.54 Arachnoid cyst in a preterm neonate of 31 weeks' gestation with rapid head growth. US on the 10th day of life. **a** Coronal scan: massive expansion of the occipital horns. Abnormal posterior fossa with a fluid-containing mass. **b** Midsagittal scan shows a cyst behind the cerebellum causing supratentorial hydrocephalus: retrocerebellar arachnoid cyst.

Vascular Anomaly

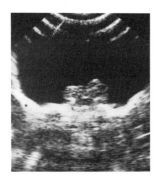

1.55

1.55 Hydranencephaly. Massive destruction of both hemispheres, probably of vascular origin. Parietal coronal scan: only the two thalami are still visible. Diagnosis confirmed by autopsy.

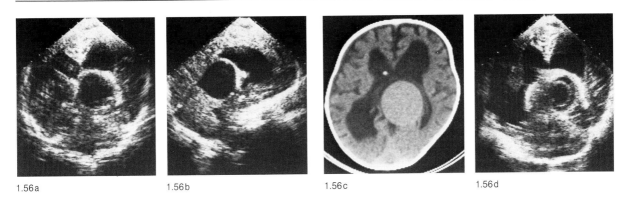

1.56a   1.56b   1.56c   1.56d

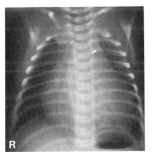
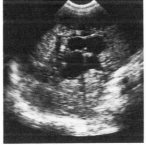
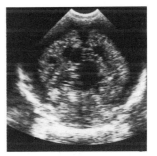

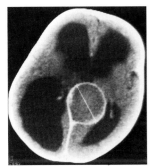

1.56e

1.56 Hydrocephalus and vein of Galen aneurysm in a 10-month-old infant with a ventriculoperitoneal shunt. **a** Coronal scans show ventricular dilatation and **b** a large, round structure below the left lateral ventricle and behind the third ventricle. **c** CT at 10 months. **d** US 3 months later: spontaneous partial thrombosis of the aneurysm, represented by an echogenic ringlike area within the lesion. **e** Findings confirmed by CT.

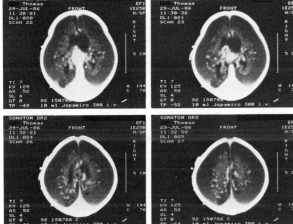

1.57a   1.57b   1.57c

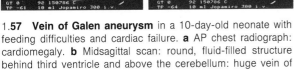
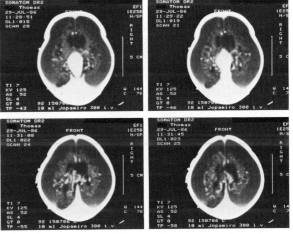

1.57d

1.57 Vein of Galen aneurysm in a 10-day-old neonate with feeding difficulties and cardiac failure. **a** AP chest radiograph: cardiomegaly. **b** Midsagittal scan: round, fluid-filled structure behind third ventricle and above the cerebellum: huge vein of Galen aneurysm. **c** Coronal scan clearly shows the cyst in the midline region. Brain parenchyma is atrophic and echogenic. Brain atrophy develops during fetal life, brought on by massive arteriovenous shunt. **d** CT: caput medusae.

Complex Malformation

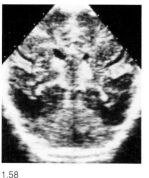

1.58

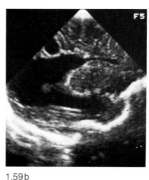

1.59a   1.59b

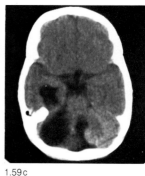

1.59c

1.58 Lissencephaly. Rare anomaly with failure of sulcal and gyral development, moderately enlarged ventricles, and incomplete insular opercularization. Lissencephaly has diverse etiologies: malformation, infection, migration defect, vascular anomaly.

1.59 Complex brain malformation in a 3-month-old infant with infantile spasms. **a** Coronal and **b** right parasagittal scans: complex cerebral anomaly with corpus callosum agenesis, asymmetric ectasia of lateral ventricles, a large third ventricle, and a presumed porencephalic cyst in the right parieto-occipital area. **c** CT findings are similar: corpus callosum agenesis, massive asymmetric ventricular dilatation, porencephalic cyst between the falx and upper portion of the right lateral ventricle. Evaluation: complex brain malformation, possibly of vascular origin.

Postnatal Infection

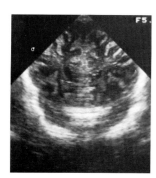

1.60a

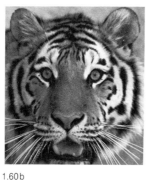

1.60b

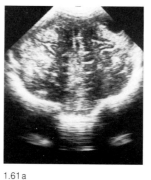

1.61a

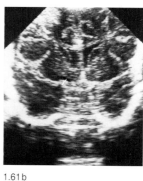

1.61b

1.60 "Tiger face" sign in a 6-month-old infant with *Hemophilus influenzae* meningitis and sepsis. **a** Parietal coronal scan: expansion of the CSF spaces and lateral ventricles, blunt-angled sulci. **b** The "tiger face" pattern is recognizable in the coronal view.

1.61 Meningitis in a 7-week-old infant; causative organism unknown. **a** Frontal and **b** parietal coronal scans: widening of the interhemispheric fissure and prominent sulci. Very marked increase of parenchymal echogenicity. Mild enlargement of lateral ventricles.

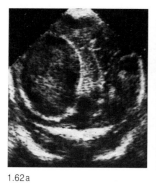

1.62a

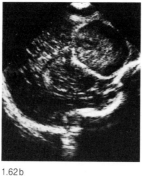

1.62b

1.62 Neonatal meningitis with abscess inadequately treated, in a 23-day-old infant. **a, b** Development of a cystic brain abscess in the right frontoparietal area. Needle aspiration under US control yielded 64 mL of sterile pus, with the subsequent collapse of the cyst. Course: development at 22 months is practically normal for that age.

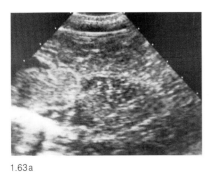
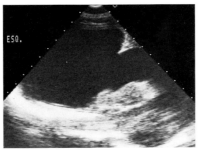
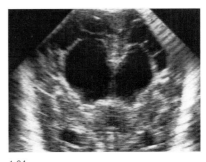

1.63a   1.63b   1.64

1.63 Gram-negative meningitis with abscess in a neonate. **a** Right parasagittal scan at 25 days: development of brain abscess in the right frontal region with prominent echogenic rim. **b** By 6 months the abscess has penetrated into the right lateral ventricle.

1.64 Neonatal sepsis and Proteus mirabilis meningitis, late stage after 2 months. Parietal coronal scan: massive ventricular dilatation accompanied by multiple periventricular foci of cystic necrosis.

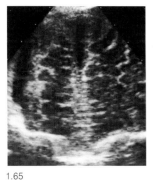
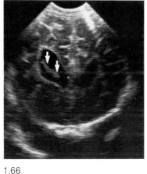
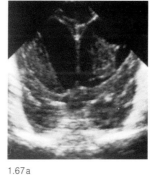
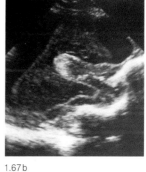

1.65   1.66   1.67a   1.67b

1.65 Meningococcal meningitis in a 4-month-old infant. Sonogram shows widening of the pericerebral CSF spaces and the interhemispheric fissure with prominent, blunt-angled sulci.

1.66 Staphylococcus epidermidis meningitis at the age of 3 months in a former preterm infant with posthemorrhagic hydrocephalus and a shunt. Frontal coronal scan: increased echogenicity in the right lateral ventricle representing a fibrin strand.

1.67 Neonatal Klebsiella meningitis. Late stage after 2 months. **a** Parietal coronal scan: massive ventricular dilatation with fibrin structures adhering to the ventricle walls (typical feature of ventriculitis). **b** Left parasagittal scan: fibrin collection forming a cast of the lateral ventricle. Third and fourth ventricles are normal: obstruction of the foramina of Monro.

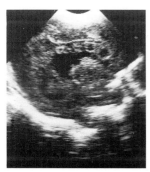
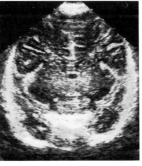
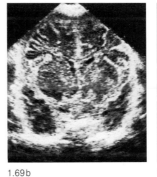
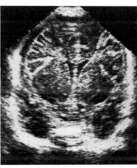

1.68   1.69a   1.69b   1.69c

1.68 Candida albicans encephalitis in a 4-week-old former preterm infant of 26 weeks' gestation. Left parasagittal scan: ventricular dilatation with an irregular outline. Multiple cysts in the cerebral parenchyma. Autopsy: multiple foci of hemorrhagic necrosis.

1.69 Meningitis in a 4-month-old infant; causative organism unknown. **a** Frontal and **b** parietal coronal scans: extracerebral effusion. **c** Marked increase of effusion 2 weeks later.

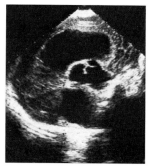

1.70

1.70 Status following meningoencephalitis in a 1-month-old infant; causative organism unknown. The sagittal sonogram shows tetraventricular enlargement.

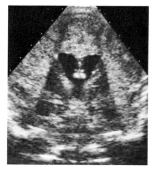 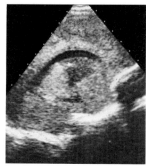

1.71a   1.71b

1.71 Herpes encephalitis in a 3-month-old infant. **a** Parietal coronal scan: multiple echogenic foci with moderate dilatation of the ventricular system. **b** Left parasagittal scan: involvement of basal ganglia.

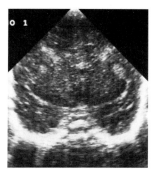

1.72a   1.72b

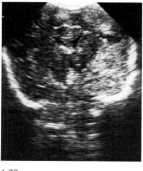

1.73

1.72 Suspected herpes encephalitis in a 3-week-old infant with convulsions. Herpes vesicles noted in the mother's mouth. **a** Frontal coronal scan: increased periventricular echogenicity, increased echogenicity about the sylvian fissure. **b** Occipital coronal scan: circumscribed echogenicity in the right periventricular area.

1.73 Herpes encephalitis in a 1-month-old infant with fever and convulsions. The lumbar puncture was normal. Parietal coronal scan: markedly increased echogenicity in the left parietotemporal region.

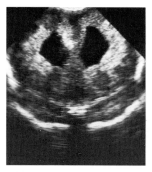 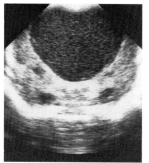

1.74a   1.74b

1.74 Shunt complications. Prenatal diagnosis of hydrocephalus prompted cesarean delivery at 29 weeks. Insertion of a ventriculoatrial shunt was complicated by choroid plexus hemorrhage and meningitis. Pyocephalus developed. **a** Parietal coronal scan at 20 days of age: strong periventricular echogenicity, enlarged ventricular system with an irregular contour. **b** Scan on day 40: increased intraventricular echogenicity due to the presence of purulent CSF (normal gain setting). Destruction of the septum pellucidum.

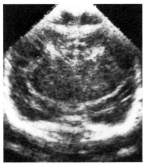
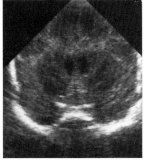
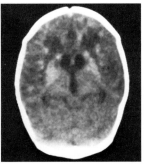
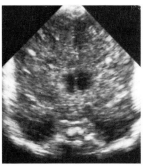

1.75a   1.75b   1.75c   1.75d

1.75 Noenatal streptococcus B meningoencephalitis. a Scan on day 12: normal. **b** Scan on day 21: disappearance of cerebral structures. Moderate enlargement of lateral ventricles. **c** Concurrent CT shows the heterogeneity of the cerebral paren-

chyma, which is permeated by areas of mixed density. **d** Scan on day 42: complete effacement of the cerebral structures and midline. Nonhomogeneous appearance of the cerebral parenchyma. Irregular ventricular enlargement.

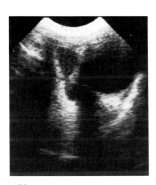
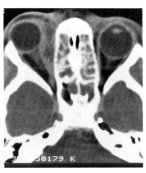

1.76a   1.76b

1.76 Orbital abscess in a 6-year-old child with palpebral edema and a low fever. **DD:** orbital cellulitis. Cavernous sinus thrombosis. **a** Scan through the right orbit shows echogenic effusion: orbital abscess secondary to ethmoiditis. **b** Confirmed by CT.

Brain Tumors

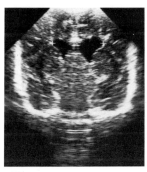
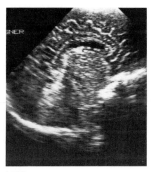
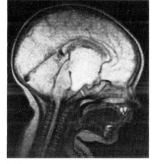

1.77a   1.77b   1.77c

1.77 Astrocytoma in a 3-month-old infant with convulsions. Patient kept head turned to the right side. EEG normal. **a** Parietal coronal scan: moderate, asymmetric dilatation of the lateral ventricles and a uniform, rhomboid hyperechogenic area in the

region of the diencephalon and third ventricle displacing the temporal lobes laterally. **b** Midsagittal scan also shows a hyperechogenic area in the region of the third ventricle. **c** MRI: tumor infiltrating the third ventricle and optic chiasm.

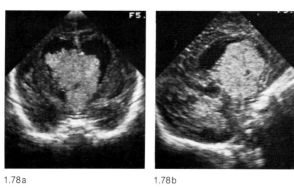

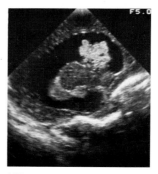

1.78a   1.78b   1.78c

1.78 Choroid plexus papilloma in a 4-month-old infant with cerebral compression signs. **a** Frontal coronal scan: a huge echogenic mass filling both ventricular lumina, which are enlarged. **b** Midsagittal scan: ingrowth of the echogenic mass into the foramina of Monro and the third ventricle. **c** Right parasagittal scan identifies the choroid plexus as the origin of the mass: choroid plexus papilloma with increased CSF production and ventricular enlargement. Treatment: total surgical extirpation, no recurrence.

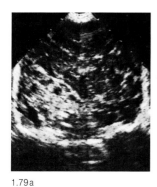

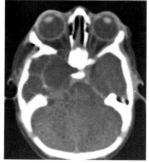

1.79a   1.79b   1.79c

1.79 Teratoma in a 12-day-old neonate delivered with the vacuum extractor. Edema of the right eyelid. Suspected oculomotor paresis. **a** Coronal scan: very echogenic area in the right temporoparietal region causing upward displacement of the sylvian fissure and expanding the right temporal fossa. No obvious mass effect. **b** Right parasagittal scan: sonolucencies within the echogenic mass. **c** CT confirms the temporal fossa expansion and demonstrates the tumor.

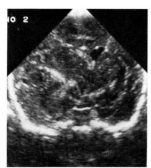

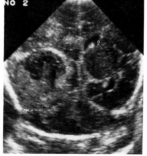

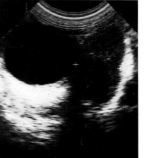

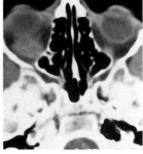

1.80a   1.80b   1.81a   1.81b

1.80 Hemorrhagic infarction in a term infant. **a** Parietal and **b** parieto-occipital coronal scans: heterogeneous, echogenic area in the left temporo-occipital region causing midline shift and obstructing the left lateral ventricle. **DD:** tumor or hemorrhage. Autopsy: hemorrhagic infarction in the territory of the right middle cerebral artery and part of the posterior cerebral artery territory in a full-term infant with neonatal asphyxia.

1.81 Embryonic rhabdomyosarcoma of the right orbit. a Sagittal scan through the right orbit: 1.3–1.5 cm, oblong, hypoechogenic mass adjacent to the eye. **b** CT.

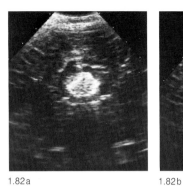
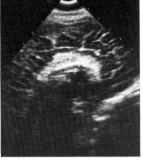
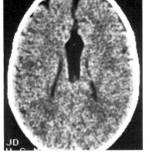

1.82a   1.82b   1.82c

1.82 Lipoma of the corpus callosum. Fortuitous US finding in a newborn with neonatal asphyxia delivered by vacuum extraction. **a** Frontal coronal scan: round, hyperechogenic mass in the midline region above the corpus callosum. **b** Midsagittal view demonstrates the lipoma as a curved, elongated, highly echogenic mass surmounting the corpus callosum. Agenesis of the corpus callosum, a frequent association, is absent here. **c** CT.

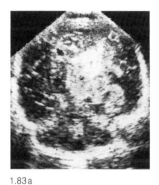
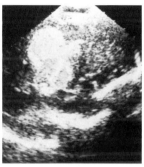
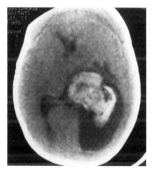

1.83a   1.83b   1.83c

1.83 Rhabdoid brain tumor in a 3-month-old sick infant with vomiting, cerebral compression signs, and a bloody spinal tap. **a** Coronal and **b** left parasagittal scans: intensely echogenic left intraventricular mass also occupying portions of the third ventricle and left thalamus. **DD:** trauma, hemorrhage, malformation, tumor. **c** CT scan: rhabdoid tumor. Infant did not survive.

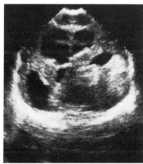
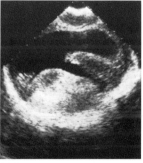
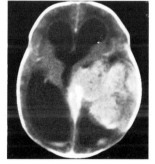

1.84a   1.84b   1.84c

1.84 Glioblastoma in a neonate with congenital hydrocephalus and left facial paresis. **a** Coronal and **b** left parasagittal scans: heterogeneous, echogenic mass in the left temporal region displacing the midline, third ventricle, and sylvian fissure. **c** CT: glioblastoma suspected. Infant survived only a short time.

2 Spinal Tract

S. Jequier

Ultrasound examination of the spinal tract is a very simple procedure in newborns and small infants as long as the neural arches are still mostly cartilaginous. The best instrument for this study is a small-head sector scanner or linear-array scanner with a near-field focus of 1−3 cm operating at a frequency of 7.5 or 10 MHz. A static compound scanner is useful for demonstrating anatomic relationships. The spinal cord can be examined from the craniocervical junction to the cauda equina with only a modest investment of time.

With advancing age and progressive ossification of the neural arches, ist becomes increasingly difficult to visualize the spinal cord. After 1 year of age, sonography of the spinal cord is limited to patients with a congenitally open neural arch and to intraoperative and postoperative cases following laminectomy.

The indications for ultrasound examination of the infant spinal cord include congenital malformations of the vertebral column, especially dysraphia of the neural arches, tumors overlying the spinal column and sacrum (Naidich et al. 1984), cutaneous anomalies (pigmented nevus, hairy nevus, pigmentary aplasia, etc.), a sacral dimple, neurogenic motor and sensory deficits in the extremities (e.g., clubfoot), and suspected Chiari II malformation. In older patients, neurosurgeons often use ultrasound to establish the intraoperative location of a lesion following laminectomy and before incision of the dura, and also to monitor the postoperative course (Raghavendra and Epstein 1985, Quencer et al. 1987).

Normal Findings

Craniocervical junction (Cramer et al. 1986). The infant is positioned on its side with the neck flexed forward (Fig. 2.**1**).

Cervical and thoracic cord. On longitudinal (sagittal) scans the spinal cord appears at all levels as a hypoechogenic structure with a bright central linear echo representing the central canal. The anterior and posterior borders of the spinal cord appear as hyperechogenic lines. The cord is surrounded by the echo-free subarachnoid space, which is bounded peripherally by the hyperechogenic dura and spinal arachnoid; these are not resolved as separate structures (Fig. 2.**2a**). The anterior spinal artery is frequently seen (Fig. 2.**2b**). On axial (transverse) scans the spinal cord appears as an elongated oval with a central dot (central canal). The dentate ligament forms an echogenic band within the echo-free subarachnoid space, as do the anterior spinal artery and other blood vessels (Fig. 2.**2c**). The cartilaginous and ossified portions of the neural arch and the paravertebral muscles can be evaluated.

Conus medullaris and cauda equina. The lumbar cord exhibits a bulbous expansion (intumescentia lumbalis) and then tapers caudally at the conus medullaris before terminating in the 1 mm−wide, hypoechogenic filum terminale. In most neonates the tip of the conus medullaris has already reached the L1/L2 level (Fig. 2.**3a**), though in some cases it may be at L3. The nerve bundles of the cauda equina produce echoes of moderate intensity about the conus and filum terminale (Fig. 2.**3b**).

References

Cramer, B. C., S. Jequier, A. M. O'Gorman: Ultrasound of the neonatal craniocervical junction. Amer. J. Neuroradiol. 7 (1986) 449

Naidich, T. P., S. K. Fernbach, D. G. McLone, A. Shkolnik: Sonography of the caudal spine and back: congenital anomalies of children. Amer. J. Neuroradiol. 5 (1984) 221

Quencer, R. M., B. M. Montalvo, T. P. Naidich, M. J. Donovan Post, A. Green, L. K. Page: Intraoperative sonography in spinal dysraphism and syringohydromyelia. Amer. J. Roentgenol. 148 (1987) 1005

Raghavendra, B. N., F. J. Epstein: Sonography of the spine and spinal cord. Radiol. Clin. N. Amer. 23 (1985) 91

Rubin, J. M., M. A. DiPietro, W. F. Chandler, J. L. Venes: Spinal ultrasonography; intraoperative and pediatric applications. Radiol. Clin. N. Amer. 26 (1988) 1–27

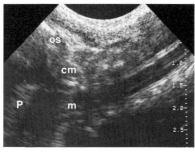
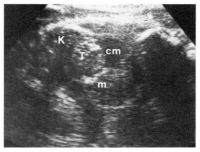

2.1a   2.1b

2.1   Normal craniocervical junction. a Longitudinal and **b** axial sonograms demonstrate the hypoechogenic cervical spinal cord with a central, linear echo representing the central canal. cm = Cisterna magna (anechogenic), m = medulla oblongata, p = pons, ci = interpeduncular cistern. Rarely can the cerebellum be seen as far as the fourth ventricle. T = Tonsils, K = portions of the cerebellar gyri, O = occipital bone.

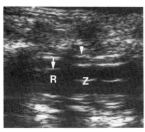
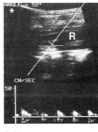
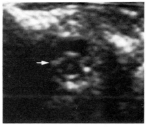

2.2a   2.2b   2.2c

2.2   Normal thoracolumbar cord. a Longitudinal scan: R = spinal cord, Z = central tract, ← = subarachnoid space, ◀ = dura. **b** Anterior spinal artery. **c** Axial scan: the arrow points to the dentate ligament.

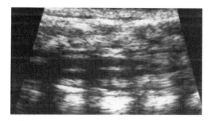
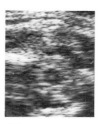

2.3a   2.3b

2.3   Normal conus medullaris and cauda equina. a Longitudinal scan. **b** Axial scan through the conus and cauda equina.

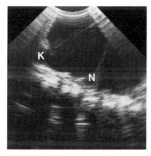
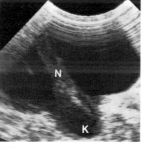
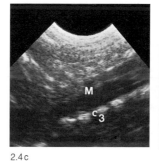
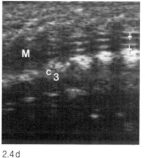

2.4a   2.4b   2.4c   2.4d

2.4   Lumbosacral myelomeningocele and Chiari II malformation. a Longitudinal scan, **b** axial scan through the lumbosacral myelomeningocele of a female infant with loss of motor and sensory innervation distal to L3. Nerve roots (N) emanate from the spinal canal (K) into the CSF-filled sac. **c, d** Longitudinal cervical scans of two patients with myelomeningoceles. Both the sector scan (**c**) and linear scan (**d**) show the distally displaced medulla oblongata (M). The cerebellum obliterates the cisterna magna. C3 = Third vertical vertebra.

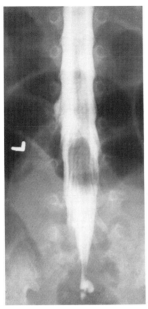 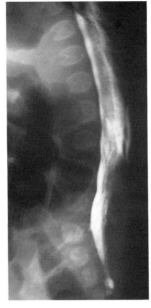

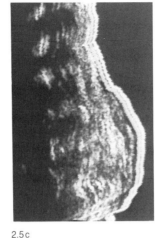 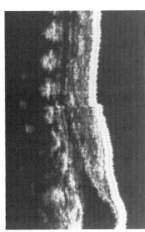

2.5a   2.5b   2.5c   2.6

2.5 Lipomeningocele (operatively confirmed) in a 2-month-old girl, neurologically normal, with a dorsal subcutaneous mass over L2–L3 and a sacral dimple. **a, b** Myelography: conus medullaris at the L3 level. An intraspinal mass displaces the cauda equina and the widened filum terminale. The small sacral cyst is visible distally. **c** Longitudinal compound scan: echogenic tissue in a subcutaneous mass, ingrowth into the spinal canal.

2.6 Meningocele in a neurologically normal newborn girl with a dorsal subcutaneous sacral mass. Longitudinal compound scan: low position of the conus medullaris, a thick filum terminale, and a CSF-filled sac containing no neural structures.

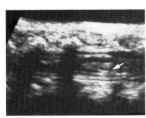 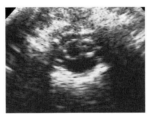

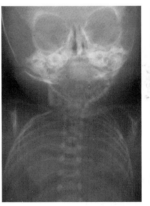  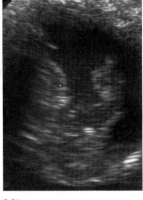

2.7a   2.7b   2.8a   2.8b

2.7 Diastematomyelia. a One-month-old boy with a hairy nevus over L4–S1 and an underlying palpable spina bifida. Motor weakness more pronounced in the right leg than in the left. Longitudinal scan: spinal cord cleft into two hemicords with an associated bone spur (arrow; visible on radiograph). **b** Twelve-month-old girl with delayed motor development in the lower extremities. Axial scan (postlaminectomy): side-by-side hemicords separated only by a membrane.

2.8 Iniencephaly (extreme case of the Klippel–Feil syndrome) in a preterm female infant of 31 weeks' gestation who died from pulmonary hypoplasia and diaphragmatic hernia shortly after spontaneous delivery. **a** Radiograph (for genetic counseling): severe malformation of the cervical spine. **b** Axial scan at the craniocervical junction: cerebellar hypoplasia, agenesis of the vermis, dilated fourth ventricle.

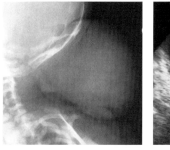
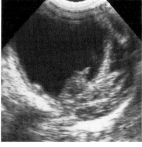
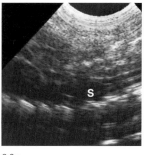
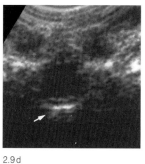

2.9a   2.9b   2.9c   2.9d

2.9 Syringomyelia. a—c Newborn male with an occipital encephalocele. **a** Radiograph: cranial defect and encephalocele. **b** Transverse scan through the encephalocele: disorganized brain tissue and a CSF-filled cyst. **c** Longitudinal scan through the spinal cord shows coexisting syringomyelia (S). Whenever a neural tube defect is recognized, examination of the entire spinal tract is advised (see **d**). d Full-term newborn male whose mother underwent myelomeningocele repair as an infant. Child born with an open myelomeningocele, Chiari II malformation, hydrocephalus, and hydromyelia. On the axial sonogram, the spinal cord is reduced to a thin rim around the enlarged central canal. Distal acoustic enhancement (arrow) does not occur behind normal cord tissue, and the usual central dot is absent. Infant died of sepsis at the age of 4 months. Autopsy confirmed syringomyelia.

2.10b

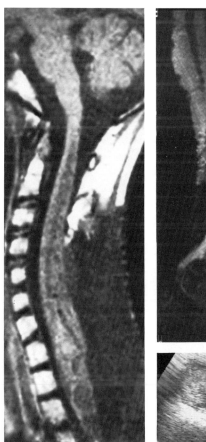
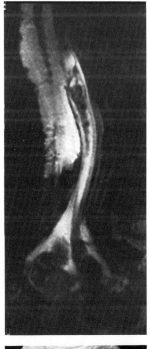

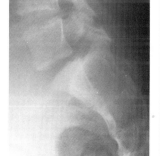
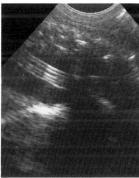

2.11a   2.11b

2.11 Sacral arachnoid cyst in a 16-year-old boy with sacral pain. **a** Lateral radiograph of the lumbosacral spine shows spondylolysis at L5 and an intrasacral space-occupying lesion. A sacral arachnoid cyst was decompressed with a lumboperitoneal shunt. **b** Postoperative scan confirms the correct placement fo the shunt in the cyst lumen.

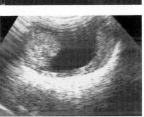

2.10a   2.10c

2.10 Cystic astrocytoma of the cervicothoracic cord in a 17-year-old boy. Neither MRI (**a:** TE 30, TR 450, **b:** TE 300, TR 2000) nor CT could distinguish solid tumor from surrounding cysts. Intraoperative US (**c**) proved extremely useful in this regard.

3 Abnormal Thoracic Findings

I. Gaßner

Although ossified ribs and aerated lung tend to block the transmission of ultrasound, the chest wall, diaphragm, mediastinum, and their lesions are accessible to sonographic scrutiny.

The mediastinum can be scanned from suprasternal (jugular fossa, also the supraclavicular fossae in newborns and infants), parasternal, and subxiphoidal sites. Transsternal scanning is possible if the sternum is still largely cartilaginous. Due to the short neck of neonates and infants, the head should be turned to the side or the shoulders elevated on a pad. The thymus makes an excellent acoustic window.

The major arteries and veins and their anomalies are easily recognized: right aortic arch (should be excluded before operation for esophageal atresia); double aortic arch or pulmonary artery sling producing a stridor; and persistent left superior vena cava.

More reliably than by the position of the liver and spleen, viscero atrial situs can be determined by the positional relationship of the aorta and inferior vena cava to each other at the level of the diaphragm and to the spinal column and also by evaluating the inferior vena cava (azygos continuation) and the hepatic venous connection (a direct connection to the atrium with no confluence between the inferior vena cava and the hepatic veins is anomalous).

With situs solitus, the aorta is located on the left and the inferior vena cava on the right. With situs inversus, these positions are reversed.

In the polysplenia syndrome (left isomerism), all the hepatic veins connect directly to the atrium, and there is almost always an azygos continuation of the inferior vena cava (the hepatic segment fo the inferior vena cava is absent). Often there is a persistent left superior vena cava that drains into the coronary sinus.

In asplenia syndrome the aorta and inferior vena cava course together on the right or left side of the spine at the level of the diaphragm (aorta is posterior, inferior vena cava is anterior). All or some of the hepatic veins connect to the inferior vena cava. Usually there is a persistent left superior vena cava that drains directly into the left-sided (morphologically right) atrium (the coronary sinus is absent!; Huhta et al. 1982).

Besides congenital defects, pericardial effusions are easily detected with ultrasound, even when small.

In patients with central venous catheters, specific complications can be quickly identified (large adherent thrombi, perforations with an "infusion thorax" or "infusion pericardium").

In patients with mediastinal masses, the echo structure of the mass (solid, cystic, mixed) and its position relative to the vessels are determined. At the level of the supra-aortic vessels, the topographic relationships and small masses (e. g., lymphomas) are sometimes perceived more clearly than on CT scans. Hilar masses, on the other hand, are poorly accessible to ultrasound due to overlying aerated lung.

The normal thymus surrounds the vessels without displacing them. Thymic lymphomas are less echogenic or sometimes exhibit a heterogeneous echo structure, may displace vessels, and may be associated with effusions.

Chest wall lesions and peripheral or superficial pulmonary densities and tumors are directly accessible to sonographic evaluation. Juxtadiaphragmatic masses are accessible via the liver and spleen or through the fluid-filled stomach. Adjacent aerated lung should not be mistaken for posterior acoustic enhancement. Motion of the mass relative to the chest wall with respirations implies that the lesion is intrapulmonary.

Diaphragm mobility can be reliably assessed, and in infants with diaphragmatic hernia and eventration, the anatomic location of the defect can be established and the herniated viscera identified.

With partial or complete opacity fo the hemithorax, sonography can differentiate among pleural effusion, tumor, and infiltrate. In atelectatic or infiltrated lung, ultrasound can demonstrate the pulsating pulmonary arteries and the echogenic bronchial tree.

Ultrasound can also be used to determine the optimum site for percutaneous biopsy or drainage of an effusion (especially in loculated effusions) and assess the efficacy of the drainage.

References

Blank, E., T. D. Michael: Muscular hypertrophy of the esophagus: report of a case with involvement of the entire esophagus. Pediatrics 32 (1963) 595–598

Gilsanz, V., D. Emons, M. Hansmann, M. Meradji, J. S. Donaldson, F. Omenaca, J. Quero, B. L. Tucker: Hydrothorax, ascites, and right diaphragmatic hernia. Radiology 158 (1986) 243–246

Huhta, J. C., J. F. Smallhorn, F. J. Macartney: Two dimensional echocardiographic diagnosis of situs. Brit. Heart J. 48 (1982a) 97–108

Huhta, J. C., J. F. Smallhorn, F. J. Macartney, R. H. Anderson, M. De Leval: Cross-sectional echocardiographic diagnosis of systemic venous return. Brit. Heart J. 48 (1982b) 388–403

Laurin, S., S. Aronson, H. Schüller, H. Henrikson: Spontaneous hemothorax from bronchopulmonary sequestration. Unusual angiographic and pathologic-anatomic findings. Pediat. Radiol. 10 (1980) 54–56

Martin, R. P., R. Bowden, K. Filly, R. L. Popp: Intrapericardial abnormalities in patients with pericardial effusion. Circulation 61 (1980) 568–572

Merten, D. F., J. D. Bowie, D. R. Kirks, H. Grossman: Anteromedial diaphragmatic defects in infancy: current approaches to diagnostic imaging. Radiology 142 (1982) 361–365

Yeager, S. B., A. J. Chin, P. S. Stephen: Two-dimensional echocardiographic diagnosis of pulmonary artery sling in infancy. J. Amer. Coll. Cardiol. 7 (1986) 625–629

Fig. 3.1e: after Swischuk, L. E.: Differential diagnosis in pediatric radiology, Fig. 1.3. Baltimore: Williams & Wilkins, 1984.

Fig. 3.4d: after Gedgaudas, E. et al.: Cardiovascular radiology, Fig. 10-9. Philadelphia: Saunders, 1985.

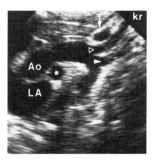
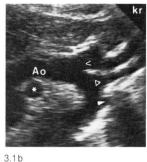
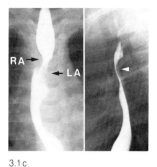
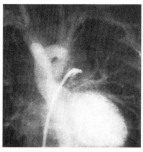

3.1a   3.1b   3.1c   3.1d

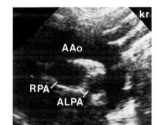

3.1e

3.1   Double aortic arch in a 14-month-old boy with inspiratory stridor since birth and recurrent episodes of bronchitis. **a** Suprasternal scan: the left aortic arch (Ao) gives off only the left carotid artery (▽) and subclavian artery (▼). ↓ = Left brachiocephalic vein. Rotating the transducer to the right demonstrates a smaller right arch with the right carotid artery and subclavian artery (not shown). **b** Normal left aortic arch. ★ = right pulmonary artery. < = innominate artery. **c** Esophagrams. Left AP projection shows a bilateral extrinsic compression of the esophagus by the right (RA) and lower-lying left (LA) aortic arch. The lateral view, on the right, shows posterior indentation of the esophagus by the aortic arch (◀). **d** Angiographic view of a double aortic arch. Each arch gives off the corresponding subclavian and carotid artery. Operation: division of the smaller right arch (in 80% of cases the right arch is larger). US localization of the aortic arch is indicated prior to any surgery for esophageal atresia! **e** Schematic drawing. Ao = Aorta, RA = right aortic arch, PA = pulmonary artery.

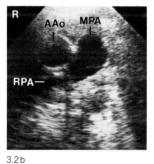
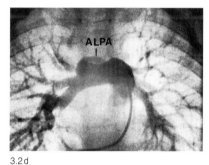

3.2a   3.2b   3.2d

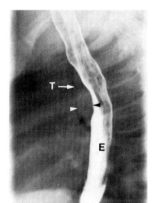
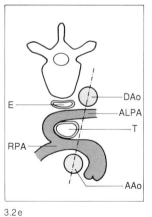
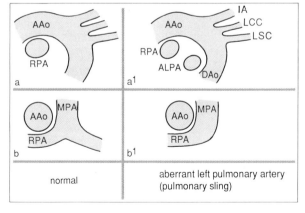

3.2c   3.2e

normal   aberrant left pulmonary artery (pulmonary sling)

3.2   Pulmonary sling in a 1½-year-old girl with exertional stridor. **a** Suprasternal scan, plane of section marked in **e** (−·−·−). Transverse views of both pulmonary artery branches within the aortic arch. **b** Axial transsternal scan: absence of the left pulmonary artery origin from the main trunk of the pulmonary artery. **c** Esophagram: aberrant left pulmonary artery (▶◀) between the trachea and esophagus. **d** Pulmonary angiogram in the semisitting position (45° caudocranial) confirms the diagnosis. **e** Schematic drawing of the pulmonary sling. The aberrant left pulmonary artery arises from the right pulmonary artery and runs to the left between the trachea and esophagus.

MPA	Main trunk of the pulmonary artery
RPA	Right pulmonary artery
ALPA	Aberrant left pulmonary artery
AAo	Ascending aorta
DAo	Descending aorta
IA	Innominate artery
LCC	Left common carotid artery
LSC	Left subclavian artery
E	Esophagus
T	Trachea

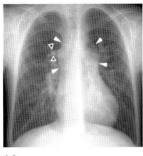
3.3a

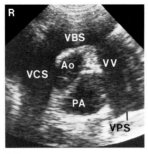
3.3b

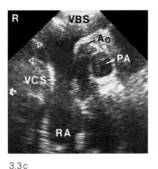
3.3c

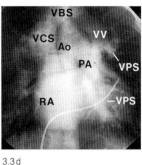
3.3d

3.3 Partial anomalous pulmonary venous drainage in an asymptomatic 8-year-old boy whose cardiac murmur was detected when he was seen for pneumonia. **a** Chest radiograph: bilateral convex widening of the superior mediastinum (▼), increased pulmonary perfusion, and an anomalous course of a right-sided pulmonary vein (▽). **b, c** Mediastinum, suprasternal coronal scan: a large vertical vein (VV) ("persistent left superior vena cava") drains through the dilated left brachiocephalic vein (VBS) into the right superior vena cava (VCS). The left pulmonary veins (VPS) drain into the VV and the right upper lobe vein (X̄) into the VCS. Right lower lobe vein connects to the left atrium. Ao = Aorta, PA = pulmonary artery, RA = right atrium. **d** Angiography. A large brachiocephalic vein always suggests anomalous pulmonary venous drainage (supracardiac type) or a cerebral arteriovenous fistula.

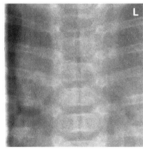
3.4a

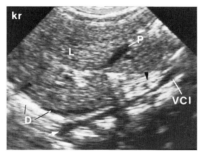
3.4b

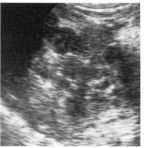
3.4c

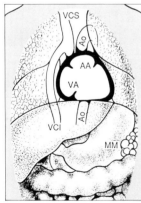
3.4d

3.4 Polysplenia syndrome with azygos continuation in a 4-month-old girl, acyanotic with a cardiac murmur. **a** Chest radiograph (detail): left isomerism of the bronchi, bilateral hyparterial (left) upper lobe bronchi. **b** Right parasagittal abdominal scan: absence of the hepatic segment of the inferior vena cava (VCI), which continues as the azygos vein (→): azygos continuation. The azygos vein apposes directly to the spinal column on traversing the diaphragm (D). Right renal artery (▼) crosses the VCI anteriorly. P = Portal vein, L = liver. **c** Left flank longitudinal scan: multiple small accessory spleens. Also, an atrial septal defect (sinus venosus defect) and nonrotation of the bowel. **d** Schematic drawing. Ao = Aorta, VCI/VCS = inferior vena cava/superior vena cava, VA = venous atrium, AA = arterial atrium, MM = multiple accessory spleens.

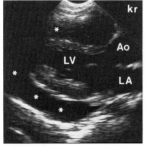
3.5a

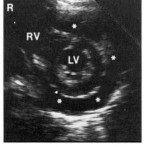
3.5b

3.5 Pericardial effusion in an 11-year-old boy 10 days after closure of an atrial septal defect (ASD II). Parasternal **a** longitudinal and **b** transverse scans show a wide echo-free zone (★) around both ventricles: pericardial effusion. Diagnosis different from pleural effusion, which is seldom retrocardiac. Pericardial effusion does not extend behind the left atrium because the pericardium is fixed there by pulmonary veins. LV = Left ventricle, LA = left atrium, RV = right ventricle, Ao = aorta.

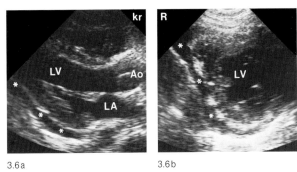
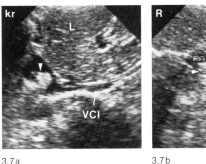
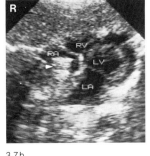

3.6a   3.6b   3.7a   3.7b

3.6 Radiation-induced pericarditis in a 15-year-old boy following resection of the left 5th rib and radiation to the chest for a
Ewing sarcoma. Chest radiograph: postoperative diaphragmatic
paresis and pleural thickening on the left side. Cardiac size and
configuration are normal. Left parasternal **a** longitudinal and **b**
transverse scans: narrow hypoechogenic zone (★) between the
epicardium and pericardium. Transverse scan shows highly
echogenic structures in the epicardial area. LV = Left ventricle,
LA = left atrium, Ao = aorta.

3.7 Floating thrombus in a 14-month-old girl with hydrocephalus secondary to a primitive neuroectodermal tumor. Ventriculoatrial shunt and chemotherapy, *Candida* sepsis, shunt
dysfunction. **a** Longitudinal epigastric scan and **b** subxiphoid
cardiac scan: large, hyperechogenic floating thrombus (▼, culture grew *Candida*) at the catheter tip in the right atrium (RA). LA
= Left atrium, RV/LV = right/left ventricle, VCI = inferior vena
cava, L = liver.

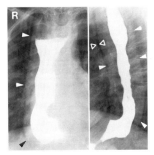
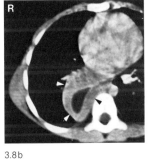
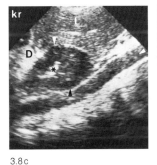
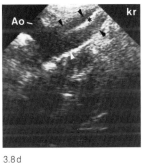

3.8a   3.8b   3.8c   3.8d

3.8 Idiopathic muscular hypertrophy of the esophagus in a
6-year-old girl who became cyanotic during a bout of febrile
bronchitis. Chest radiograph showed sharply defined mediastinal
widening toward the right side to the level of the diaphragm. **a** AP
and lateral esophagrams: dilated esophagus with a greatly thickened wall (▲), tertiary contractions, and delayed emptying.
Severe tracheal compression (▷◁). **b** Thoracic CT: concentric

thickening of the esophageal wall (▲), which projects to the right
paravertebral region. **c** Longitudinal epigastric scan and **d** suprasternal scan show the greatly tickened (approximately 1 cm),
hypoechogenic esophageal musculature (▼). The cardia projects
well below the diaphragm (D). The stomach wall is not thickened.
Ao = Aortic arch, L = liver, ★ = esophageal lumen.

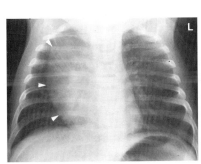
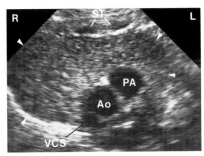

3.9a   3.9b

3.9 Normal thymus in a 5-month-old boy X-rayed for recurrent bronchitis: mediastinal tumor suspected. **a** Chest radiograph: significant mediastinal widening toward the right side
(▶)—probably thymus. **b** Transverse thoracic scan: retrosternal

mass (ST = sternum) of uniform moderate echogenicity (▼)
surrounds the great vessels (VCS = superior vena cava, Ao =
aorta, PA = pulmonary artery) and extends far toward the right
side. Position and echo pattern consistent with normal thymus.

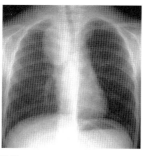
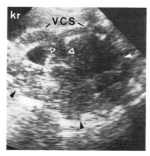
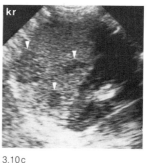
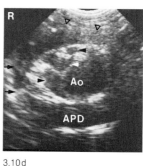

3.10a   3.10b   3.10c   3.10d

3.10 Hodgkin disease with cervical, mediastinal, and abdominal (spleen) involvement in a girl of 7 years, 9 months with 3-month history of fatigue and abdominal pain. Cervical lymphomas. **a** Chest radiograph: sharply marginated mediastinal mass, more prominent on the right side. **b** Right parasternal longitudinal scan: nonhomogeneous mass 5 cm in diameter (▼) displacing the superior vena cava (VCS) anteriorly and encasing

the azygos vein (▷◁). **c** Left flank coronal scan: hypoechogenic foci in the spleen (▼). Lymphomas in the splenic hilum. Histology: Hodgkin disease, nodular sclerosing type. **d** Suprasternal coronal scan after 4 month's chemotherapy still shows residual lymphomas (◄) between the ascending aorta (Ao) and left brachiocephalic vein (▽), superior vena cava (→) and right pulmonary artery (APD).

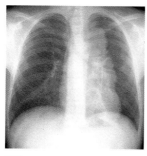
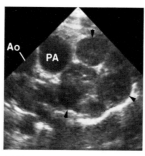
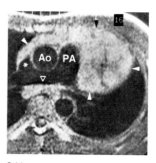

3.11a   3.11b   3.11c

3.11 Hodgkin disease with splenic involvement in an 14½-year-old boy with a 4-day history of night sweats and stabbing chest pain. **a** Chest radiograph: polycyclic mediastinal widening to the left and bowing of the trachea to the right. **b** Left parasternal transverse thoracic scan: multiple spherical, hypoechogenic masses (lymphomas, ▼) bordering on the pulmonary artery (PA).

There were also lymphomas in the retrosternal and suprasternal regions and hypoechogenic lesions in the spleen. **c** Thoracic MRI: tumor mass (▼) around the superior vena cava (★), ascending aorta (Ao), and pulmonary artery (PA). ▽ = Right pulmonary artery.

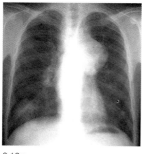
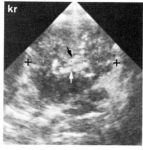
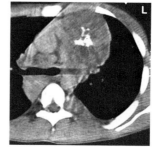

3.12a   3.12b   3.12c

3.12 Hodgkin disease with mediastinal and pulmonary involvement, predominantly nodular type (calcification unusual) in a boy of 13 years, 3 months with a 3-month history of chest pain and cough. **a** Chest radiograph: bilateral mediastinal mass with calcifications on the left side. Densities are also visible in the right and left power pulmonary lobes. **b** Left parasternal longitu-

dinal scan: solid retrosternal mass with irregular margins (+···+) and central hyperechogenic areas (arrows indicate calcifications). **c** CT: left anterior mediastinal mass with central calcification and extension to the right paravertebral region. Large intrapulmonary mass in the lower right field and multiple small round foci in both lungs.

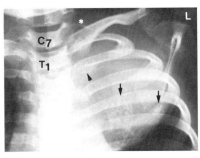
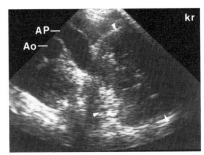
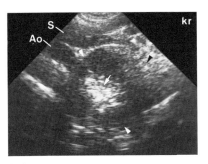

3.13a   3.13b   3.13c

3.13 Ganglioneuroma in an 8½-year-old girl with a 3-week history of slight cough and left shoulder pain. Neurologically normal. **a** Chest radiograph (detail): sharply marginated posterior mass with patchy foci of calcification (↑). The left pedicle of the C7 vertebra is destroyed, that of T1 is deformed. The left transverse process of C7 is thinned (★), the head of the 2nd rib is expanded (▼). **b** Left parasternal longitudinal scan and **c** suprasternal olique scan show a moderately echogenic mass (▼)

with hyperechogenic areas (↓, calcifications) bordering on the main trunk of the pulmonary artery (AP) and aortic arch (Ao) and displacing the brachial vessels (here the subclavian artery, S) anteriorly and superiorly. **DD:** ganglioneuroma, neuroblasoma, neurofibroma. CT following i.v. and intrathecal contrast showed intraspinal tumor extension from C7 to T3 with no cord compression. Histology: ganglioneuroma.

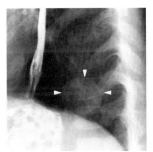
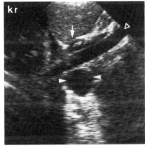
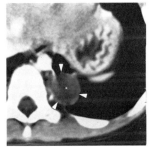

3.14a   3.14b   3.14c

3.14 Bronchogenic cyst in a 5½-year-old boy asymptomatic except for adenoids. Preoperative chest film showed a spherical (2.5-cm) soft-tissue density in the left basal paravertebral region with no apparent vertebral deformity. **a** Contrast study of the esophagus, stomach, and duodenum: spherical density in the posterior mediastinum (▼) abutting on the diaphragm and show-

ing no communication with the GI tract. **b** Longitudinal epigastric scan: 2.5-cm cystic mass (▼) posterior to the aorta (▽) causing acoustic enhancement. ↓ = Esophagus. **c** Contrast-enhanced CT: only the thin cyst wall (▼) shows enhancement. **DD:** bronchogenic cyst or esophageal duplication cyst.

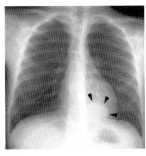
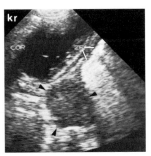

3.15a   3.15b

3.15 Leiomyoma in a 6-year-old boy with septic fever, anemia (Hb 64 g/L), ESR 140/170 mm/h. **a** AP chest radiograph: spherical, sharply marginated 4-cm opacity in the left retrocardiac area (▼). No spinal abnormality. **b** Left subcostal longitudinal scan: moderately echogenic 4.5-cm mass (▼) posterior to the heart (COR) abutting widely on the diaphragm (ZF). Connection with the diaphragm is unclear; no evidence of feeding vessel. Upper

GI series showed no communication with the GI tract. CT showed nonenhancing lesion (not sequestration or abscess). Catecholamines normal (not neuroblastoma). No response to antibiotic therapy. Operation: leiomyoma of the posterior mediastinum, fused to the visceral pleura. The patient's temperature normalized after surgery; hemogram returned to normal.

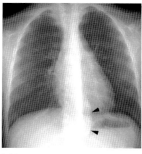
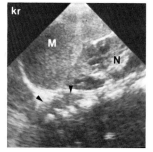
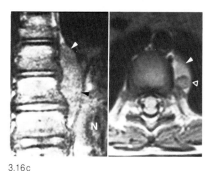

3.16a   3.16b   3.16c

3.16 Ganglioneuroma with neuroblastoma in an asymptomatic 6-year-old girl undergoing a preimmigration medical exam. **a** Chest radiograph: spindle-shaped density in the left paravertebral region (▼), no osteolysis. **b** Left flank coronal scan: paravertebral, retrocrural hypoechogenic mass (▼) that does not move with respiration. **DD:** sympathetic tumor, pulmonary sequestration, lymphoma, abscess (cathecholamines and bone

scan normal). Aortic aneurysm excluded by US. **c** MRI: paravertebral mass (▼) with posterosuperior low-signal-intensity inclusion 1 cm in diameter (▽). No infiltration of vertebral bodies or the spinal canal. Myelogram normal. Operation and histology: ganglioneuroma with neuroblastomatous inclusion and extensions in the intervertebral foramina. N = Kidney, M = spleen.

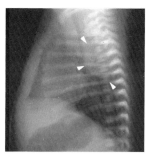
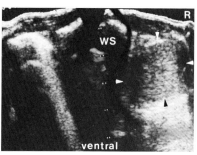

3.17a   3.17b

3.17 Pulmonary sequestration in a 6-day-old girl who had a chest X-ray for cardiac murmur (atrial and small ventricular septal defect). **a** Lateral chest radiograph: sharply defined spherical opacity (▼) posteriorly. **b** Transverse thoracic scan in the prone position: 2.5-cm spherical mass of uniform moderate echogenicity (▼) against the posterior chest wall (static B-scan poor for

determining intrapulmonary or extrapulmonary location, i.e., mobility relative to the chest wall or lung). WS = Spinal column. **DD:** neuroblastoma (catecholamines normal), enterogenous or bronchogenic cyst (echogenic due to hemorrhage or inspissated secretions). Operation: sequestered accessory upper lobe.

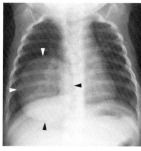
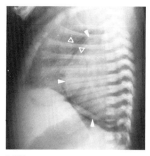
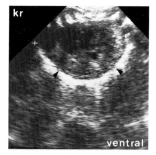
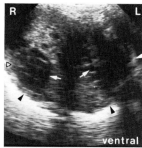

3.18a   3.18b   3.18c   3.18d

3.18 Diffuse neonatal hemangiomatosis with retinal hemangiomas in a mature newborn girl with postpartum dyspnea and diminished breath sounds on the right side; multiple bluishred cutaneous nodules up to 5 mm in diameter. Catecholamines and platelets normal. **a, b** PA and lateral chest radiographs: right intrachoracic mass (▼) based broadly on the posterior chest wall and displacing the right main bronchus anteriorly (▽). No spinal abnormality or calcification. **c** Longitudinal and **d** transverse thoracic scans in the prone position: moderately echogenic mass (▼) that moves with respiration (intrapulmonary), abuts broadly

on the posterior chest wall, and contains echo-free septated areas (↓; vessels?). Following an i.v. plasma bolus, abundant contrast echoes appear in the right atrium and ventricle but none in the tumor. CT showed marked contrast enhancement (indicating systemic arterial or very slow pulmonary arterial perfusion). Aortography showed no systemic supply. Pulmonary angiography was unsuccessful. Lung perfusion scan showed no isotope uptake. Operation: intrapulmonary cavernous hemangioma of the right lower lobe.

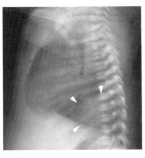

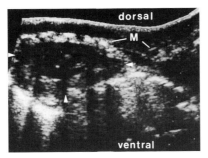

3.19a

3.19b

3.19 **Intrathoracic kidney** in a newborn boy who underwent repair of a right diaphragmatic hernia and reduction of an intrathoracic kidney on his 1st day of life. **a** Lateral chest radiograph 2 weeks postoperatively: sharply marginated density (▼) posteriorly (medial on AP film) with nondelineation of the right posterior portion of the diaphragm. **b** Right posterior longitudinal thoracic scan: intrathoracic kidney (▼) located well above the quadratus lumborum muscle (M). **DD:** recurrent hernia, eventration.

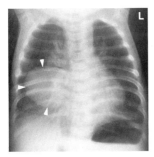

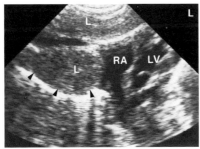

3.20a

3.20c

3.20 **Anteromedial diaphragmatic defect** in a 2-year-old boy with trisomy 21 and a febrile respiratory tract infection. **a, b** AP and lateral chest radiographs: sharply marginated elliptical mass in the anterior cardiophrenic angle with patchy opacification in the right hilar and left retrocardiac regions. **c** Transverse epigastric scan angled cranially and **d** right longitudinal scan: liver (L) herniates anteriorly into the chest (▲), abutting on the anterior chest wall and right atrium (RA). LV = Left ventricle, ↓ = hepatic vessel. **DD:** Morgagni hernia (herniated liver covered only by pleura and peritoneum) or partial eventration (hypoplastic diaphragm between the peritoneum and pleura).

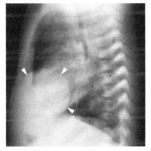

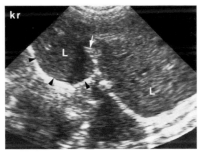

3.20b

3.20d

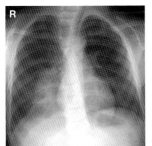

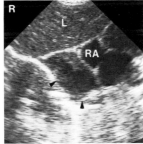

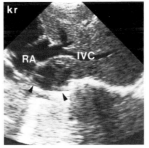

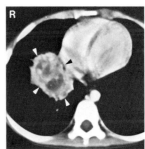

3.21a

3.21b

3.21c

3.21d

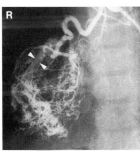

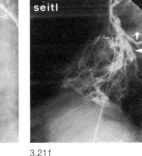

3.21e

3.21f

3.21 **Pulmonary sequestration** in a boy of 5 years, 9 months with intractable "pneumonia". **a** Chest radiograph: well-defined opacity in the medial portion of the right lower lung field (persistent). **b** Transverse epigastric scan angled cranially and **c** longitudinal scan: mass of mixed echogenicity (▼) bordering on the diaphragm and right atrium (RA). In **c**, nondelineation of the diaphragm just behind the inferior vena cava (IVC). L = Liver. **d** CT: enhancing mass (▼) with solid and cystic components bordering on the RA. Suspected pulmonary sequestration. **e** PA and **f** lateral angiograms: sequestrum is supplied chiefly by a collateral vessel arising high on the descending aorta (and by smaller collaterals from the descending aorta). Venous drainage is via the right lower lobe artery (◄) and upper lobe vein (▼). Operation: sequestered middle lobe.

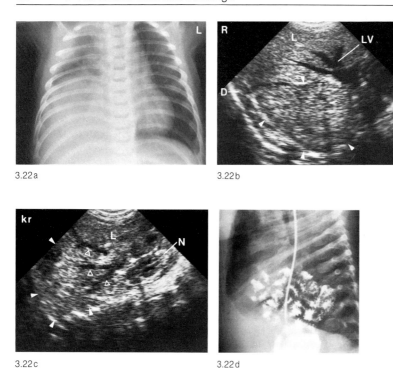

3.22a

3.22b

3.22c

3.22d

3.22 Bochdalek diaphragmatic hernia in a 2-month-old boy with a 1-week history of tonic postprandial vomiting and decreased breath sounds on the right side. **a** Supine chest radiograph: opacity of the right lower- and midlung fields with nondelineation of the diaphragm and pleural effusion. **b** Right subcostal transverse scan and **c** longitudinal scan: mass (▼) of mixed echogenicity between the chest wall and the anteriorly displaced liver (L). Mass exhibits peristalsis and caudally converging veins (▽) and communicates with the peritoneal cavity. LV = Hepatic veins, L = liver, D= diaphragm, N = kidney. The cranial border of the mass is polycyclic and surrounded by a small amount of free intrathoracic fluid. The superior mesenteric artery runs to the right over the inferior vena cava. **d** UGI series: intrathoracic small bowel. Operation: right diaphragmatic hernia with incarceration of the small bowel and ascending colon and edematous mesentery (intrathoracic fluid due to the compression of mesenteric veins).

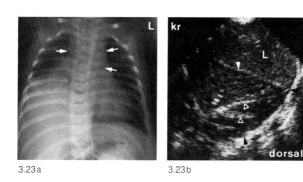

3.23a

3.23b

3.23 Tuberculous primary complex in a 5-month-old boy with a 4-week history of respiratory tract infection. Despite antibiotic therapy, the patient had a low-grade fever, progressive tachypnea, and persistent density in the right lower lobe, as well as hepatosplenomegaly and leukocytosis. Tuberculin reaction was initially negative (not BCG-inoculated). **a** Chest radiograph: dense opacification of the right lower- and midlung fields, hilar enlargement on the right side, enlarged paratracheal nodes (arrows). **b** Right subcostal oblique scan: good sound transmission through all of the right lower lobe (▼) and hyperechogenic bronchi (▽; filled with secretions). Bronchoscopy showed compression of the right upper mainstem bronchus by the enlarged lymph node that penetrated the bronchial lumen. The distal bronchial tree was filled with secretions, from which tubercle bacilli were isolated. Tuberculous primary complex with atelectasis and presumed perifocal exudate in the right lower lobe.

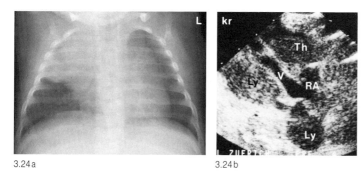

3.24a

3.24b

3.24 Tuberculous primary complex in a 2½-month-old boy (not BCG-inoculated) with a cough, splenomegaly, and a strongly positive Moro test. **a** Chest radiograph: uniform, sharply marginated opacification of the right upper- and midlung fields; thymus on the left. **b** Right parasternal longitudinal scan: thymus (Th) anterior to the superior vena cava (V) and giant lymphoma (Ly) posterior to the vena cava and right atrium (RA). Tuberculous primary complex: enlarged hilar lymph nodes with atelectasis and/or infiltration of the right upper lobe ("epituberculosis"). Bronchial secretions yielded acid-fast rods.

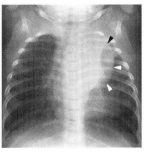
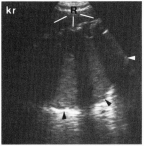
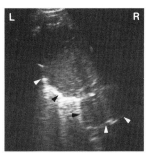

3.25a   3.25b   3.25c

3.25 Neuroblastoma in a 4½-month-old girl with a 3-day history of fever and progressive dyspnea. Mild cyanosis. Neurologically normal. **a** Chest radiograph: large intrathoracic mass (▼) compressing and displacing the trachea, atelectasis of the left upper lobe. The third intercostal space is widened; erosion of the 2nd and 3rd vertebral pedicles and rib. **b** Left posterior longitudinal and **c** transverse thoracic scans: moder-

ately echogenic mass (▼) composed of two different-sized nodes abutting broadly on the chest wall (R = ribs). Fixed position implies extrapulmonary mass: neurogenic tumor with intraspinal extension (pedicles!), most likely a neuroblastoma. CT myelography (obligatory study) showed extradural extension with no cord compression. Bone marrow involvement: neuroblastoma IV-S.

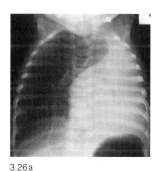
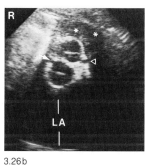

3.26a   3.26b

3-26 Bland—White—Garland syndrome in a 3-month-old girl with a febrile airway infection and cardiac decompensation. **a** Atelectasis of the left lung (compression of the left main bronchus by the dilated left atrium). **b** Left parasternal transverse scan through the valvular plane of the aorta (posterior) and pulmonary artery (anterior): right coronary artery (→) arising from the aorta, left (▽) arising from the pulmonary artery. LA = Dilated left atrium, ★ = atelectatic lung.

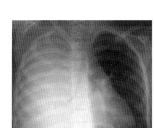
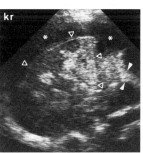
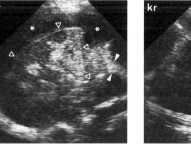
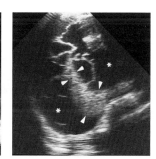

3.27a   3.27b   3.27c   3.27d

3.27 Lobar pneumonia with serofibrinous effusion in a 7½-year-old girl with severe abdominal pain (appendicitis suspected) and right upper lobar pneumonia. **a** Chest radiograph (on the 3rd day of illness): uniform opacity of the right hemithorax. Right thoracic, **b, c** longitudinal and **d** basal transverse scans: con-

gested upper lobe (▽) with blunt border and heterogeneous echo pattern swaying in the effusion (★). Lower lobe (▼) is completely collapsed and floats in the effusion (★). Echogenic membranes (presumably fibrin) float between the lower lobe and diaphragm (D).

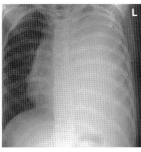 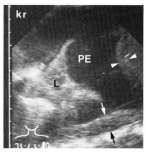

3.28a   3.28b

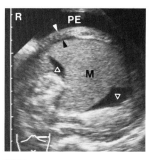 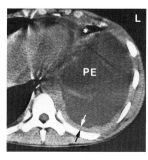

3.28c   3.28d

3.28 Acute lymphocytic leukemia in a 12-year-old girl with a 1-week history of exertional dyspnea, left thoracic dullness, and generalized lymph node swelling; abdomen could not be evaluated. **a** Chest radiograph: complete opacification of the left hemithorax with a shift of the midline shadow to the right and downward displacement of the diaphragm. Left thoracic **b** coronal and **c** transverse scans at the level of the sinus: massive pleural effusion (PE) containing fine mobile particles (cells). The

lung (L) is completely collapsed. The whole pleura (↓) and diaphragm (🗶) are greatly thickened (suggesting subpleural infiltration). M = Spleen, ▽ = ascites. **d** Thoracic CT: pleural effusion (PE), pleural tickening (⊦), compressed lung (★). Mediastinal and mesenteric lymph node enlargement, hepatosplenomegaly, adnexal infiltration. Pathologic cells in pleural effusion and CSF. Bone marrow aspiration: pre-TALL.

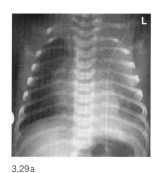 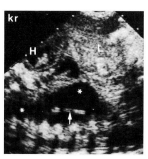

3.29a   3.29b

3.29 Malposition of a subclavian catheter in a 7-day-old girl with *d*-transposition. Subclavian catheter insertion (no position check) was followed within hours by tachypnea and increased cyanosis. **a** Chest radiograph: left-sided pleural effusion and a malpositioned subclavian catheter. **b** Left longitudinal subcostal scan: catheter (arrow) in the pleural cavity, "infusion thorax" (★). H = Heart, L = liver. The effusion was catheter-drained under US guidance.

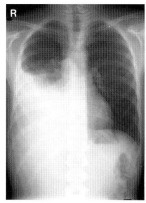

3.30a

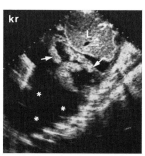 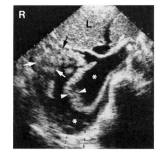

3.30b   3.30c

3.30 Bleeding extralobar sequestration in a 13-year-old boy with stabbing right chest pain 10 days before, admitted with 1-day history of recurrent pain and exertional dyspnea. Anemia (Hb 98 g/L). **a** Chest radiograph: uniform opacity of the right lower- and midlung fields. Aspiration: hematothorax. Right thoracic **b** longitudinal and **c** basal transverse scans: massive pleural effusion (★), complete collapse of the lower lobe (🗶),

mobile echogenic mass (blood clots = ↓), L = liver. CT: no additional information. Aortography raised suspicion of pulmonary sequestration. Operation: spontaneous hematothorax caused by a small, bleeding extralobar sequestration in the right mediobasal region. Organized hematoma was adherent to the sequestrum.

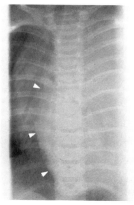

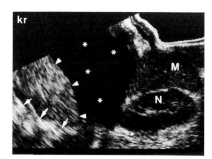

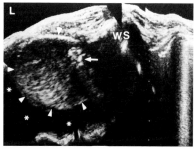

3.31a   3.31b   3.31c

3.**31** **Neuroblastoma** in a 9-month-old girl with a longstanding protuberance in the left thoracic and paravertebral region; sudden dyspnea, no fever. Dullness and decreased breath sounds on the left side, splenomegaly. Neurologically normal. **a** Chest radiograph (detail): complete opacity of the left hemithorax with faint calcifications and a mediastinal shift to the right (▼); erosion of the 5th–9th ribs on the left side. **b** Left flank longitudinal scan

and **c** posterior transverse thoracic scan: extensive pleural effusion (★) and a solid paravertebral mass (▼) with calcifications (↓) adherent to the posterior chest wall. N = Kidney, M = spleen, WS = spinal column. Neuroblastoma (positive vanillylmandelic acid test, bone marrow involvement). Operation and histology: poorly differentiated neuroblastoma with extensive soft-tissue infiltration and bloody pleural effusion.

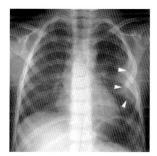

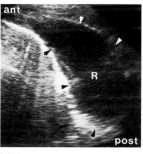

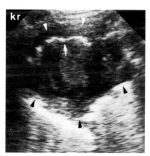

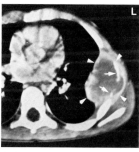

3.32a   3.32b   3.32c   3.32d

3.**32** **Histiocytosis X** in a 3½-year-old boy with a 6-week history of left-sided chest pain on the left side. **a** Chest radiograph: osteolytic erosion of the left 5th rib posterolaterally with extrathoracic and intrathoracic expansion (▼) and plaquelike calcification. Small pleural effusion on the left side. Sonograms of the left chest wall **b** longitudinal and **c** transverse to the rib show tumorous expansion of the rib (R; ▲). The tumor is heteroge-

neous with bright linear echoes (↓; calcifications) and a knobby surface; does not move with the lung. **d** Postcontrast thoracic CT: extensive rib destruction by a nonhomogeneous tumor (▼) with calcifications (↓). **DD:** Ewing sarcoma, less likely histiocytosis X. Histology: histiocytosis X. Subsequent skeletal radiographs showed sharply circumscribed osteolysis in the left parietal region.

4 Abdominal Pain

R. D. Schulz

Abdominal pain is among the most common symptoms that move parents to seek medical attention for their child. Unfortunately, the examining physician is often unable to establish a cause, especially when the pain is chronic and recurring. This is frustrating for the child, the parents, and the physician. The value of diagnostic ultrasound in these cases depends on various factors: acute abdominal pain; localizable pain; the patient's age and gender; accompanying symptoms such as fever, vomiting, anemia, and failure to thrive; or postoperative states. Even diseases remote from the abdomen (e. g., pneumonia, tonsillitis) can be a source of abdominal pain in infants and young schoolchildren.

Conversely, pain outside the abdomen may be symptomatic of intra-abdominal disease, such as shoulder pain due to splenic rupture or groin pain due to ureteral colic. Even older children may have difficulty reporting the exact location of their abdominal pain. Infants and young schoolchildren tend to localize their pain to the umbilical area ("umbilical colic"), although it is very rare for objective evidence of disease actually to be found in the umbilical region. School and family problems or other emotional factors may cause youngsters to complain of abdominal pain. In all cases, a detailed history of the pain should be elicited, from the patient, even though this is time-consuming.

In children with chronic recurring abdominal pain, clinical examination reveals an organic lesion in only 5–10% of cases, and only a small percentage of these can be objectively documented with ultrasound. Some clinical problems are reflected only partially, transiently, or not at all in sonographic findings. Sometimes there is a morphologic correlate that is easily recognized but perhaps nonspecific, so that ist significance is not appreciated. A structure found to be abnormal may indeed be the offending lesion, such as a cystic lesion of the spleen following splenic trauma, or the finding may be symptomatic of an underlying disorder, such as ascites secondary to an abdominal lymphoma.

Sonography is most often rewarding in patients with acute abdominal pain due, for example, to a ureteral stone, gallstone, pancreatitis, blunt organ trauma, acute urinary tract infection, hematocolpos, torsion of ovarian cyst, intussusception, perityphlitic abscess, or appendicitis. Ultrasound is less frequently rewarding in children with recurrent abdominal pain, although conditions such as ureteropelvic junction obstruction, organic lesions developing weeks or months after trauma (e. g., splenic and pancreatic cysts), postoperative scar abscesses (sometimes forming years after abdominal surgery), gallstones, Meckel diverticulum, abdominal tumor, and Crohn disease (circumscribed or long segmental thickening of the bowel wall) are

detected with greater frequency than might be assumed. Ureteropelvic junction obstruction in particular may go undetected for years. A posttraumatic splenic or pancreatic cyst may remain silent for a prolonged period until the child finally presents with abdominal pain, and careful questioning may be needed to elicit an antecedent trauma. In a number of patients examined for chronic abdominal pain, we have diagnosed Crohn disease by noting a persistent thickening of the bowel wall, although sonographic findings permit only a presumptive diagnosis of this condition.

The symptom of abdominal pain plays a role in many disorders—abdominal mass, renal disease, hydronephrosis, blunt abdominal trauma, gastrointestinal disease, pediatric gynecologic problems—so it will be dealt with in those chapters as well.

The sonographic evaluation of recurrent abdominal pain should always be performed with a full urinary bladder (good acoustic window) so that abnormalities in the lesser pelvis can be recognized. Experience shows that sonograms of a schoolchild with chronic abdominal pain demonstrating normal internal organs can have a profoundly reassuring effect on the child and his or her parents and can even lead to a regression of symptoms in some patients.

Although a complete overview of pediatric abdominal pain and its manifold causes is beyond our scope, we shall present illustrative cases that will familiarize the examiner with the sonographic features of important diseases.

References

Alpern, M. B., M. A. Sandler, G. M. Kellman, B. L. Madrazo: Chronic pancreatitis: ultrasonic features. Radiology 155 (1985) 215–219

Fawcett, H. D., C. K. Hayden, L. E. Swischuk, et al.: Spontaneous extrahepatic biliary duct perforation in infancy. J. Canad. Ass. Radiol. 37 (1986) 206

Henschke, C. I., R. L. Teele: Cholelithiasis in children: recent observations. J. Ultrasound Med. 2 (1983) 481–484

Jeffrey, R. B., F. C. Laing, F. R. Lewis: Acute appendicitis: high resolution real-time US findings. Radiology 163 (1987) 11–14

Laing, F. C., R. B. Jeffrey jr.: Ultrasound versus excretory uropathy in evaluating acute flank pain. Radiology 154 (1985) 613–616

McGahan, J. P., H. E. Phillips, R. C. Stadalnik et al.: Ultrasound and radionuclide biliary scanning in acute pediatric abdominal pain. Radiology 152 (1984) 549

Peters, H., K. H. Deeg, D. Weitzel: Die Ultraschalluntersuchung des Kindes. Springer, Berlin 1987

Urinary Tract

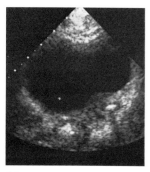
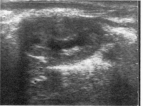
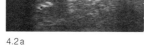

4.1   4.2a

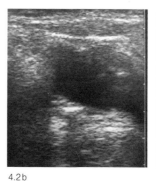
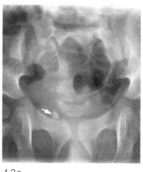

4.2b   4.2c

4.1   Left ureteral stone in an 8-year-old boy with acute left lower abdominal pain and hematuria. Transverse scan of the left lower abdomen: single elliptical echo with a hypoechogenic rim and acoustic shadow posterior to the echo-free urinary bladder: distal ureteral calculus, without evidence of stasis. The stone was passed spontaneously.

4.2   Right ureteral stone with urinary statis in a 2-year-old boy with recurrent, sometimes paroxysmal abdominal pain; no hematuria. **a** Right posterior paravertebral longitudinal scan: kidney with mild ectasia of the renal pelvis: urinary stasis. **b** Transverse lower abdominal scan: ureteral stone appears as a solitary echo of moderate intensity in the right paramedian area, posterior to the anechogenic urinary bladder. **c** Detail of a pelvic radiograph: triangular calculus above the right pubic bone (arrow).

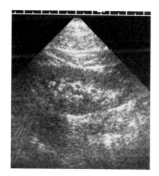
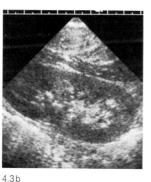

4.3a   4.3b

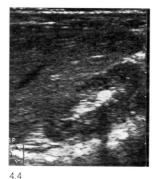

4.4

4.3   Reflux nephropathy of the right kidney in a 9-year-old boy with a long history of recurrent abdominal pain. Urine studies reportedly negative. **a** Right paravertebral posterior longitudinal scan: small right kidney (length 5.5 cm) with concentric parenchymal reduction. **b** Left paravertebral posterior longitudinal scan: normal left kidney (length 8.5 cm). VCUG confirmed the suspicion of a grade III vesicoureteral reflux on the right side.

4.4   Renal pelvic stone in a 10-month-old boy with several weeks' history of abdominal cramps and two episodes of microhematuria. Admitted with acute abdominal pain. Right flank longitudinal scan: large solitary echo in the renal pelvis, slightly below center, with associated acoustic shadow. No urinary stasis. Renal pelvic stone.

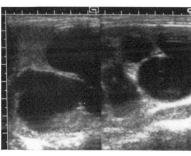
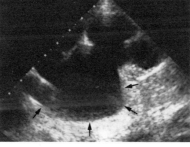

4.5a   4.5b

4.5   Left ureteropelvic junction obstruction in a 7-year-old girl with a long history of abdominal pain that became predominantly left-sided in the last 6 months. Urine studies negative. Negative US elsewhere 6 months before. **a** Left flank longitudinal scan: thin renal parenchyma with multiple round and mushroom-shaped anechogenic areas filling the pyelocaliceal system. **DD:** multicystic dysplastic kidney, hydronephrosis of other etiology.

b Left flank coronal scan: massive dilatation of the collecting system with a balloon-like protrusion of the anechogenic renal pelvis past the medial renal contour (arrows). A large extrarenal protrusion of the pelvis having no communication with the ureter is pathognomonic for uteropelvic junction obstruction. Renal scintigraphy still indicated 27% activity on the left side. The patient became asymptomatic following surgery.

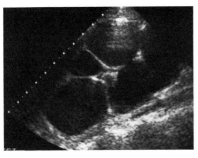
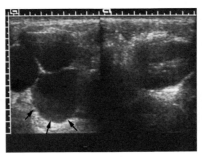
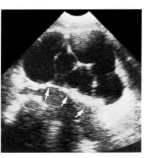

4.6a   4.6b   4.7

4.6   Left ureteropelvic junction obstruction in a 15-year-old girl with a long history of abdominal pain, at times more pronounced on the left side. Her pediatrician regarded her symptoms as psychogenic. Negative US by the urologist 6 months before. **a** Left flank longitudinal scan: multiple echo-free areas of varying size in the renal collecting system with severe parenchymal narrowing. **DD:** multicystic dysplastic kidney, hydronephrosis of other etiology. **b** Posterior transverse scans over the spinal column: Right side: normal renal cross section. Left side: anechogenic areas completely fill the renal collecting system. Also a typical balloon-like expansion of the extrarenal pelvis (arrows). Ureteropelvic junction obstruction. Intravenous EU confirmed diagnosis with contrast retention for 12 hours on the left side. Isotope scan showed left renal function impairment. The patient was asymptomatic following an Anderson—Heynes operation.

4.7   Ureteropelvic junction obstruction in a pelvic kidney. A 14-year-old boy with recurrent periumbilical pain admitted with acute colicky pain in the lower abdomen and a palpable lower abdominal mass. Midlongitudinal scan of the lower abdomen: "septated" echo-free mass with scalloped borders anterior to the promontory and sacrum (arrows). Urography showed no excretion on the left side, even after 20 hours. Isotope scan showed a silent kidney with normal function on the right side. **DD:** multicystic displastic left kidney, extreme hydronephrosis. Operation: nephrectomy due to a nonfunctioning pelvic kidney with ureteropelvic junction stenosis.

Biliary Tract

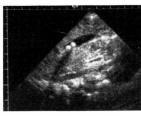
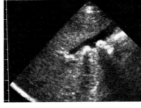
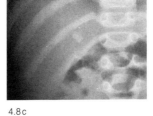

4.8a   4.8b   4.8c

4.8   Gallstones in a 5-month-old boy, restless since birth with cramping abdominal pain. The infant would not become quiet when held by the mother, who felt rejected by her child. **a** Parasagittal scan of the right upper abdomen: two coarse solitary echoes in the gallbladder lumen, at the neck of the gallbladder, with associated shadows. No hydrops. **DD:** bowel gas. **b** On upright examination the coarse echoes move toward the fundus but remain intraluminal: two gallstones. **c** Abdominal radiograph: faintly opaque calculi in the right upper abdomen. Elucidation of the etiology of stone formation: hemolytic disease, metabolic disease, cystic fibrosis?

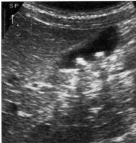

4.9

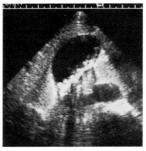

4.10

4.9   Gallstones in a 14-year-old girl with known cystic fibrosis, who presented with acute right upper abdominal pain that was most severe after fatty meals. Right upper abdominal longitudinal scan: two relatively large, solitary echoes in the gallbladder with associated acoustic shadows; cholecystolithiasis. Symptoms regressed after operative removal.

4.10   Gallstones in a 14-year-old boy with sickle cell anemia, admitted with acute right upper quadrant pain. Parasagittal scan of the right upper abdomen: numerous echoes of varying size on the floor of the gallbladder, some with acoustic shadows: multiple gallbladder calculi. This complication is more common in the setting of certain hematologic disorders. Sometimes an acute event of this kind is the first sign of underlying disease.

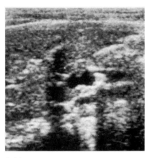
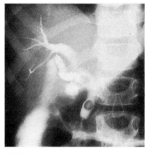
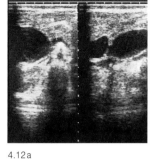
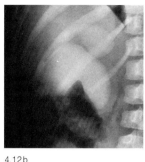

4.11a   4.11b   4.12a   4.12b

4.11 Common duct stone in an 8-year-old girl with recurrent, poorly localized abdominal pain and jaundice. **a** Right flank longitudinal scan of the upper abdomen: widened common bile duct containing a single echo that spans the whole lumen and casts an acoustic shadow: common duct stone. **b** Cholangiography shows an oval-shaped filling defect in the common bile duct caused by a prepapillary calculus: common duct stone (Dr. Winkielman, Essen).

4.12 Two choledochal cysts in a 2-year-old girl with recurrent, sometimes colicky upper abdominal pain. **a** Transverse and longitudinal scans of the upper abdomen: spherical, anechogenic, right paramedian lesion in the area of the pancreatic head; longitudinal scan shows two ovoid, echo-free structures anterior to the vena cava: choledochal cysts. **b** Cholangiography 3 hours postcontrast: one small and one very large biliary tract cyst. Surgery (Dr. Tröger, Heidelberg).

Posttraumatic Lesions

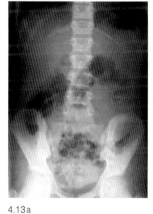
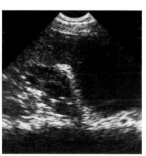

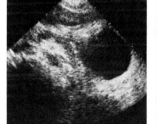
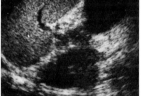

4.13a   4.13b   4.14a   4.14b

4.13 Posttraumatic splenic cyst in a 10-year-old girl with recurrent, predominantly left-sided abdominal pain. **a** Plain abdominal radiograph: large, rounded soft-tissue density in the left middle and lower abdomen displacing the intestinal tract. The mass cannot be assigned to a specific organ. **b** Left flank coronal scan: large, echo-free lesion at the lower pole of the spleen partly overlying the inferior renal pole. Posttraumatic splenic cyst situated low on the inferior pole of the spleen. Several weeks earlier the patient had sustained blunt trauma to the left side of the abdomen. Cyst removed operatively.

4.14 Posttraumatic pseudocyst of the pancreatic tail in a 15-year-old boy with a 2-month history of abdominal pain. The patient was a motocross cyclist who claimed no ill effects from repeated previous falls **a** Upper abdominal transverse scan: 4-cm echo-free structure with acoustic enhancement in the tail of the pancreas: posttraumatic cyst of the pancreatic tail. Appearance of this lesion is often delayed weeks or months after trauma. Clinical symptom: abdominal pain. **b** Left upper abdominal longitudinal scan angled to the left: echo-free cyst caudal to the splenic pole and lateral to the left kidney, partially cut by the scan. Also, an anechogenic crescent-shaped area in the epidiaphragmatic region: low-lying pancreatic cyst and left-sided pleural effusion. The cyst was percutaneously aspirated under US guidance, partially refilled, then gradually resolved over a period of weeks.

Tumor

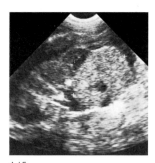 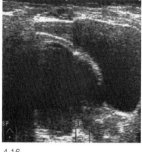 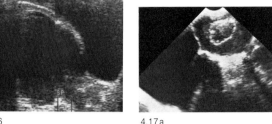 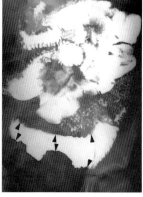

4.15   4.16   4.17a   4.17b

4.**15** **Wilms tumor** in a 4½-year-old girl admitted with sudden postprandial pain and pallor; no shock. Right flank longitudinal scan: echogenic mass in the lower half of the right kidney with scattered foci of necrosis (hypoechogenic). Operation: Wilms tumor.

4.**16** **Torsion of a right ovarian cyst** in an 11-year-old girl with right lower abdominal pain of sudden onset. Oblique scan of the lower abdomen: a large, almost echo-free mass with scalloped margins indenting the posterior bladder wall: ovarian cyst. **DD:** abscess, teratoma.

4.**17** **Non-Hodgkin lymphoma of the small bowel** in a 12-year-old boy with occasional upper abdominal pain and a 3-year history of declining activity level. Anemia, palpable lower abdominal mass. **a** Oblique scan of the left lower abdomen: large cranial anechogenic area representing ascites; below is a hypoechogenic target pattern with a central echo-free lumen sourrounded by small bowel wall thickened by tumor infiltration. **b** UGI series: rigid segment of small bowel with thickened wall (▼) and coarse mucosal folds in the lower abdomen: tumor infiltration of the bowel wall and mesentery.

Infection

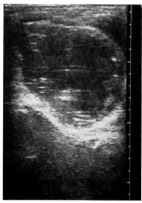 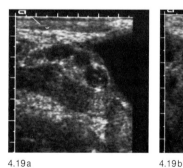

4.18   4.19a   4.19b

4.**18** **Perityphlitic abscess** in a 9-year-old girl with a 10-day history of abdominal pain and low-grade fever. No leukocytosis. Swelling in the right lower abdomen was noted clinically. Parasagittal scan of the right lower abdomen: large mass with a moderately echogenic periphery and nonhomogeneous center. Part of the mass is retrovesical and part extends past the upper border of the bladder to a point directly beneath the abdominal wall: abscess. **DD:** ovarian cyst, cystic teratoma (hematocolpos). Operation: perityphlitic abscess involving loops of the small bowel.

4.**19** **Loop abscess** in a 7-year-old boy who had enteritis with severe abdominal pain and fever 8 days before, was asymptomatic for 6 days, then suffered increasing diffuse abdominal pain. Elevated ESR and WBC. **a** Longitudinal scan of the right lower abdomen: partly chainlike, partly bandlike hypoechogenic structures, reasonably well defined, located behind the bladder. Suspected perityphlitic abscess with bowel wall infiltration in the lower abdomen. **DD:** lymph node tumors in the mesentery. **b** Right midabdominal longitudinal scan: three intestinal target patterns below the abdominal wall with bowel-wall tickening and "stagnant" intraluminal fluid: atonic loops of the small bowel. Operation: lops abscess. US features of perityphlitic abscess are highly variable. A nonhomogeneous hypoechogenic pattern is most common, but some lesions are moderately echogenic, like a solid tumor, usually signifying that the abscess hat not yet liquefied or has a creamy-purulent composition.

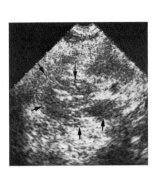
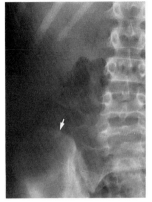

4.20a   4.20b

4.20 Phlegmonous appendicitis in a 14-year-old boy with noncharacteristic abdominal pain, slight tenderness in the right lower quadrant, negative rectal findings, no peritonism. **a** Longitudinal scan of the right lower abdomen: curved hypoechogenic structure in the lower abdomen (arrows), tender to pressure: inflamed appendix. Also a moderate collection of free fluid in the lower abdomen: appendicitis with exudation suspected. **b** Abdominal radiograph: fist-sized soft-tissue density in the right lower quadrant with a padding effect on the surrounding bowel and a pea-size stone within the density: fecolith. Operation: phlegmonous appendicitis with impending perforation.

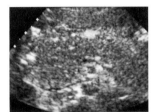

4.21

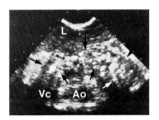
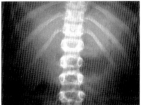

4.22a   4.22b

4.21 Pancreatitis in a 5-year-old girl with acute onset of upper abdominal pain, elevated ESR, elevated amylase and lipase. Transverse epigastric scan: moderate diffuse swelling of the pancreas with a slightly increased echogenicity: acute pancreatitis. Coexisting non-Hodgkin lymphoma.

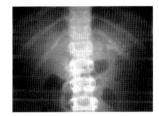

4.22c

4.22 Hereditary clacifying pancreatitis in a 9-year-old girl with recurrent abdominal pain. Known maternal and sibling history of pancreatitis. **a** Transverse epigastric scan: moderate diffuse enlargement of the pancreas (arrows) with multiple coarse echoes, some with associated shadowing: calcifications. L = Liver, Ao = aorta, Vc = vena cava. Normal pancreatic structure has largely disappeared. Calcifying pancreatitis. **b** Detail of an abdominal radiograph at the age of 7 years: no abnormalities 2 years prior to US. **c** Radiograph at the time of US (**a**) shows multiple plaquelike calcifications in the upper midabdomen following the anatomic course of the pancreas (Dr. Richter, Hamburg).

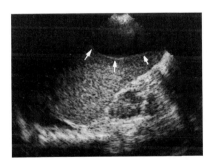

4.23

4.23 Splenic abscess in an 8-year-old girl who had an upper airway infection with fever and diarrhea 2 weeks before, improved with supportive care. Admitted with high fever, abdominal pain, vomiting. Left flank longitudinal coronal scan: oval echo-free area in the lateral subcapsular part of the spleen, well demarcated (arrows). Also a crescent-shaped anechogenic zone over the diaphragm: left pleural effusion. **DD** of cystic splenic lesion: posttraumatic splenic cyst (despite no apparent trauma history), splenic abscess (consistent with clinical picture). US-guided splenic aspiration: abscess. Treatment: emergency splenectomy. Infectious swelling of the spleen can lead to rupture with subcapsular hemorrhage. *Caution:* needle aspiration in a patient with splenic abscess or subcapsular hemorrhage can cause profuse and potentially fatal bleeding.

Other Causes

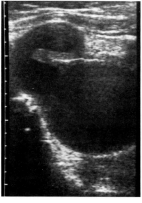
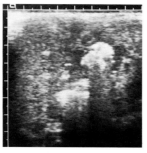
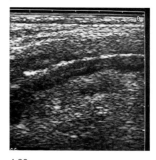

4.24   4.25   4.26

4.24 Hematocolpos in an 11-year-old girl (premenarchal) with a 5-week history of lower abdominal and back pain. Lower midabdominal longitudinal scan: large anechogenic structure in the lesser pelvis with a hooklike anterior extension (anteflexed uterus): hematocolpos.

4.25 "Adult" type pyloric stenosis in a 6-month-old girl with occasional vomiting since the age of 4 weeks. Presented with a 2-week history of colicky abdominal pain and profuse vomiting, cessation of weight gain. Parasagittal scan of the upper abdomen: large subhepatic target pattern (diameter > 3 cm, wall thickness 7 mm). Pyloric stenosis, which became clinically manifest at a relatively late stage ("adult" type). Treatment: pylorotomy. "Ordinary" pyloric stenoses that are clinically and sonographically apparent at 2–6 weeks, like intussusception (see chapter 7), belong to the symptom of abdominal pain.

4.26 Crohn disease in a 15-year-old girl with recurrent abdominal pain for months. Oblique scan of the right mid- to lower abdomen: two parallel, relatively wide hypoechogenic bands, tender and rigid on palpation. The bands represent a longitudinal section through the terminal ileum, which shows marked wall thickening. Impression of Crohn disease requires confirmation by a GI series and clinical tests. Here the suspicion was confirmed. US alone cannot provide a definitive diagnosis of Crohn disease but in confirmed cases is useful for investigating complications: peforation, recurrence, abscess formation.

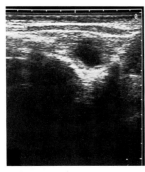
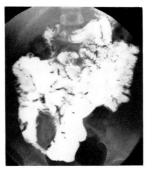
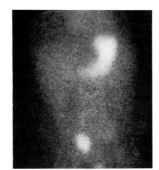

4.27 a   4.27 b   4.27 c

4.27 Meckel diverticulum in a 4½-year-old boy with a 3-week history of abdominal pain, sometimes colicky. One occasion of fresh blood in the stool. **a** Longitudinal scan of the right lower abdomen: peripherally sonodense, centrally anechogenic feature at the level of the promontory. The lesion cannot be assigned to a specific organ. Repeat scan on the following day showed the same findings. Enteric duplication, such as a Meckel diverticulum, suspected. **b** Small bowel series shows filling

defect in the right lower abdomen displacing the terminal ileum. Space-occupying lesion, such as a Meckel diverticulum. **c** ^{99m}Technetium scan, 90 minutes after isotope administration. Uptake in the right lower abdomen signifies ectopic gastric mucosa. Suspicion was confirmed at the operation, which relieved the patient's complaints. In retrospect, the small bowel contrast study was unnecessary.

5 Abdominal Masses

U. V. Willi

An abdominal mass can arise in association with a neoplastic, inflammatory, traumatic, malformative, metabolic, or iatrogenic disorder. As a result, abdominal masses are presented in various sections of this book. Many examples in this chapter are tumors in the strict sense, e.g., malignancies. But the majority of pediatric abdominal masses are benign, and cystic masses in children are almost invariably benign. Many pediatric abdominal masses are characteristic for a specific age group.

Sonography, radiography (including CT), radionuclide scanning, and magnetic resonance imaging must be coordinated to ensure a maximum gain of diagnostic information. The *plain supine abdominal radiograph* gives information on the location of the *mass*, its size, and its effect on adjacent structures (with a possible disturbance of *bowel* motility). This may help in establishing its origin. The film can be examined for possible *calcifications* and any associated malformations of the *skeleton*. Knowledge of these simple X-ray findings (like any useful preliminary information) can make the subsequent ultrasound examination simpler, faster, and more rewarding. We also reemphasize the importance of a detailed history and clinical examination, giving attention to general and special symptoms, clinical findings, and simple laboratory tests.

Lesions ot the peritoneal cavity or retroperitoneum can be difficult for the clinican to localize to a particular space, so "abdomen" frequently refers to both compartments. In most cases sonography is an effective localizing tool, especially when the examiner notes *differences in the mobility* of different structures *with respiration*. For example, free motion of the liver over a neuroblastoma implies a free inner gliding surface of the peritoneum. Mobility between a retroperitoneal tumor and kidney suggests that there should be no difficulty separating the tumor from the kidney. Of course, such criteria may not be useful if the mass is very large or if pain limits respiratory excursions.

Change in the location, size, shape, or echo pattern of a mass in serial examinations, or the absence of such change, is an important diagnostic criterion. If the appearance and especially the echo pattern of a mass remain unchanged over a period of days, the lesion is definitely not a hematoma. "Classic" presentations do exist, but the "classic triad" of a palpable mass, abdominal pain, and jaundice, for example, is rarely seen in a child with a choledochal cyst. Each of these symptoms alone, possibly combined with an acholic stool, may suggest the diagnosis.

Essentially a *morphologic* study, sonography should be used first and foremost to ascertain the location or origin of a mass, i.e., identify it as retroperitoneal (renal/nonrenal) or intraperitoneal (pelvis/anterior abdomen and spleen/liver).

The *functional* (pathophysiologic) behavior of a mass can be demonstrated by simple *conventional radiographic contrast studies* or by the more sophisticated process of *scintigraphy* (radionuclide scanning). In the case of a cystic mass of the liver (of the choledochal cyst type) where there is a question of biliary tract obstruction, biliary scintigraphy can be informative. Hepatic scintigraphy using various markers is employed with advantage for the differentiation of (malignant) hepatic tumors (see examples in this chapter). Skeletal scintigraphy in patients with neuroblastoma can demonstrate even subtle lesions, and it offers an alternative to excretory urography when applied as a function test in the early phase of renal excretion. The combined use of metaiodobenzylguanidine (MIBG) and iodine-123 scintigraphy is a superior technique for demonstrating neuroblastoma and its metastases both in solid bone and in the bone marrow (relies on the labeling of neurosecretory granules in tumor tissue, though their quantum is highly variable).

The diagnosis of possible spinal canal involvement by neuroblastoma is often academic, as it is seldom relevant to therapy. Nevertheless, *magnetic resonance imaging* may one day become a routine investigation when this question arises.

In most cases sonography will either confirm and clarify or else refute the clinical suspicion of an abdominal mass, the latter by demonstrating normal findings or by establishing a different diagnosis or suspicion. This may in turn lead to the institution of other diagnostic procedures. Repetition of the ultrasound examination in patients with equivocal findings is often the simplest approach and is frequently rewarding.

References

A modern approach to the abdominal mass in children. Semin. Roentgenol. 23 (1988)

Hartman, G. E., S. J. Shochat: Abdominal mass lesions in the newborn: diagnosis and treatment. Clin. Perinatol. 16 (1989)

Miller, J. H., B. S. Greenspan: Integrated imaging of hepatic tumors in childhood. Part 1: Malignant lesions. – Part 2: Benign lesions. Radiology 154 (1985) 83–90; 91–100

Reiman, T. A. H., M. J. Siegel, G. D. Shackelford: Wilms tumor in children: abdominal CT and US evaluation. Radiology 160 (1986) 501–505

Retroperitoneum, Renal
(Differential Diagnosis of Wilms Tumor)

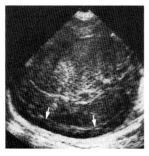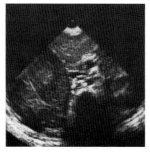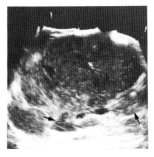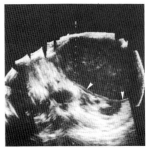

5.1a   5.1b   5.2a   5.2b

5.1 Stage I Wilms tumor in a girl of 3 years, 4 months with a right flank mass noted incidentally in a routine examination. **a** Longitudinal and **b** transverse scans: solid, relatively homogeneous, sharply marginated renal mass on the right side, hypoechogenic to the liver. Renal tissue is visible posteriorly (arrows): characteristic of a stage I Wilms tumor. Respiratory dynamics show movement of the liver relative to the tumor. Nephrectomy. Histology confirmed US diagnosis. Chemotherapy. No complications at 7 years of age.

5.2 Stage I Wilms tumor in a 12-year-old girl who had noticed a left upper quadrant mass 1 month before and had stabbing pains for 1 week prior to admission. "Splenic tumor." **a** Longitudinal and **b** transverse scans: large, predominantly solid, well-defined mass arising from the anterior portion of the left kidney, which is expanded longitudinally and transversely by tumor. Pseudomembrane (▸), renal pole (→): stage I Wilms tumor. Nephrectomy. Histology confirmed US diagnosis. Chemotherapy. 4½ years later, local irregularity of the hepatic echo structure. Clinical and CT findings normal, patient healthy.

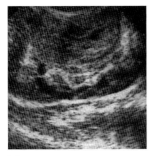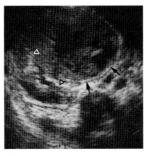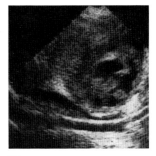

5.3a   5.3b   5.3c

5.3 Stage I Wilms tumor in a 4-year-old girl with a right-sided abdominal mass, tumor suspected. **a** Right longitudinal scan: exophytic growth of a predominantly hypoechogenic, solid / cystic, well-defined tumor from an anterior part of the kidney toward the abdominal wall. Posterior renal echo structure is normal. **b** Transverse scan demonstrates separation between the tumor and the transversely extending posteroinferior part of

the kidney with al slight cavitary dilatation; pseudomembrane of tumor (→). ■. **c** Right flank coronal scan: indentation and medial displacement of the caudal portion of the inferior vena cava, characteristic of stage I Wilms tumor. Nephrectomy. Histology confirmed US impression. Chemotherapy. No complications at the age of 6½ years.

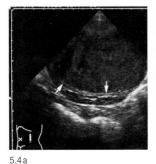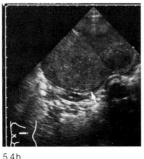

5.4a   5.4b

5.4 Stage I Wilms tumor in a 14-month-old girl with congenital bilateral aniridia and central cataract as well as a left-sided abdominal mass suspected of being a Wilms tumor. **a** Left flank coronal and **b** transverse scans confirm the suspicion: typical solid, well-demarcated stage I renal tumor showing exophytic growth in an anterolateral direction. Pseudomembrane (←). Nephrectomy. Histology confirmed US diagnosis. Chromosomes: deletion of the short arm of chromosome 11. Chemotherapy. 7 months later sepsis. Recovery.

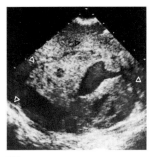

5.5

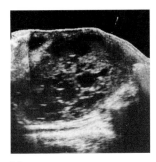 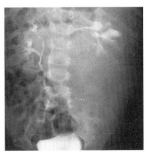

5.6a   5.6b

5.5 Sarcomatous form of Wilms tumor in a 10-month-old boy (North Africa) with a facial cleft, VSD, and "massive hepatomegaly"; tumor? Longitudinal scan: large, heterogenic, predominantly solid tumor of the right kidney containing relatively large, lacuna-like cystic areas. Relation to the parenchyma is unclear, appears limited to the intracapsular space. Endophytic growth? Renal function (left kidney unenlarged)? EU showed "normal" function of the anterior part. Sarcomatous form of a Wilms tumor? Nephrectomy. Histology confirmed suspicion. Chemotherapy. Patient lost to follow-up.

5.6 Suspected Wilms tumor in a 1-year-old girl with an abdominal mass. **a** Longitudinal scan of the left hemiabdomen: large, solid tumor permeated by numerous cysts; Wilms tumor suspected, possibly sarcomatous. **b** 15-minute EU consistent with a Wilms tumor. Nephrectomy. Histology showed congenital mesoblastic nephroma. No chemotherapy. No complications at 7 years of age.

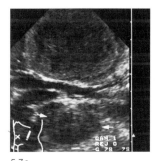 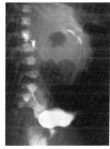

5.7a   5.7b

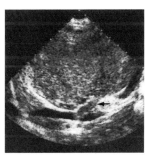 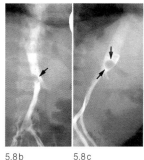

5.8a   5.8b   5.8c

5.7 Suspected congenital mesoblastic nephroma in a 1-day-old boy with a solid tumor of the left kidney diagnosed by US 7 weeks prenatally. **a** Left coronal scan: solid, heterogeneous, sharply demarcated tumor of approximately the same size; "double rim effect" on the inferior half; apparent absence of normal renal tissue. Normal right kidney (arrow). **b** EU, lateral projection: "normally" functioning anteriorized renal segments. Suspicion of congenital mesoblastic nephroma (statistics; virtually no growth in 7 weeks). **DD:** nephroblastomatosis; classic Wilms tumor; sarcomatous renal tumor; sympathetic tumor invading the kidney; prenatal renal vein thrombosis unlikely (absence of change). Nephrectomy. Histology: confirmatory. No further treatment (4 months).

5.8 Stage I Wilms tumor in a 9-months-old boy with a right-sided abdominal mass. Tumor? **a** US findings characteristic of a solid stage I Wilms tumor on the right side. Right flank coronal scan: tumor thrombus in the right renal vein projecting into the inferior vena cava (←). Cavography under general anesthesia. **b** Anteroposterior and **c** lateral views demonstrate the filling defect due to the thrombus (arrows). Kidney and thrombus removed without difficulty. Histology: confirmatory. Chemotherapy. No complications at 3 years of age.

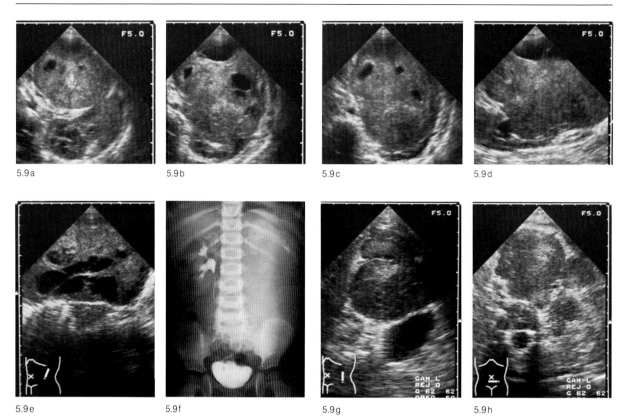

5.9a   5.9b   5.9c   5.9d

5.9e   5.9f   5.9g   5.9h

5.9 Fragile stage I Wilms tumor and secondary metastases in a girl of 2 years, 7 months with a large left-sided abdominal mass: Wilms tumor? **a–c** Transverse and **d** longitudinal scans: progressive reduction of normal renal parenchyma posteriorly in a cranial to caudal direction. Solid, moderately echogenic, well-demarcated tumor growing exophytically from the anteroinferior part of the kidney. **e** Left flank longitudinal scan angled anteromedially: multiple large, lacuna-like cystic areas, most conspicuous anteromedially. **f** 15-minute EU: persistent left renal opacification signifying mild outflow obstruction or renal artery compression: fragile stage I Wilms tumor? **DD:** cystic/rhabdoid/sarcomatous variant? Nephrectomy; intraoperative rupture of the tumor (iatrogenic conversion of stage I to stage III).

Histology: Wilms tumor with a "favorable" histology. Chemotherapy administered as for stage I disease. **g, h** Scans 5 months later show extensive secondary solid/polycyclic metastases from the left flank to the pelvis. Secondary subtotal resection (involvement of the left uterine tube, left ovary, colon, and abdominal wall). More chemotherapy, radiation. Scintigraphy showed cold spots in the liver: metastases? Sonograms at age 4 years: irregular hepatic echo structure. *Note:* presumed "veno-occlusive disease" of the liver secondary to the combination of Fluothane (anesthesia), chemotherapy, and irradiation. Isotope and US findings consistent with this assumption (the patient had 3 Fluothane anesthesias).

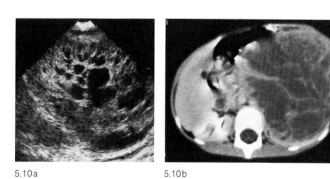

5.10a   5.10b

5.10 Suspected stage III Wilms tumor in a 5-year-old boy who had fallen from a sofa 2 months before; presented with an abdominal mass. **a** Left longitudinal scan: very large, solid tumor containing numerous rounded cysts of moderate size: suspicion of nephroblastoma: sarcomatous or unusually cystic due to trauma? EU showed no apparent contrast excretion on the left side. **b** CT: faint enhancement of the left kidney posteriorly. Right kidney normal. Operation: nephrectomy, splenectomy, removal of the pancreatic tail and para-aortic and mesenteric nodes. Histology: metastases in the adrenal gland, peripancreatic fat and lymph nodes; spleen negative. Stage III nephroblastoma (possibly posttraumatic expansion). Chemotherapy, radiation. The patient is doing well at the age of 8 years, 9 months.

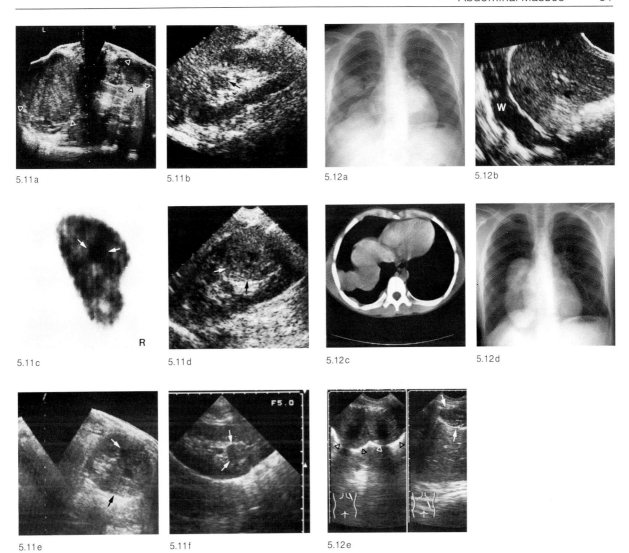

5.11a 5.11b 5.12a 5.12b

5.11c 5.11d 5.12c 5.12d

5.11e 5.11f 5.12e

5.**11** **Bilateral Wilms tumor** in a 10-month-old boy with a left-sided abdominal mass: splenomegaly? tumor? **a** Posterior transverse scan: large, predominantly solid left-sided tumor with posterior exophytic growth (△), smaller inferolateral tumor on right side (△): bilateral Wilms tumors. Nephrectomy on the left, tumor enucleation on the right. 1-year course of chemotherapy. **b** Right flank longitudinal scan at 28 months: pseudotumor (arrow), confirmed by **c** posterior DMSA scintigram: increased uptake by prominent Bertini column (arrows); kidney shape altered by previous tumor enucleation. **d** Right flank longitudinal scan and **e** posterior transverse scan at the age of 3½ years: tumor recurrence inferolaterally on the right side (arrows). Extirpation, 1 year chemotherapy. **f** Posterior longitudinal scan at 5 years, 4 months: second tumor recurrence inferiorly (arrows). Extirpation, 1 year chemotherapy. Fourteen months later, the patient is "healthy". Right kidney shows irregular compensatory hypertrophy and increased echogenicity. Creatinine normal (6½ years). *Note:* EU also performed initially, EU and CT with each recurrence. Primary tumors and recurrences were all diagnosed by US.

5.**12** **Metastatic Wilms tumor** in a 4-year-old boy (North Africa) who had undergone a right nephrectomy. **a** Chest radiograph at 7 years of age: multiple pulmonary metastases in both lungs. **b** Longitudinal scan of the right upper abdomen: extensive supradiaphragmatic metastasis (M) in close contact with the diaphragm. **c** CT scan after 1 month of chemotherapy: shrinkage of metastases. Two-stage removal, starting on the left side; removal on the right side was incomplete due to the involvement of the diaphragm. Chemotherapy continued for 1 year. **d** Radiograph 3½ years later: recurrent metastasis in the basal posteromedial area of the right thorax. **e** Posterior longitudinal thoracic scan: solid, bilobed metastasis (▽); slightly lower, at the retrohepatic level, is a smaller retroperitoneal metastasis (←). Reoperation with radical removal. Chemotherapy. 16 months postoperatively the patient is "well" at the age of about 12 years).

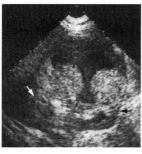
5.13a

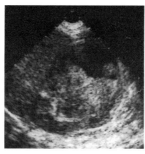
5.13b

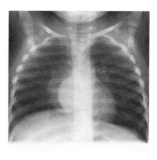
5.13c

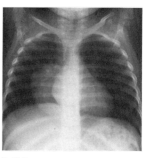
5.13d

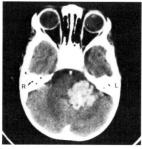
5.13e

5.13   Malignant rhabdoid renal tumor with metastatic complications in an 8-month-old boy with a 2-week history of progressive gross hematuria, otherwise healthy. **a, b** Right flank longitudinal scans give the impression of a very heterogeneous renal tumor (→ renal pole) with extensive peripheral cystic components, exhibiting both exophytic and endophytic growth.

Tumor confined to the right kidney? Massive necrotic / hemorrhagic degeneration? Sarcomatous form? Renal-invasive form of neuroblastoma? Status of inferior vena cava was further investigated by cavography, which was equivocal in terms of assessing patency. Nephrectomy uneventful. Histology: malignant rhabdoid renal tumor, partially calcified, with large necrotic foci. Local lymph nodes negative. Chemotherapy. **c** Radiograph 1 year later, right pulmonary metastases suspected. **d** Rapid progression in 3 weeks. Right lower and middle lobectomy followed by progressive vomiting. **e** CT 2 weeks postoperatively: cerebellar tumor, presumably metastatic. Palliative treatment. Patient died a few weeks later. No autopsy. *Note:* This case is unusual in its clinical presentation, US features, diagnosis, and course. With this histologic diagnosis, CT monitoring of the lungs and brain is advised. High malignancy (approximately 4% of nephroblastomas).

Retroperitoneum, Extrarenal
(Differential Diagnosis of Neuroblastoma)

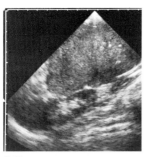
5.14a

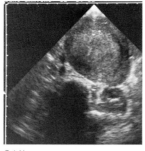
5.14b

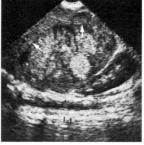
5.15a

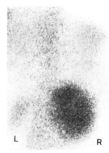
5.15b

5.14   Ganglioneuroma in a boy of 3 years, 4 months with a large mass in the left hemiabdomen found incidentally during an examination for enteritis and fever. **a** Longitudinal an **b** transverse scans: large, solid, well-defined, moderately echogenic, relatively homogeneous retroperitoneal mass with small calcifications in the left prerenal and infrarenal areas. **DD:** extrarenal neuroblastoma, ganglioneuroma, etc.; less likely teratoma, sarcoma, inflammatory pseudotumor, etc. Laboratory tests showed moderate elevation of catecholamines. Operation: removal. Catecholamines normalized in 3 weeks. *Note:* catecholamines were elevated by presumed small neuroblastomatous elements missed in the histologic examination.

5.15   Stage I neuroblastoma in a preterm male of 28.5 weeks' gestation, suspected abdominal tumor at the age of 13 months. **a** Right longitudinal scan: large, solid, sharply marginated, very heterogeneous prerenal mass containing highly echogenic elements and distorting the kidney superiorly. With respirations, high mobility is noted between the tumor and kidney and between the liver and tumor (arrows). **b** Bone scintigraphy shows normal low activity in the left kidney and spine. Very high, abnormal activity in the tumor (calcium metabolism): stage I neuroblastoma, confirmed by operation and histology. Chemotherapy. The patient is free of complications at the age of 3 years, 7 months.

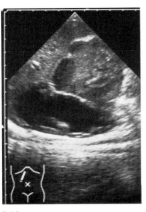
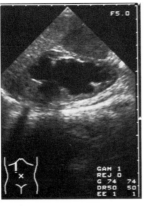
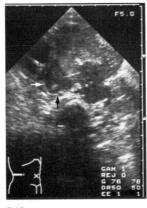
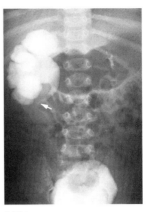

5.16a   5.16b   5.16c   5.16d

5.**16** **Stage III neuroblastoma** in a 10-month-old boy with a right upper quadrant mass found fortuitously in a routine examination. **a, b** Longitudinal and **c** right flank transverse scans: solid, heterogeneous mass with scalloped borders and calcifications (visible on radiographs) in the right prerenal area with extension between the lower renal half and the spinal column (arrows) causing extrinsic compression of the upper urinary tract and obstructive hydronephrosis. Renal size, parenchymal thickness, and echo pattern imply adequate function. **d** EU 2 hours postcontrast confirms US findings; ureteral compression (arrow). Presumed extrarenal neuroblastoma. Subtotal operative removal (lesion was partly intraspinal). Prompt regression of hydronephrosis. Histology: confirmatory. The patient is on chemotherapy at 1 year of age.

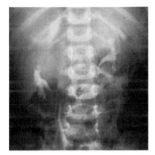
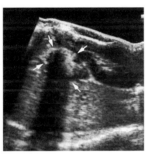
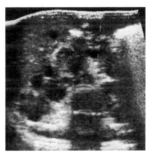
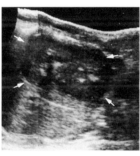

5.17a   5.17b   5.17c   5.17d

5.**17** **Recurrent stage III neuroblastoma** in a boy of 3 years, 9 months with thalassemia minor and bilateral oculomotor paresis. Presumptive US diagnosis of a neuroblastoma made elsewhere. **a** EU: suprarenal calcifying lesion on the right side with caudal displacement of the kidney and flattening of the upper pole. **b** Appearance of a lesion on a posterior longitudinal scan (arrows). **c** Transverse scan: multiple solid retroperitoneal / peripancreatic nodular lesions of varying size and echogenicity, characteristic of stage III neuroblastoma. Skeletal scintigraphy showed massive activity in the primary tumor with no osseous lesions. Laboratory tests showed massive elevation of catecholamines. Operation: removal of the tumor and multiple lymph node metastases adherent to the renal arteries, inferior vena cava, diaphragm, and inferior hepatic surface. Persistent renal ischemia necessitated nephrectomy. Histology: confirmatory. Chemotherapy. **d** Posterior longitudinal scan 7 months later: large recurrent (metastatic) tumor (arrows) in the right renal fossa. Subtotal removal was again followed by progressive recurrence, cachexia. The patient died at the age of 5 years, 3 months.

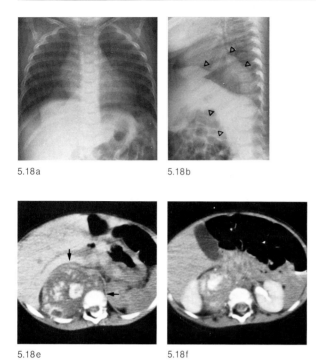
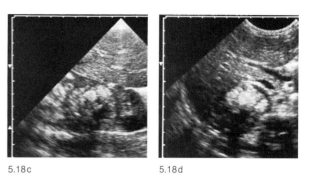

5.18a   5.18b   5.18c   5.18d

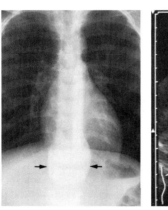
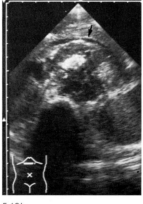

5.18e   5.18f

5.18 Stage III neuroblastoma in a 9-month-old boy with a 2-month history of recurrent cough and fever: "pneumonia." **a** AP and **b** lateral radiographs: right basal paravertebral density (△), unusual for pneumonia; nonvisualization of the right posterior diaphragm contour; possible dorsal excavation of several vertebral bodies; calcifications in the right paravertebral area at the level of T12−L1 are visible on original films. **c** Longitudinal an **d** transverse scans: solid, heterogeneous, mostly echogenic posterior tumor with a compact multinodular appearance; lesion grows cephalad from above the kidney by a transdiaphragmatic or retrodiaphragmatic route, or vice-versa, and contains calcifica-

tions. **e** Noncontrast and **f** contrast-enhanced CT: retrocrural process (arrows point to diaphragm) growing toward the renal hilum: stage III neuroblastoma. Operative removal by a thoracoabdominal route, subtotal (paraspinal / intraspinal). Histology confirmatory; ganglionic differentiation. Chemotherapy. Tumor recurred at 23 months. Two-stage operative removal: abdominal, thoracic, each subtotal. Histology: neuroblastoma with ganglionic differentiation (abdominal), ganglioneuroma (thoracic). Chemotherapy. US showed a small, fixed, solid structure between the spine and the right kidney. Patient is "well" at 3 years.

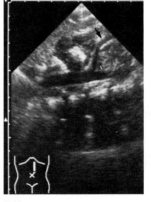
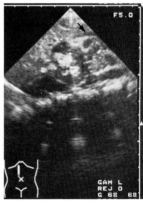

5.19a   5.19b   5.19c   5.19d

5.19 Neuroblastoma in a boy aged 4 years, 3 months with an abdominal mass. **a** Radiograph shows local bilateral paraspinal density (arrows) at T10−12, consistent with a lesion of the sympathetic system. **b** Transverse and **c, d** longitudinal scans: multinodular mass with scalloped borders and a very heterogeneous echo pattern, probably containing calcific foci. The pancreas and splenic artery (arrow in **b**) are displaced anteriorly. Lesions cranial and caudal to the superior mesenteric

artery (arrow in **c**); extension toward the porta hepatis with anterior displacement of the superior mesenteric artery (arrow in **d**). Operation: partial tumor removal. Histology confirmatory. Chemotherapy. Radical removal was attempted 1 month later, resulting at the age of 5 years, 4 months in total obstructive hydronephrosis on the left side with a nonfunctioning kidney. Nephroureterectomy. Course satisfactory until 5 years, 8 months; then, reactivation of residual tumor.

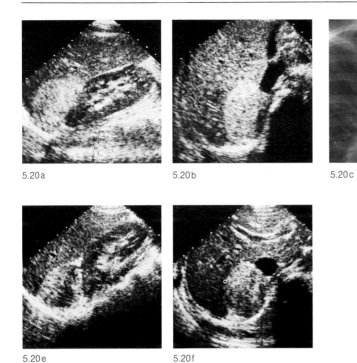

5.20a   5.20b

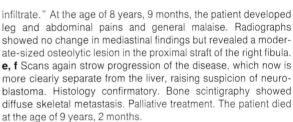

5.20c   5.20d

5.20e   5.20f

5.20 Neuroblastoma in an 8½-year-old girl with fever, hip pain, and diffuse abdominal pain. **a** Longitudinal and **b** transverse scans: erroneous impression of a well-demarcated, uniformly echogenic hepatic lesion in the right suprarenal area. **c** Radiograph: hemispheric density of moderate size in the left paramediastinal area: suspected leukemia with hepatic infiltrate and possible skeletal involvement. Multiple suboptimum bone marrow biopsies: consistent with leukemia. Chemotherapy. **d** Longitudinal scan 1 month later: partial regression of the "hepatic

infiltrate." At the age of 8 years, 9 months, the patient developed leg and abdominal pains and general malaise. Radiographs showed no change in mediastinal findings but revealed a moderate-sized osteolytic lesion in the proximal straft of the right fibula. **e, f** Scans again strow progression of the disease, which now is more clearly separate from the liver, raising suspicion of neuroblastoma. Histology confirmatory. Bone scintigraphy showed diffuse skeletal metastasis. Palliative treatment. The patient died at the age of 9 years, 2 months.

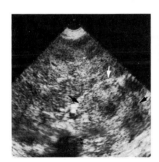
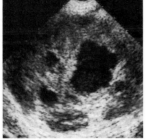
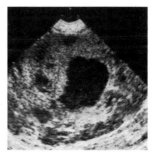

5.21a   5.21b   5.21c

5.21 Stage IV-S neuroblastoma in a 4-month-old girl with a mass in the right hemiabdomen. EU elsewhere showed downward and lateral displacement of the left kidney with normal renal function and anatomy. **a** Transverse and **b, c** left flank longitudinal scans: large, rounded prerenal / suprarenal, retrohepatic mass with large cystic components (arrows in **a**), whose separateness from the kidney is best appreciated during respirations on real-time scans. Highly irregular, diffuse increase of echogenicity in

the enlarged liver. Stage IV-S neuroblastoma with diffuse hepatic metastases suspected. Laboratory tests show massive elevation of catecholamines and moderate elevation of alpha-fetoprotein. Bone marrow normal. Operative removal of an adrenal tumor, easily separated from the kidney. Liver biopsies confirmed diagnosis. Chemotherapy. No complications. US showed incomplete regression of hepatic changes at the age of 2 years, 9 months.

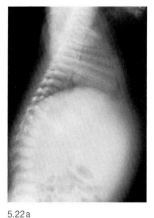
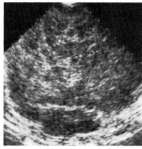
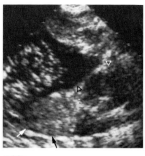
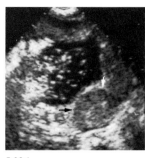

5.22a   5.22b   5.22c   5.22d

5.22 Stage IV-S neuroblastoma in a 3-month-old boy with a hard, distended abdomen. **a** Lateral radiograph: consistent with a very large liver. **b** Longitudinal scan of the right upper abdomen: very heterogeneous, enlarged right hepatic lobe with irregular hyperechogenicity. Right kidney is partially visualized. Left flank **c** coronal and **d** transverse scans: relatively small, solid suprarenal primary tumor (←) surrounded by fluid contents of the adjacent stomach. Left kidney is marked superolaterally (△).

Findings are characteristic of stage IV-S neuroblastoma (hepatic and/or bone marrow and/or cutaneous metastases). Laboratory tests showed massive elevation of catecholamines and moderate elevation of alpha-fetoprotein. Operative removal of adrenal tumor; lymph node, liver and bone marrow biopsies confirmed diagnosis (hepatic and bone marrow metastases). Chemotherapy. No complications. Slow, incomplete regression of abnormal hepatic echo structure at the age of 3½ years.

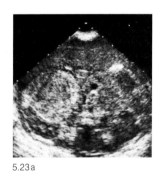
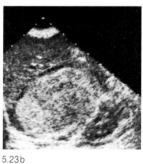

5.23a   5.23b

5.23 Stage IV-S neuroblastoma in a 12-day-old boy with a palpable mass noted in a routine examination. Laboratory tests showed very high catecholamines. CT elsewhere confirmed suspicion of neuroblastoma. Faint calcifications. **a** Transverse and **b** longitudinal scans: relatively homogeneous, well-defined, echogenic tumor in the right prerenal area. Tumor is freely mobile relative to the kidney and liver during respirations. Hypoechogenic rim, pseudomembrane-like: stage I neuroblastoma suspected. Operative removal of an adrenal tumor. Histology confirmatory. Bone marrow aspiration yielded tumor cells indicating IV-S neuroblastoma. No chemotherapy. Catecholamines normalized after surgery.

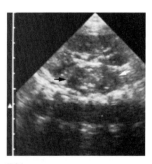
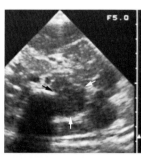
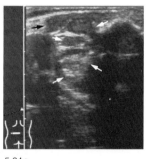
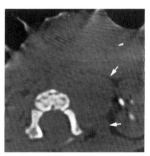

5.24a   5.24b   5.24c   5.24d

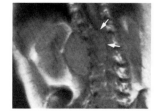
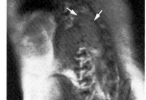
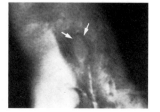

5.24e   5.24f   5.24g

5.25 **Adrenal hemorrhage** in a 7-day-old boy referred with a US diagnosis of "suprarenal process" at 2 days of age: adrenal hemorrhage? Adrenal tumor? **a** Transverse and **b** longitudinal scans: rounded, sharply marginated mass in the right suprarenal area with a dense, echogenic rim and small hypoechogenic center. **DD:** ganglioneuroma, neuroblastoma, adrenal hemorrhage, malformation. Laboratory tests showed normal catecholamines, and hematocrit. US 5 weeks later: reduction in size and sonodensity (more cystic), consistent with adrenal hemorrhage. Scans 1 year later showed a small, triangular residual sonodensity different from the opposite side. X-rays showed no calcification.

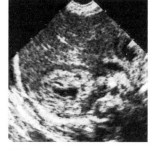 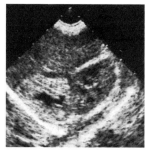

5.25a   5.25b

Pelvis

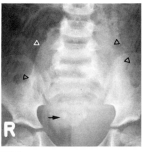 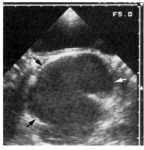 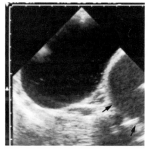 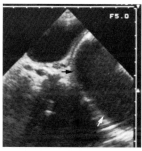

5.26a   5.26b   5.26c   5.26d

5.26 **Coccygeal teratoma** in a 4-year old girl with an approximately 2-year history of alternate constipation and diarrhea. Acute urinary retention. **a** Pelvic radiograph: mass (△) and absence of the coccyx (S5: ←); no abnormal calcification. **b** Transverse scan, **c** longitudinal scan, and **d** longitudinal scan after catheterization: hypoechogenic (predominantly cystic) retrovesical mass (arrows) with an echogenic rim and faint evidence of septation. **e** Excretory urograms, **f** with endorectal contrast, demonstrate a retrorectal mass. Anterosuperior displacement of the urinary bladder obstructs bladder emptying and drainage of the upper urinary tract. **DD:** teratoma, neuroblastoma/ganglioneuroma. Operation: total extirpation. Histology: differentiated coccygeal teratoma, nonmalignant. No chemotherapy.

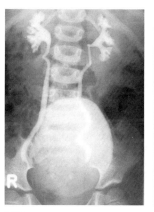 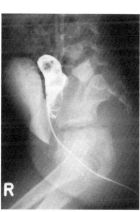

5.26e   5.26f

◀ **5.24** **Neuroblastoma** in a 3-month-old boy whose mother noticed a nodular mass in the left paravertebral area. **a** Left flank coronal scan and **b** transverse abdominal scan: solitary pararenal hilar spindle-shaped mass (arrows) that may communicate with a palpable posterior lesion. **c** Left posterior transverse scan: multinodular structures of varying echogenicity (arrows). **d** Corresponding CT appearance (arrows). **e–g** Longitudinal MRI scans in an oblique position: tumor in the renal hilum contrasting sharply with the kidney; intraspinal extensions; local intraspinal expansion (arrows in **e**) that is subcutaneous posteriorly. Findings consistent with neuroblastoma. Operative removal of the pararenal component. Biopsy confirmed invasion of the psoas muscle, local lymph nodes, and liver. Histology confirmatory. Psoas, lymph node, and hepatic metastases indicate stage IV-S disease. Chemotherapy. Transient paraparesis. No evidence of recurrence at the age of 1½ years.

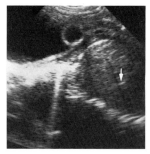

5.27

5.**27 Malignant coccygeal teratoma** in a 5-month-old girl with urinary retention. Longitudinal scan: solid, well-demarcated retrovesical/infravesical mass (balloon catheter in the bladder). Calcification (arrow)? Radiographs showed that the mass was retrorectal: coccygeal teratoma? Operative removal. Histology: malignant coccygeal teratoma (trace evidence of yolk sac tumor). Chemotherapy. Patient is well at the age of 3 years, 8 months.

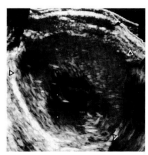 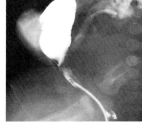

5.29a   5.29b

5.**29 Sacrococcygeal neuroblastoma** in a 2½-month-old boy first hospitalized at the age of 6 weeks for a "bloody stool." Low hematocrit! Palpation "normal." Interpretation "anal fissures." At 2½ months, the patient had a tumorlike mass in the pelvis. **a** Transverse scan: predominantly solid retrovesical mass (△) with fairly large cystic components; urinary bladder is almost empty (←). **b** Lateral projection EU with endorectal contrast: retrorectal mass with compression-induced stasis of the upper urinary tract. **DD:** sacrococcygeal teratoma, neuroblastoma, anterior myelomeningocele. Operation: extirpation. Histology: neuroblastoma. Chemotherapy. Postoperative neurogenic bladder with hypertonic external sphincter; urine dribbling, urinary tract infections: absent Achilles tendon reflexes. These problems largely regressed over time. The patient is well at the age of 6½ years.

5.**30 Rhabdomyosarcoma of the prostate** in a boy aged 4 years, 4 months with acute urinary retention. Repeated attempts at catheterization were unsuccessful. **a** Initial midsagittal scan: massively distended urinary bladder. VCUG in **b** longitudinal and **c** transverse projection: infravesical, preurethral mass. **d** Longitudinal and **e** transverse scans following suprapubic catheter insertion and drainage: preurethral / prevesical mass (arrows), prostatic rhabdomyosarcoma suspected. CT: no additional information; mass not separable from the rectum. Operation: subtotal resection. Histology confirmatory. Chemotherapy. Suspected recurrence at the age of 5½ years disproved by negative biopsy: cystitis. The patient is "well" at 6 years, 10 months of age (same patient as in Fig. 17.**24**). *Note:* An overdistended urinary bladder can hamper or prevent US diagnosis.

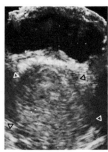 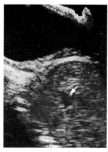

5.28a   5.28b   5.28c

5.**28 Yolk sac tumor** in a 17-month-old girl with a 6-week history of constipation and painful defecation with a pencil-thin stool; 5-day history of fecal retention. Firm pelvic mass with a knobby surface. **a** Transverse and **b** longitudinal US scans: solid retrovesical mass (△) with a small cystic component (←). **c** EU, lateral projection, with endorectal contrast demonstrates a retrorectal mass. **DD:** teratoma, neuroblastoma. Alpha-fetoprotein greatly elevated. Histology: yolk sac tumor, malignant. Chemotherapy (bleomycin, cisplatin). Subsequent episodes of severe malaise with anorexia. Patient died at the age of 4½ years. Autopsy: diffuse pulmonary fibrosis, atrophic kidney (both presumably a result of chemotherapy); papillary carcinoma of the thyroid (second malignancy? metastasis?).

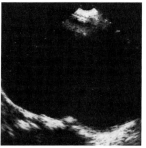

5.30a

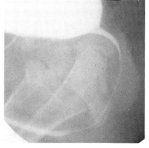 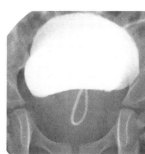

5.30b   5.30c

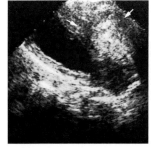 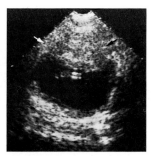

5.30d   5.30e

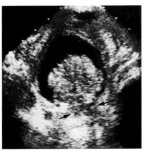 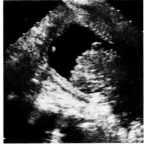 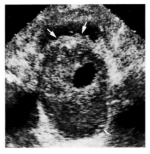 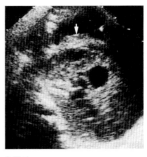

5.31a   5.31b   5.31c   5.31d

5.31 Rhabdomyosarcoma in an 11-month-old boy who had painful, difficult micturition 1 month before. Local treatment for "balanitis" produced no clinical improvement. Presented with urinary retention and postrenal renal failure. **a** Transverse and **b** longitudinal scans: solid intravesical mass with a cauliflower-like contour. Origin in trigone region or retrovesical component (arrows)? Rhabdomyosarcoma (sarcoma botryoides) suspected. Operation: transvesical subtotal resection (removal of all tumor mass from the bladder lumen and posterior urethra; tumor origin or extension prostatic?). Histology confirmatory. Chemotherapy. Four small recurrent growths removed at cystoscopy 5 months later; 3 months later, urinary retention recurred. **c** Transverse and **d** longitudinal scans demonstrate large prostatic recurrence. Irregular contour of the inner bladder wall (arrows). Operation: removal of a large tumor mass. Infiltration of the distal ureter. Bilateral nephrostomy. Rapid tumor growth resumed despite radiation and chemotherapy. The patient died at the age of 1 year, 9 months.

Anterior Abdomen

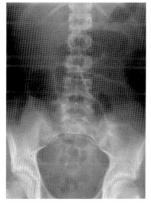 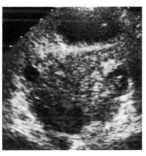

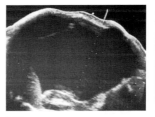 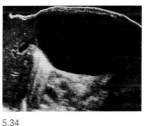

5.32a   5.32b   5.33   5.34

5.32 Loop abscess in a 12-year-old girl admitted 3 days earlier with abdominal pain, diarrhea, and a temperature of 38.5°C: "gastroenteritis." Rehospitalized due to vomiting. **a** Supine AP radiograph: ileus. **b** Transverse scan: predominantly solid, well-defined retrovesical mass. **DD:** abscess, Crohn disease. Operation: perforated appendix located near the cul-de-sac and "loop abscess"; severe hemorrhagic inflammation of the distal ileum.

5.33 Full urinary bladder in an 8-day-old girl with a congenital myelomeningocele repaired at the age of 2 days. Two days postoperatively: hydrocephalus, bilateral hydronephrosis. Four days postoperatively: lower limb swelling. Inferior cava thrombosis? Longitudinal scan: massively distended urinary bladder. Catheterization yielded 220 mL, followed by regression of hydronephrosis and leg swelling.

5.34 CSF pseudocyst in a 14-month-old girl with myelomeningocele. Massive neonatal hydrocephalus prompted insertion of a ventriculoperitoneal shunt. Shunt infection at 11 months. Moderately sized intraperitoneal CSF pseudocyst. Child presented with a strong acute increase in abdominal volume. Longitudinal scan: massive ascites-like intraperitoneal fluid collection. Exploration: giant CSF pseudocyst. Peripheral membrane prevents absorption of CSF.

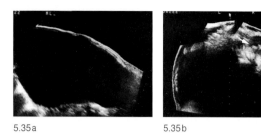

5.35a   5.35b

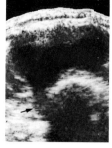
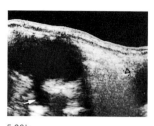

5.36a   5.36b

5.36 Ganglioneuroma in a girl of 3 years, 4 months with a soft abdominal mass found fortuitously during examination by a pediatrician. **a** Transverse and **b** longitudinal scans: anterior cystic mass with right paraspinal extension (←). Urinary bladder (△). **DD:** intestinal, neuroenteric duplication, chyle cyst. CT yielded no additional information. Operation: removal with paraspinal pedicle at L4−5, subtotal. Histology: ganglioneuroma.

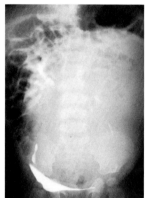
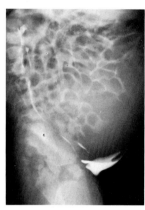

5.35c   5.35d

5.35 Bladder diverticulum in a 1-year-old boy who had suffered neonatal asphyxia with shock. At 4 months, soft mass at the center of the abdomen, regressed spontaneously in 2 weeks. Presented at the age of 1 year with large, tense midabdominal swelling. **a** Longitudinal and **b** posterior transverse scans: giant cystic mass. **DD:** intraperitoneal or retroperitoneal. Left kidney not visible (arrows indicate right kidney). **c** EU, anteroposterior view at 15 minutes and **d** lateral view at 20 minutes: possibly a retroperitoneal mass (affecting the ureter position); small dysplastic (?) left kidney. Operation: giant posterobasal bladder diverticulum. Resection followed by neurogenic bladder disturbance. *Note:* first mass intermittent due to the emptying of the diverticulum, later decompensation; second speculative: atrophic left kidney secondary to neonatal ischemia?

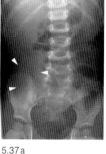
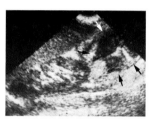

5.37a   5.37b

5.37 Abscess in a boy of 2 years, 9 months with an acute abdomen. Appendicitis? **a** Radiograph: mass in the right hemiabdomen (▲), lumbar scoliosis. **b** Right longitudinal scan: heterogeneous, predominantly cystic infrarenal mass (arrows). Operation: appendicitis with perforation and a large perityphlitic abscess.

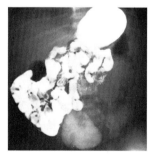
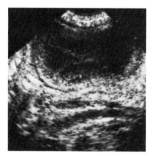

5.38a   5.38b

5.38 Hemorrhagic ovarian cyst in a 3-day-old girl diagnosed at 2 and 1 weeks prenatally with a "cystic structure in the left renal area." No palpable mass at birth, normal EU. **a** UGI series: bowel displacement by a mass in the left hemiabdomen. **b** Left flank longitudinal scan: cystic mass with scattered internal echoes and a relatively thick, echogenic border. **DD:** malformation (lymphogenous, intestinal mesenteric, omental, ovarian) tumor (neurogenic, teratoma), etc. Operation: large, soft, left-sided hemorrhagic ovarian cyst ("chocolate cyst").

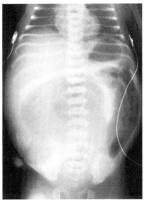
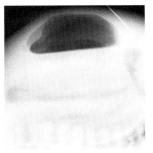
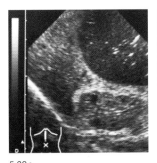
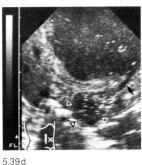

5.39a   5.39b   5.39c   5.39d

5.**39   Pseudocyst** in a 1-day-old girl with a marked increase in abdominal volume on her 1st day of life. **a** AP and **b** lateral radiographs: large extraintestinal air collection in the anterior abdomen. **c** Sagittal and **d** coronal scans: "cystic" encapsulated structure containing diffuse echoes and numerous air bubbles, communicating by a channel (←) with the bowel (△). Operation: removal of a pseudocyst with small bowel perforation; resection included several centimeters of damaged ileum; ileostomy. Histology: (focal) neuronal intestinal dysplasia. Course favorable after reconstruction.

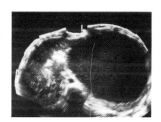

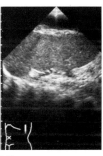

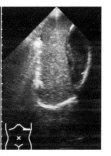
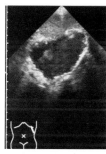

5.40   5.41a   5.41b   5.41c

5.**40   Splenic cyst** in a 14-year-old asthmatic girl who had been hospitalized several times. Chest normal at age 5, 7, and 10 years. Onset of precordial pain at age 12. Appendectomy (mesenteric lymphadenitis). Chest (in retrospect) abnormal due to a left-sided infradiaphragmatic mass. New: recurrent left-sided thoracic pain, swelling in the region of the left thoracic outlet. Radiograph showed left-sided infradiaphragmatic mass. Transverse scan: cystic mass with fine internal echoes: splenic cyst. Operation: removal. Histology: presumed lymphangiectatic splenic cyst with organizing hematoma (endothelium-like epithelium).

5.**41   Parasplenic abscess** in a girl of 10 years, 9 months with recessive polycystic renal disease who underwent renal transplantation; transplant was removed due to nonperfusion and necrosis; patient now on peritoneal dialysis. Presented with recurrent fever, abdominal pain, and a mass in the left lateral hemiabdomen. **a** Left flank longitudinal scan, **b** lateral transverse scan of the left upper abdomen, and **c** longitudinal oblique scan: parasplenic abscess with extensive wall calcification. Aspiration yielded sterile pus. Secondary removal by laparotomy (same patient as in Fig. 10.**6**, 14.**23**, and 14.**60**).

5.**42   Rhabdomyosarcoma** in a 2-year-old boy (North Africa) with a very large, hard abdominal mass. Pollakiuria, circulatory impairment in the right leg, general malaise. **a** Transverse infrarenal scan and **b** right longitudinal scan medial to the kidney: compact tumor mass in the left hemiabdomen and a heterogeneous mass in the right hemiabdomen. Not shown: nondelineation of the left kidney, massive bilateral hydronephrosis. EU showed massive obstructive uropathy due to compression of both ureters by tumor. Pulmonary metastases. Hypertension. **DD:** Wilms tumor, rhabdomyosarcoma. Chemotherapy. Rapid tumor enlargement. The patient was lost early to follow-up.

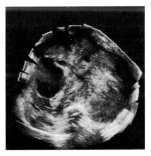
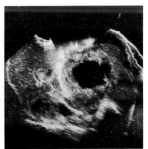

5.42a   5.42b

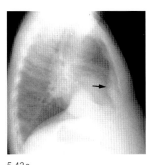 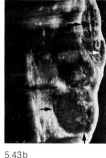 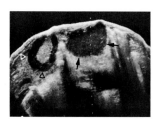

5.43a   5.43b   5.43c

5.43 Non-Hodgkin lymphoma in a boy of 4 years, 7 months (North Africa) with a 7-month history of recurrent abdominal pain. Appendicitis suspected 7 months before, X-rays showing bowel motility disorder (in retrospect, possible intermittent intussusception). **a** Radiograph: distortion of the right hemidiaphragm by a hepatic tumor; tumor also retrosternal (arrow) and subcutaneous, infrasternal. **b** Midanterior sagittal thoracoabdominal scan:

subcutaneous tumor correlating with **a** (▲) and large tumor mass in the midcaudal portion of the liver (←). **c** Transverse scan shows lesion in **b** (←) as well as bowel wall involvement (△). Not shown: multiple nodular intrahepatic and presumably mesenteric lesions. **DD:** non-Hodgkin lymphoma more likely than neuro-

blastoma. Biopsy (infrasternal / subcutaneous, axillary): non-Hodgkin lymphoma, B-cell type, lymphoblastic, highly malignant. Chemotherapy. The patient did well for 8 months, then was lost to follow-up.

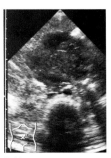 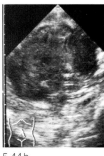 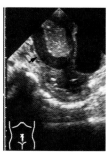   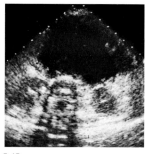

5.44a   5.44b   5.44c   5.45

5.44 Non-Hodgkin lymphoma in a boy of 5 years, 3 months with acute abdomen, colicky pains. Intussusception? Ascites? Tumor? Disease of kidney, urinary tract, pancreas? **a** Transverse, **b** longitudinal oblique, and **c** midsagittal (pelvic) scans: large, solid, relatively hypoechogenic intra-/abdominal mass with involvement of the bowel wall (arrow). Not shown: multiple nodular mesenteric and retroperitoneal lesions; massive ascites. Questionable diffuse renal involvement. Right pleural effusion: non-Hodgkin lymphoma suspected. Pleural aspiration: B-cell lymphoma. Chemotherapy. After initial renal insufficiency (high uric acid), patient has done well for 9 months.

5.45 Malignant lymphoma in a girl of 2 years, 8 months (North Africa) with about a 3-week history of progressive abdominal pain and vomiting; 3-kg weight loss. Transverse scan: extensive, moderately well-defined, relatively hypoechogenic mass in the midabdomen. **DD:** neuroblastoma, lymphoma, infected malformation cyst. Pancreatic pseudocyst or choledochal cyst unlikely. CT appearance suggested a solid mass (approximately 70 HU) with local involvement of the left kidney. Laparotomy / biopsy. Histology: malignant lymphoblastic lymphoma. Chemotherapy. Rapid downhill course with vomiting, aspiration, respiratory / circulatory failure. The patient died 10 days after diagnosis.

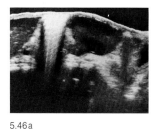 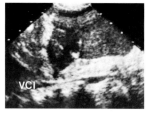 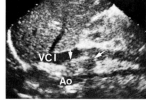   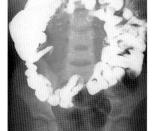

5.46a   5.46b   5.46c

5.46 Inflammatory pseudotumor in a girl of 4 years, 9 months with a 3- to 4-month history of abdominal distention and pain and a 3-week history a fever of 38−39.5 °C. Large, knobby abdominal mass. **a, b** Right parasagittal scans: relatively hypoechogenic, predominantly solid tumor with fine extensions toward the inferior vena cava (VCI). **c** Right flank longitudinal scan: enlarged lymph nodes (arrows) between the inferior vena cava and the aorta (Ao). **d** Contrast film of the small bowel and colon: central mass effect from the tumor. **DD:** malignant lymphoma; sympathetic nerve cell tumor (neuroblastoma, ganglioneuroma); teratoma; maldevelopmental tumor of the mesentery of omentum, etc. Laparotomy / biopsy. Histology: benign inflammatory pseudotumor. Subsequent extirpation of the tumor

5.46d

(total?). The patient did well for 2 years and 4 months, then there was a recurrence. Extirpation repeated. Histology: inflammatory pseudotumor. *Note:* Tumor may be of the xanthogranulomatous (histiocytic), plasmacell−rich, or sclerosing type depending on the composition of the tumor or the main cellular component. Differentiation from malignant fibrous histiocytoma is very difficult.

Liver

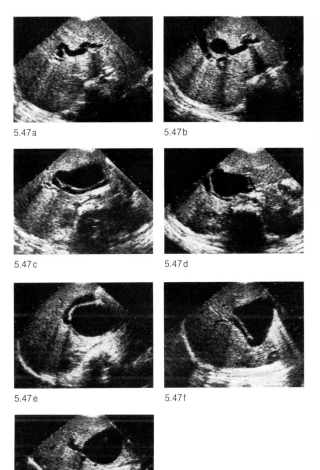

5.47a

5.47b

5.47c

5.47d

5.47e

5.47f

5.47g

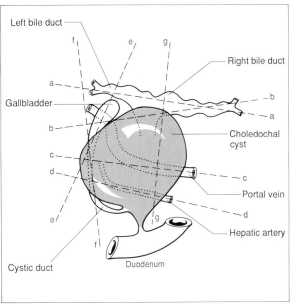

5.47h

5.47 Cyst of the common bile duct and common hepatic duct in a 14-month-old girl with jaundice and hepatomegaly. Hepatitis? **a–d** Transverse oblique and **e–g** longitudinal oblique sonograms (**h**: diagram of the scan planes) show a large common bile duct and common hepatic duct cyst with massive ectasia of the right and left hepatic ducts and milder ectasia of the more intrahepatic ducts. Operation: portoenterostomy (Kimura–Kasai modification); followed by bouts of cholangitis and moderate hepatic fibrosis. The patient improved following reexposure and shortening of the hepatojejunal connection. The patient is well at 5½ years, developing appropriately for her age.

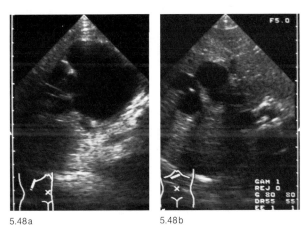

5.48a

5.48b

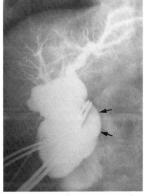

5.48c

5.48 Choledochal cyst in a 6½-year-old girl who underwent US elsewhere for a urinary tract infection; "questionable hepatic cyst" noted as an incidental finding. **a** Right flank coronal and **b** transverse scans: choledochal cyst with biliary tract ectasia. Operation: excision of the cyst and the gallbladder, "porto"- enterostomy (anastomosis to the common hepatic duct). **c** Radiograph (intraoperative retrograde cholangiogram via gallbladder) shows the gallbladder (arrows) clamped off after contrast injection. Satisfactory postoperative course.

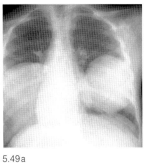
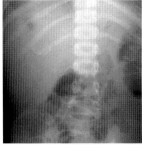

5.49a   5.49b

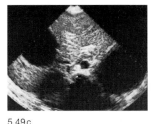
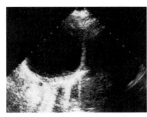

5.49c   5.49d

5.49   Echinococcal cysts in a 7-year-old boy (North Africa) with a progressive dry cough. **a** Chest and **b** abdominal radiographs: large spherical density in the right lower pulmonary lobe, similar lesion on the left. **c** Upper abdominal transverse scan: large cyst in the liver and left lower pulmonary lobe. **d** Coronal scan of the right chest wall: cyst in the right lower pulmonary lobe and liver (corresponding to **c**). **e, f** Right transverse and longitudinal scans: one large and one smaller (with calcified shell, see film **b**) cyst in the liver. Operation: pulmonary cysts enucleated in two sittings, hepatic cysts excised in a third. No complications.

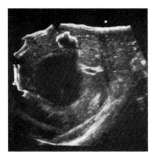
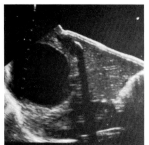

5.49e   5.49f

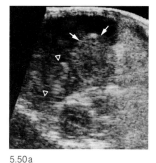
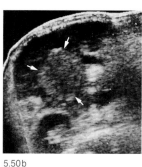

5.50a   5.50b

5.50   Regenerative hepatic nodule in a 2½-year-old boy with a type I hereditary tyrosinosis (same patient as in Fig. 14.**11**). Last US scan at 17 months showed a normal-appearing liver. Right **a** longitudinal and **b** transverse scans: rounded, uniformly echogenic solid mass (←) and a less well-defined smaller, irregular sonodensity (△): hepatoma(s)? The patient died 1 month later from an acute cardiopulmonary insufficiency associated with sepsis and pneumonia Autopsy: coarsely nodular cirrhosis and fatty degeneration of the liver; suspected hepatoma was a regenerative nodule; portal congestion; kidney: mesangial sclerosis, fatty infiltration of the tubules.

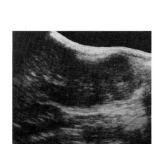
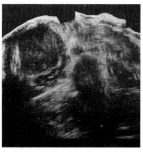
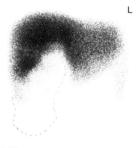
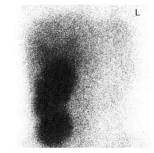

5.51a   5.51b   5.51c   5.51d

5.51   Hepatocellular carcinoma in a 13½-year-old girl whose parents had chronic subclinical hepatitis B. The patient and her two younger brothers were congenital hepatitis carriers. The girl was admitted with a 2-month history of fatigue, anorexia, malaise, and weight loss. A nontender mass in the right hemiabdomen. **a** Right longitudinal and **b** transverse scans: tumorous process extending from the right hepatic lobe to an infraumbilical site. The lesion has a rounded cross section and is approximately isoechogenic to the liver: hepatic tumor. **c** Sulfur-colloid liver scan: tumor (– – –) devoid of activity (no normal reticuloen-

dothelium). **d** Gallium-citrate scan: uptake is very high in the tumor, relatively low in the normal liver (corresponding to the excess of hepatocytes in the tumor): characteristic of hepatocellular carcinoma. CT scans were nonspecific; extensive right portal vein thrombosis; probable malignant tumor. Biopsy. Histology confirmed hepatocellular carcinoma. Preoperative hepatic arteriography. Operation two-thirds hepatectomy. Chemotherapy. Pulmonary metastases and cachexia ensued; the patient died at the age of 15 years.

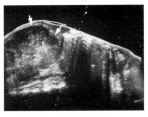
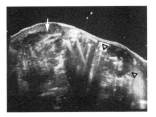
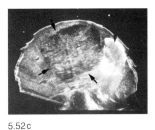

5.52a   5.52b   5.52c

5.52 Malignant lymphoma in a boy of 3 years, 7 months with a 10-day history of acholic stool. Presented with hepatomegaly and a lower abdominal mass. **a, b** Midsagittal / parasagittal and **c** transverse scans: solid, heterogeneous tumor in the left hepatic lobe (←). Bowel involvement (△)? **d** Sulfur-colloid scintigram shows a defect in the tumor area. **e** Gallium-citrate scan: very intense uptake in the tumor with abnormal accumulation in the right lower abdomen and left hemiabdomen. Radiographs raised suspicion of a pulmonary metastasis. **DD:** hepatoblastoma (bowel involvement unusual), lymphomatous process. Biopsy. Histology: consistent with hepatoblastoma (unusual). Alpha-fetoprotein normal. Preoperative hepatic arteriography. Operation: left hemihepatectomy with resection of metastases from the left mesenterery and right ileum (lower abdomen). Histology: malignant lymphoma of B-cell type (revision of the primary diagnosis). Chemotherapy, radiation. Gastrointestinal bleeding. Blood transfusion. Diffuse dermatologic complications (graft-versus-host? Medical allergy? Toxic?). Cachexia. Patient died at the age of 3 years, 11 months.

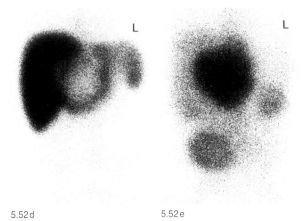

5.52d   5.52e

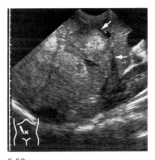
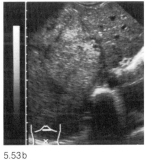
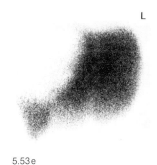

5.53a   5.53b   5.53e   5.53f

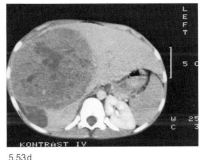

5.53c   5.53d

5.53 Hepatoblastoma in an 11-year-old boy with a 6-week history of fatigue, angina, fever, weight loss (2 kg), and recurrent epistaxis. Presented with hepatomegaly. **a** Longitudinal oblique and **b** transverse scans: large, solid, well-defined, heterogeneous, relatively echogenic hepatic tumor (arrows) with sinusoidal zones. **DD:** probably malignant: hepatocellular carcinoma; undifferentiated small cell sarcoma, rhabdomyosarcoma, possibly hepatoblastoma (relatively old); mixed form; mesenchymal hamartoma; hemangioendothelioma unlikely. **c, d** CT: moderate perfusion, local calcification; probable malignancy. **e** Sulfur-colloid scintigram: photopenic area in the mass. **f** Gallium-citrate scan is negative, ruling out hepatocellular carcinoma. Preoperative hepatic arteriography. Operation: two-thirds hepatectomy (right/middle trisegmentectomy). Histology: pure epithelial hepatoblastoma. Alpha-fetoprotein level, previously very high, normalized shortly after surgery. Uncomplicated course. The patient is well at the age of 12½ years.

6 Blunt Abdominal Trauma

R. D. Schulz

After the abdominal plain film, sonography is the imaging procedure of first choice in patients who have sustained blunt abdominal trauma. It can be performed even in severely injured children whose circulatory status is stable. The plain abdominal radiograph can provide important preliminary information in preparation for sonography: bony injury, mass effect, gas distribution in the bowel, free fluid, free air, soft-tissue contours, organ enlargements, pleural effusion. Pediatric blunt abdominal trauma may be broadly classified as adequate, inadequate, or perinatal. Organ damage can result from injuries sustained during play or automobile accidents, birth trauma (predisposing factors: high birth weight, bleeding tendency, asphyxia, direct trauma), or child abuse, especially in younger children. Affected organs in order of decreasing frequency are the kidney, spleen, liver, pancreas, gastrointestinal tract, and urinary bladder. Hematomas of the abdominal wall and retroperitoneum are also observed. The organs most commonly affected by birth trauma, in order of frequency, are the liver, adrenal gland, spleen, and kidney. In 18% of cases more than one abdominal organ is injured.

The ultrasound evaluation of abdominal trauma begins over the pelvis and proceeds to the flanks to check for free intraperitoneal fluid (scant, moderate, or massive). This is followed by a systematic examination of the parenchymatous abdominal organs. Note: a very small amount of retrovesical free fluid may be physiologic. The urinary bladder should be satisfactorily distended, as either overdistention or underdistention can hamper the detection of free fluid. Free intraperitoneal fluid generally represents blood, less frequently bile or bowel contents, or perhaps urine when following a renal injury with peritoneal damage. Free retroperitoneal fluid consists of blood and/or urine; these cannot be differentiated. Where there is free blood, an injury must be present. A laceration of the liver or spleen may be difficult to visualize by ultrasound during the first 24 hours postinjury, so scans should be repeated the following day. Fresh hematomas of the liver and spleen can often be identified by their nonhomogeneous, typically more echogenic structure. Subcapsular hematomas, on the other hand, are usually hypoechogenic to anechogenic.

Pancreatic lesions may commence with a localized swelling from which one or more pseudocysts may develop within days or weeks through autolysis. These lesions may reach considerable size, and they may form a relatively thick cyst wall. The echo pattern of these cysts can change as a result of internal hemorrhage. Echogenic sequestra or hemorrhagic debris may be visible on the floor of the hematoma or cyst. Pancreatic pseudocysts usually resolve spontaneously over a period of weeks or months. Operative treatment is seldom necessary and will depend on the patient's clinical status and sonographic follow-up.

Renal injuries, even when minor, can be detected with ultrasound at a relatively early stage. They may present as subcapsular hematomas with or without parenchymal tears or as renal ruptures with a breach of the fibrous capsule leading to a perirenal hematoma, possibly combined with penetration of the collecting system: urinoma.

Perirenal fluid may consist of blood and/or urine. If there is no hematuria and the kidneys appear sonographically normal, it is unnecessary to proceed with intravenous pyelography (IVP). If gross hematuria is present, IVP should be performed whether or not sonography demonstrates urinary tract lesions; conversely, this study is indicated in the absence of macrohematuria if sonograms show relatively large lesions. IVP yields information on partial or global function deficits and the degree of injury to the collecting system.

The sonographic features of hematomas can vary with the age and location of the lesion. The initially fast-changing picture of an organ lesion is characteristic. The course is not uniform. Hematomas may be permeated by echogenic septa belonging to uninjured portions of the organ. Given the current tendency to manage blunt abdominal trauma conservatively, serial ultrasound scans have assumed major importance. Sonographic monitoring coupled with clinical findings can greatly assist decision making.

Radionuclide imaging of the liver and spleen is superior to sonography but is not consistently available at all centers. It should be requested, however, in patients who have copious intraperitoneal fluid despite negative ultrasound findings. CT scanning is indicated in patients with unexplained complications or associated fractures.

The protracted course of a pancreatic or splenic injury is well known (development of pancreatic pseudocyst or two-stage splenic rupture). Intrahepatic biliomas can develop as a sequel to penetrating hepatic injuries.

The pediatric urinary bladder is more intra-abdominal than intrapelvic, so it is vulnerable to blunt abdominal trauma. Extravesical fluid may signify a hemorrhage and/or the extravasation of urine. Injuries of the gastrointestinal tract can result in hypoechogenic hematomas of the bowel wall. In the absence of a mechanical ileus, the location of the hematoma should be established by contrast examination.

In children with multiple injuries, intra-abdominal lesions are often less clinically conspicuous than extra-abdominal injuries. Thus, careful ultrasound scanning of the abdomen is essential in these cases to ensure that significant intra-abdominal trauma is not overlooked and that potentially life-saving interventions are not withheld. One possibility to be considered, especially with inadequate trauma, is that a preexisting but previously unrecognized disease could be mimicking an organic injury, e.g., a dystopic spleen, abscess, situs inversus, hepatic hemangioma, or a minor injury causing significant damage due to preexisting disease: hydronephrosis with hematuria, an enlarged fragile spleen in leukosis, free fluid associated with malignant lymphoma (mistaken for hematoperitoneum).

Diagnostic peritoneal lavage is inferior to sonography because it covers only the abdominal cavity and can give false-positive results. Neither can exploratory laparotomy be reasonably justified in a child with a stable circulation. Other diagnostic procedures such as CT, urography, scintigraphy, and angiography are not obviated by sonography but should be applied more selectively.

Role of sonography in patients with blunt abdominal trauma:

– detection of free intraperitoneal or retroperitoneal fluid;

– detection of organic lesions;
– follow-up of lesions, such as pancreatic pseudocysts;
– detection of lesions not apparent until 24 hours, days, or weeks postinjury, such as pancreatic pseudocysts;
– detection of non−trauma-related disorders such as hydronephrosis, tumor, splenomegaly;
– assistance in planning further diagnostic strategy and treatment.

References

Amparo, E. G., C. K. Hayden, M. Z. Schwartz, T. E. Lobe: Computerized tomography and ultrasonography in evaluation blunt abdominal trauma in children. In Brooks, B. F.: The Injured Child. University of Texas Press, Austin 1985 (pp. 61–70)

Filiatrault, D., D. Longpré, H. Patriquin, G. Perreault, A. Grignon, J. Pronovost, J. Boisvert: Investigation of childhood blunt abdominal trauma: a practical approach using ultrasound as the initial diagnostic modality. Pediat. Radiol. 17 (1987) 373

Gelfaud, M. J.: Scintigraphy in upper abdominal trauma. Semin. Roentgenol. 19 (1984) 296–307

Giedion, A.: Die geburtstraumatische Ruptur parenchymatöser Bauchorgane (Leber, Milz, Nebenniere und Niere) mit massivem Blutverlust und ihre radiologische Darstellung. Helv. paediat. Acta 18, (1963) 349–370

Hayden, C. K., L. E. Swischuk: Pediatric Ultrasonography. Williams & Wilkins, Baltimore 1987

Schulz, R. D., U. Willi: Ultraschalldiagnostik nach stumpfem Bauchtrauma im Kindesalter. Ultraschall 4 (1983) 154–159

Adequate Trauma of the Abdomen

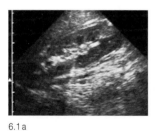
6.1a

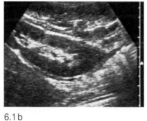
6.1b

6.1 Renal hematoma and perirenal hematoma in an 11-year-old girl who sustained a right flank injury in a bicycle fall; microhematuria. **a** Right flank scan: triangular echo-free zone inferolaterally: intraparenchymal hematoma. EU demonstrated normal function of the right kidney. **b** Longitudinal prone scan: caplike hypoechogenic zone at the lower renal pole with an intact fibrous capsule: perirenal hematoma. Treatment: conservative.

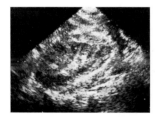
6.2a

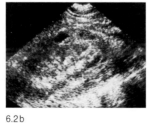
6.2b

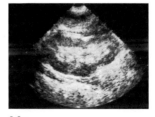
6.2c

6.2 Perirenal hematoma in an 8-year-old boy who sustained a left renal contusion when struck by the ski of another skier; gross hematuria. **a** Left flank scan: lower renal pole is not delineated due to a nonhomogeneous feature covering the lower half of the kidney: perirenal hematoma. Initial EU showed silent lower renal pole. **b** Left flank scan 4 days later: nonhomogeneous echogenic feature at the lower renal pole: parenchymal hemorrhage. Small echo-free area lateromedially in the perirenal, more echogenic hematoma: incipient liquefaction. Conservative treatment. **c** Posterior longitudinal scan 11 months later: complete smoothing of the organ contours but marked parenchymal narrowing in the lower half of the kidney.

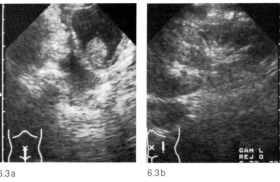
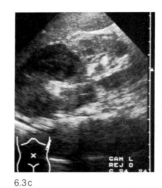
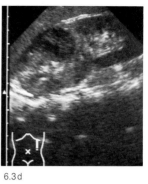

6.3a   6.3b   6.3c   6.3d

6.3   Left renal rupture in an 8-year-old boy who fell from a second-story railing. Remained conscious. Gross hematuria. **a** Longitudinal scan of the lower abdomen on the day of injury: free retroperitoneal fluid and an intravesical, elliptical echogenic area representing clotted blood within the bladder. AP abdominal radiograph showed unspharpness of the left psoas contour. EU showed rupture at the junction of the upper renal pole and the middle third with contrast extravasation. **b** Sonogram of the day of injury: lateromedially oriented elliptical area with a

hypoechogenic rim separates the kidney into an upper third and lower two-thirds: renal fracture. **c** Left flank scan 14 days later: continued disruption of the kidney, now with a hypoechogenic, swollen upper pole, a hypoechogenic hematoma centrally, and a perirenal capsular hematoma in the upper renal half. Also, splenic lesion suspected. **d** Flank scan 10 days later: reabsorption of the perirenal hematoma and regression of upper pole swelling. Hematoma is nonuniformly hypoechogenic. Persistence of microhematuria.

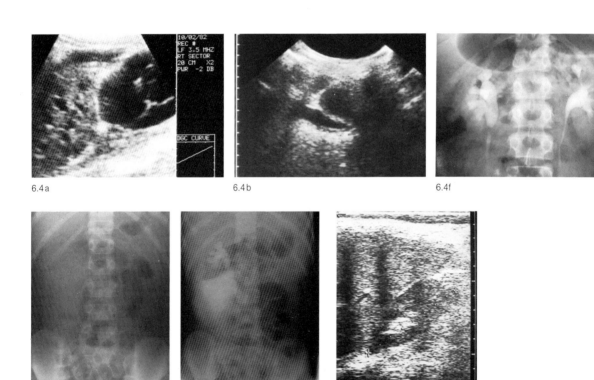

6.4a   6.4b   6.4f

6.4c   6.4d   6.4e

6.4   Right renal trauma, urinoma, renovascular avulsion at the lower pole. Seven-year-old boy caught by an automobile and dragged along the street. Initial loss of consciousness, cerebral contusion, dilatation of internal and external CSF spaces, bilateral frontal hygroma, oculomotor paresis, and right hemiparesis. Supracondylar fracture of the right femur. Hb 10.6 g%, white blood cell count 28 100. First treated neurosurgically elsewhere for 10 days, then transferred to us. Palpable mass in the right upper abdomen; increasing responsiveness. **a**

Right flank scan 10 days postinjury: echo-free perirenal area with nondelineation of the lower pole. Caudally there is a large, anechogenic feature permeated by echogenic septa: perirenal hematoma/urinoma and free retroperitoneal fluid extravasating from the renal hilum. Urinoma. **b** Longitudinal scan of the lower abdomen: retrovesical, bandlike, tapering anechogenic feature representing the lower portion of the urinoma or hematoma. **c** Plain abdominal radiograph 10 days postinjury: nonvisualization of the psoas muscle on the right side, nondelineation of the right

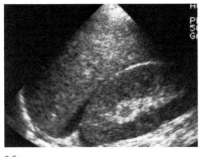 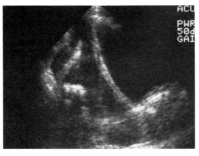 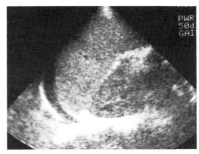

6.5a   6.5b   6.5c

6.5 Small subcapsular right renal hematoma, subcapsular hepatic hematoma, left pleural effusion, copious free intraperitoneal fluid; example of lesions coexisting in multiple abdominal organs. Thirteen-years-old boy injured in a fall from a bicycle; nausea, bruise on the right abdomen, multiple abrasions on the right side of the body. Hb 11.4 g%, white blood count 12 600, hepatic enzymes markedly elevated. Microhematuria. **a** Right flank scan: small echo-free area posteriorly on the right hepatic lobe: subcapsular hepatic hematoma. Small subcapsular

hematoma at upper pole of kidney. **b** Longitudinal scan of the lower abdomen: considerable free intraperitoneal fluid behind the bladder, consistent with intraperitoneal organ injury. **c** Upper left flank scan: crescent-shaped anechogenic area directly above the spleen but projecting medially past it: free intraperitoneal fluid. **DD:** subcapsular splenic hematoma. Twelve days later, the laboratory tests are normal; there is no further evidence of organ injury with conservative treatment.

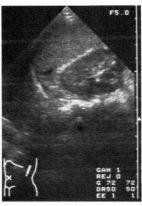 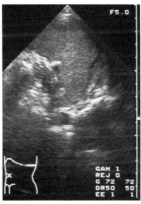

6.6 Splenic tear with small subcapsular hematoma in a 6-year-old boy who fell flat onto the abdomen; felt well initially, later developed abdominal pain. **a** Left flank longitudinal scan at 10 hours postinjury: narrow, anechogenic band in the upper pole of the spleen: splenic tear and a small capsular hematoma. Unusual to find a splenic tear at the initial examination. Also moderate free intraperitoneal fluid. Conservative therapy. **b** Left coronal scan: oblique echo-free line at the site of the tear: splenic rupture.

6.6a   6.6b

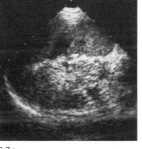 

6.7a   6.7b

(Fig. **6.4** cont.)

renal contour. Soft-tissue density in the right midabdomen with displacement of the bowel. **d** EU shows good excretory function in both kidneys with mild ectasia of the right pyelocaliceal system. Large perirenal and subrenal contrast extravasation in the midabdomen: urinoma. Treatment: based on US and EU findings. Operation: double-fist–sized urinoma protruding from the right retroperitoneum into the lesser pelvis. Avulsion of right ureter at ureteropelvic junction. Necrosis at lower pole due to torn blood vessels. Lower pole resection with anastomosis of the ureter to the renal pelvis. Nephrostomy and ureteral splint. **e** Right flank sonogram 5 years later: small right kidney with no outflow obstruction. **f** EU 2½ years later: good excretory function in both kidneys. Note smaller right kidney with mild pyelocaliceal dilatation. Right ureter opacifies after 5 minutes.

6.7 Transverse splenic rupture in a 10-year-old boy after a flank trauma. Initial US scans showed much free intraperitoneal fluid, presumably blood; a splenic lesion could not be identified. **a** Left flank coronal scan 1 week postinjury: a vertical hypoechogenic to anechogenic zone at the level of the splenic hilum marks the blood-filled rupture site; the cause of bleeding was detectable relatively late with US. **b** Spleen scan 14 days later: complete division of the organ. Conservative treatment, since the patient was clinically stable.

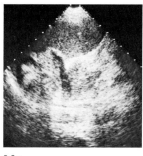

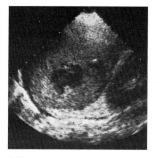

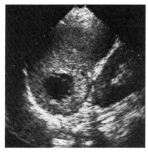

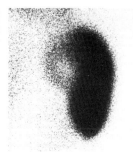

6.8a   6.8b   6.8c   6.8d

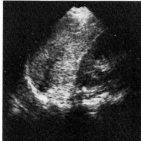
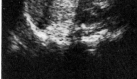

6.8e

6.8 Splenic rupture with posttraumatic cyst in a 13-year-old boy with flank trauma and upper abdominal pain. **a** Left flank coronal scan 2 days postinjury: nonhomogeneous echo structure at the upper pole: splenic rupture. **b** Scan 4 days later: echo-free crescent about the upper half of spleen, extending past the splenic contour. Free intraperitoneal fluid. **c** Left flank coronal scan 19 days later: rounded anechogenic zone signifying development of a posttraumatic cyst. Conservative treatment. **d** Spleen scintigram taken at the same time with incubated red cells: circular photon-deficient area medially in the upper half of the spleen: cyst formation. **e** Left flank coronal sonogram 5 months postinjury: an approximately 4-mm hypoechogenic area; virtually complete regression of the cyst with conservative treatment.

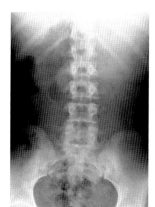

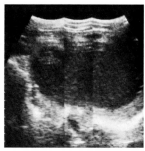

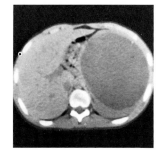

6.9a   6.9b   6.9c

6.9 Posttraumatic splenic cyst in a 12-year-old girl with abdominal pain 1 year after a skiing accident with respiration-dependent left upper quadrant pain. US not performed initially; X-rays and US ordered for persistent, recurrent abdominal pain. **a** Abdominal radiograph: uniform soft-tissue density occupying the left upper abdomen and displacing the stomach and bowel to the right past the midline: tumor? **b** Left anterior transverse scan on the same day: elliptical hypoechogenic mass in the spleen with numerous, evenly scattered echoes. Might be a solid tumor, but the posterior acoustic enhancement is more consistent with a cyst (internal echoes probably caused by cholesterol crystals). **c** Concomitant CT: large, low-density mass almost completely filling the spleen—most likely a splenic cyst. Liver–spleen scan showed a large, isotopically cold mass almost completely filling the spleen. Operation: splenectomy. Connective-tissue–lined pseudocyst 15 cm in diameter. Case illustrates how recurrent abdominal pain may be trauma-related.

Birth Trauma

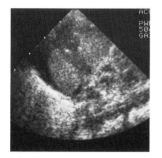

6.24

6.24 Splenic rupture in a 4-day-old girl. Erythroblastosis, exchange transfusion, repeated clots in the catheter. Abdominal distention and shock 4 days after birth. Left flank scan: subcapsular splenic hematoma and hypoechogenic bandlike structure in midspleen: splenic laceration with hematoma. Also moderate free intraperitoneal fluid. Operation: multiple small splenic lacerations, repaired with fibrin adhesive. Rapid improvement.

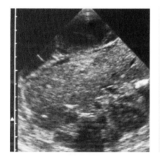

6.25a

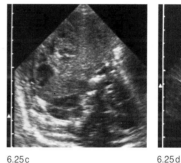

6.25b

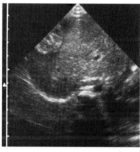

6.25c   6.25d

6.25 Subcapsular hepatic hematoma in an 8-day-old girl with a high birth weight (4600 g). **a** Upper abdominal transverse scan 8 days after birth: septated, subcapsular, anechogenic hematoma, well demarcated from the parenchyma, anterior to the hepatic surface. Conservative treatment. **b** Same view 6 days

later: subcapsular hepatic hematoma now nonhomogeneous due to coagulation (change in hematoma over time). **c** Nine days later: hematoma echo structure nonhomogeneous except for small echo-free areas. **d** By 10 weeks the hematoma has reabsorbed to a diameter of 2 cm.

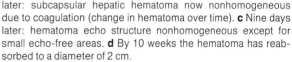

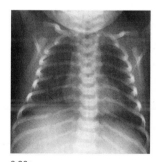

6.26a

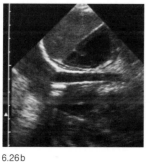

6.26b

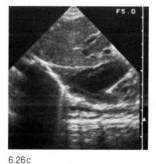

6.26c

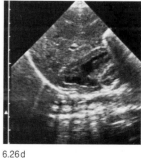

6.26d

6.26 Traumatic bilateral adrenal hemorrhage with serial rib fractures following a traumatic delivery by vacuum extraction. High birth weight (4450 g), green amniotic fluid. Postpartum respiratory distress syndrome. Multiple rib fractures on the right side, icterus praecox, hypoglycemia. **a** Chest radiograph on day 10: serial fractures of ribs 4–11. **b** Left flank scan on day 4:

caplike, echo-free adrenal hematoma on the left side. **c** Right anterior longitudinal scan on the 4th day of life: subhepatic, ovoid right-sided adrenal hematoma. **d** Same view on day 11 shows considerable regression of the hemorrhage. Conservative treatment.

7 Gastrointestinal Diseases

I. Gaßner

Ultrasound can be used to evaluate the wall thickness, wall structure, contents, and function of the pediatric gastrointestinal tract. In most situations that call for plain abdominal radiographs, abdominal sonography is also indicated. In cases where ultrasound is the primary examination, the additional information provided by abdominal plain films (and possibly a contrast series) should be considered. The sonographic findings associated with various diseases of the gastrointestinal tract are outlined below.

- *Esophagus:* visible at the level of the aortic arch and diaphragm. Gastroesophageal reflux can be detected, but not quantified, anterior to the aorta on the epigastric longitudinal scan. Reflux esophagitis is not detectable.
- *Stomach and pylorus:* partial gastric filling with fluid (tea, etc.) is advantageous. The gastric wall is thickened with an ulcer (antral thickening, sometimes with a visible ulcer crater), Schönlein−Henoch purpura, Crohn disease, lymphoid hyperplasia, septic granulomatosis, protein-losing gastropathy (coarse folds with thickened mucosa), ectopic pancreas (Hayden et al. 1987).
  Hypertrophic pyloric stenosis: examination in the right lateral decubitus may be helpful. Normal pyloric muscle thickness (distance from the submucosa to the outer muscle boundary) is no more than 2 to 3 mm. With pyloric stenosis, the muscle thickness exceeds 3 mm (measured in longitudinal and transverse section) and the length of the pyloric canal is over 17 mm (normal maximum 14 mm); hypertrophied muscle bulges into the antrum; increased gastric peristalsis, no pyloric relaxation.
- *Duodenum:* dilatation with collapse of the aboral bowel loops seen in duodenal atresia, duodenal diaphragm, possibly in malrotation with volvulus. Duodenal wall thickening in association with varices due to portal hypertension, pancreatitis, duodenal ulcer, cystic fibrosis.
- *Small intestine:* normally thin-walled with a facetted cross section and visible peristalsis. Ileus: fluid-filled bowel loops with a circular cross section. Even in mechanical ileus, peristalsis may be absent. Ultrasound often demonstrates the cause of the ileus. Free fluid seen in association with seepage peritonitis and/or perforation.
  Thickened bowel wall: diffuse thickening seen with hypoproteinemia, celiac disease, portal hypertension, irradiation, protein-losing enteropathy, etc. Localized thickening seen with Schönlein−Henoch purpura, Crohn disease, adjacent inflammatory lesion (e. g., perityphlitic abscess), trauma. Lymphoma causes very hypoechogenic wall thickening with a propensity for aneurysmatic bowel dilatation due to ulceration.

- *Colon: acute appendicitis:* with compression of the abdominal wall toward the iliopsoas muscle, the appendix appears as a tubular structure terminating in a blind pouch. The lumen is dilated (> 3 mm), usually hypoechogenic, is surrounded by a thin echogenic line (mucosa) and hypoechogenic muscle wall (> 2 m thick). The appendix is rigid and poorly compressible. Intraluminal echogenic structure with or without an acoustic shadow (appendicolith). Often there is edematous thickening of the cecal pole.
  Perforated appendix: asymmetric wall thickness, perityphlitic abscess (may also be infrahepatic and periumbilical), perhaps with appendicolith (may migrate in the abdomen); free intraperitoneal fluid. Postoperative cul-de-sac infiltrate may remain visible for 2 months (Baker et al. 1986).
  Intussusception: usually ileocolic. Transverse section in the apical part of the intussusceptum is disk-shaped. Scans farther orally show concentric rings of low echogenicity surrounding a very echogenic center and separated from one another by moderately echogenic lines (see Fig. 7.**20c**). Longitudinal scan shows three parallel, hypoechogenic bands separated by two echogenic stripes. The head of the intussusceptum can be located, and lymph nodes embedded between the layers of the intussusceptum can often be identified. Successful ileocolic reduction can be sonographically confirmed by demonstrating the free leaves of the ileocecal valve.
  Necrotizing enterocolitis: gas microbubbles flowing in the portal venous system give positive evidence of necrotizing enterocolitis. With a patent ductus venosus, microbubbles may also enter the right atrium and right ventricle through the inferior vena cava. Embolized gas bubbles produce echogenic foci in the liver (Merritt et al. 1984).
  Anal atresia: US cannot reliably distinguish between high and low anal atresia. The distance from the rectal blind pouch to the perineal fossa is over 1.5 cm with high atresia. Look for associated anomalies of the urinary tract and female internal genitalia (uterine and vaginal duplications).
- *Duplication cysts:* gastric involvement at the greater curvature, bowel involvement on the mesenteric side (usually about the ileum). The cyst is often very mobile, so US is inferior to contrast radiography as a localizing study. Duplication cysts may be echofree or echogenic (hemorrhage, secretion; Littlewood-Teele et al. 1980).

References

Babcock, D. S.: Ultrasound diagnosis of portal vein thrombosis as a complication of appendicitis. Amer. J. Roentgenol. 133 (1979) 317–319

Baker, D. E., T. M. Silver, A. G. Coran, K. I. McMillin: Postappendectomy fluid collections in children: incidence, nature, and evolution evaluated using US. Radiology 161 (1986) 341–344

Bar-Ziv, J., Y. Barki, Z. Weizmann, J. Urkin: Transient protein-losing gastropathy (Menetrier's disease) in childhood. Pediat. Radiol. 18 (1988) 82–84

Hayden, C. K., L. E. Swischuk, J. E. Rytting: Gastric ulcer disease in infants: US findings. Radiology 164 (1987) 131–134

Holthusen, W., T. Birtel, B. Brinkmann, J. Gunkel, C. Janneck, E. Richter: Die Currarino-Triade. Ein autosomal-dominant erblicher Komplex von anorektaler Mißbildung, Sakrokokzygealdefekt und präsakralem Tumor. Beobachtung von 9 weiteren Fällen. Fortschr. Röntgenstr. 143 (1985) 83–89

Littlewood-Teele, R., C. I. Henschke, D. Tapper: The radiographic and ultrasonographic evaluation of enteric duplication cysts. Pediat. Radiol. (1980) 9–14

Merritt, C. R. B., J. P. Goldsmith, M. J. Sharp: Sonographic detection of portal venous gas in infants with necrotizing enterocolitis. Amer. J. Roentgenol. 143 (1984) 1059–1062

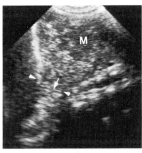
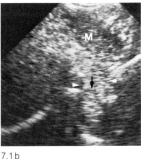
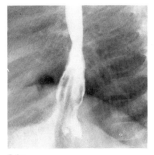

7.1a   7.1b   7.1c

7.1 Hiatal hernia, dehiscent fundoplication in a 5-month-old boy who underwent fundoplication for hiatal hernia and peptic esophageal stricture. Vomiting persisted postoperatively. Epigastric scans in **a** longitudinal and **b** transverse projection: regurgitation (↓) of gastric contents (M) through gaping hiatus (▶◄) into the esophagus. **c** Esophagram and operation confirmed diagnosis.

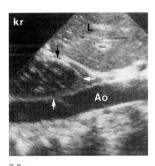
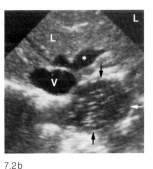

7.2a   7.2b

7.2 Achalasia in a boy aged 14 years, 3 months with a 5-year history of swallowing difficulties and regurgitation. Adrenal function normal. Epigastric scans in **a** longitudinal and **b** transverse projection, angled cranially: markedly dilated fluid-filled esophagus (arrows); despite vigorous peristalsis, no apparent relaxation of low-sited cardia. L = liver, Ao = aorta, V = inferior vena cava, * = hepatic vein. Operation. (Achalasia sometimes associated with adrenal insufficiency.)

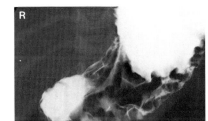
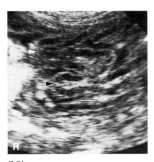
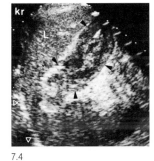

7.3a   7.3b   7.4

7.3 Protein-losing gastropathy (Ménétrier disease) in a 2-year-old boy with generalized hypoproteinemic edema. Urine and renal function normal. Suspicion of protein-losing enteropathy. **a** Barium radiograph: considerable thickening of the gastric rugal folds. **b** Left subcostal transverse scan: polypoid rugal folds in the gastric fundus with thickened, hypoechogenic submucosa (▼). Distention of the stomach with fluid can mask rugal fold enlargement. Protein-losing gastropathy (Ménétrier disease) associated with cytomegalovirus infection. Spontaneous remission after 4 weeks.

7.4 Malignant lymphoma in a 14-year-old girl with a 7-year history of epigastric pain unrelated to meals and a 4-year history of postprandial vomiting. Lymphoplasmocytic lymphoma of the gastric wall was diagnosed after multiple gastroscopies with biopsy. Epigastric longitudinal scan: the antral lumen is narrowed by massive, hypoechogenic gastric wall thickening (▼) of 1.5 cm; no peristalsis. L = liver, △ = diaphragm.

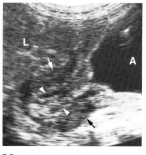
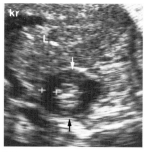

7.5a   7.5b

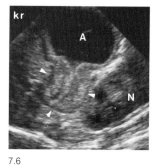
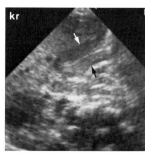

7.6   7.7

7.5   Idiopathic hypertrophic pyloric stenosis in a 6-week-old boy with a 3-week history of projectile vomiting, dehydration, hypokalemic alkalosis. Right upper abdominal **a** oblique and **b** longitudinal scans in the right lateral decubitus after tea ingestion: hypoechogenic, thickened, elongated pylorus muscle (↓) in longitudinal (**a**) and transverse section (**b**). Prominent mucosa (▼). The pylorus remains closed despite vigorous gastric peristalsis. A = antrum, L = liver.

7.6   Idiopathic hypertrophic pyloric stenosis in a 5½-week-old girl with projectile vomiting and the clinical picture of pyloric stenosis. Right oblique scan of the upper abdomen: hypertrophied pylorus muscle (▼) in longitudinal section. Muscle is isoechogenic to mucosa (transverse section of muscle appears anechogenic in these cases). A = antrum, N = kidney.

7.7   Idiopathic hypertrophic pyloric stenosis in an 11-week-old girl with a 3-week history of regurgitation progressing to projectile vomiting. Oblique epigastric scan: hypertrophied pylorus (arrows; 15 mm diameter), also elongation (3.3 cm).

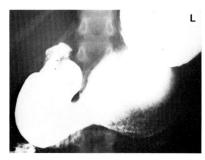
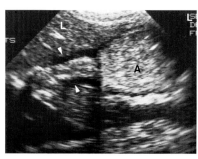
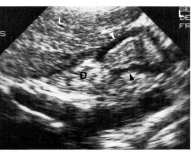

7.8a   7.8b   7.8c

7.8   "Adult type" hypertrophic pyloric stenosis in a 12-year-old boy with a 1-year history of foul eructation after meals, heartburn. Never vomited as an infant. **a** Gastroduodenal contrast film: distended stomach with vigorous peristalsis and an elongated pyloric canal; no clear evidence of an ulcer. **b, c** Transverse scans of the right upper abdomen: dilated stomach and an elongated pyloric canal with a moderately thickened,

hypoechogenic muscular layer (▼) and thick mucosa (echogenic). A = antrum, D = duodenum, L = liver. Endoscopy demonstrated reflux esophagitis and erosive antral gastritis. Pylorus could not be traversed with the scope. Gastric juice: hyperacid. "Adult type" hypertrophic pyloric stenosis with antral gastritis; in rare cases it results from undetected hypertrophic pyloric stenosis in childhood.

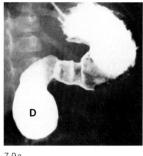
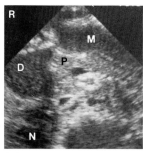
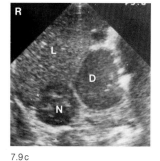

7.9a   7.9b   7.9c

7.9   Duodenal stenosis in a 7-month-old boy with trisomy 21, initially thriving; presented with a 2-month history of refusal to eat, occasional vomiting, weight loss. **a** Gastroduodenal contrast series: pear-shaped dilatation of the descending duodenum with hyperperistalsis and slight but continuous progression of the

contrast medium: "wind sock" type of duodenal stenosis. Transverse scans of **b** epigastrium and **c** right upper abdomen: markedly dilated first and second portions of the duodenum (D). No annular pancreas. M = stomach, P = pancreas, N = kidney.

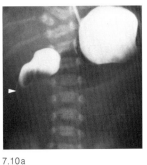
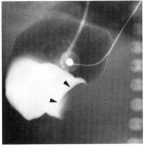

7.10a   7.10b

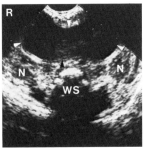
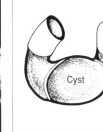

7.10c   7.10d

7.10 Double duodenal atresia with cyst formation in a preterk male neonate of 34 weeks' gestation weighing 1840 g. First day: prenatal sonogram showed polyhydramnios with a severe dilatation of the fetal stomach and small bowel loop; postpartum plain abdominal radiograph showed the double bubble sign. **a, b** Gastroduodenal radiographs: complete blockage of the contrast medium in the dilated duodenum by a spherical mass (▼). **c** Transverse epigastric scan: elliptical cystic structure (▼) that is mobile relative to the liver and kidneys (N). WS = spinal column. **DD:** duplication cyst, choledochal cyst. **d** Operation: double duodenal atresia with cyst formation in the third portion of the duodenum.

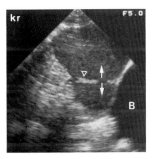
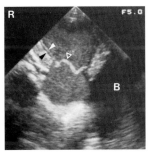

7.11a   7.11b

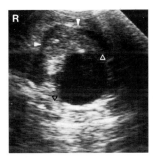
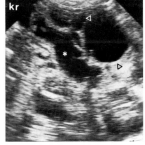

7.12a   7.12b

7.11 Small-bowel duplication cyst in a 2-year-old girl with recurrent abdominal pain, vomiting, and urinary tract infections. **a** Coronal and **b** oblique scans of the right lower abdomen: mobile, septated (▽), cystic mass with a thin, hypoechogenic wall (▮). The moderately echogenic contents of the cyst flow back and forth through a central aperture in the membrane (⫿). B = bladder. UGI series showed nonrotation, nonopacification of the cyst, no apparent pad effect. **DD:** duplication cyst (peristalsis in cyst wall!), cystic Meckel diverticulum, less likely mesenteric, omental, or ovarian cyst. Operation: small-bowel duplication cyst with poorly differentiated gastric mucosa and segments with respiratory epithelium. Cyst contents may be echo-free or echogenic as a result of hemorrhage or inspissated secretions. Ectopic gastric mucosa can be detected by ^{99m}Tc−pertechnetate scanning.

7.12 Enteric duplication in a male newborn who began vomiting on the 3rd day of life; abdominal distention, meconium passage. Spherical, movable mass palpated in the right midabdomen. **a** Transverse and **b** longitudinal scans of the right lower abdomen: cystic mass 2.5 cm in diameter (▽) bordering on the cecum (▼) medially and dilated fluid-filled small bowel loop (★) anteriorly. Small bowel dilated and fluid-filled with vigorous peristalsis: mechanical obstruction. Suspected enteric duplication. UGI series: extrinsic ileocecal compression. Operation: duplication of the terminal ileum.

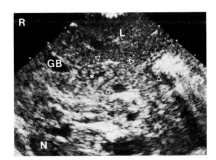

7.13

7.13 Annular pancreas in an 11-day-old girl with a history of vomiting, at times bilious, since birth. Epigastric transverse scan: duodenum (★) encircled anteriorly and posteriorly by the pancreas (▽). L = liver, N = kidney. Annular pancreas in itself cannot cause duodenal obstruction. UGI series showed coexisting malrotation. Diagnosis confirmed at operation.

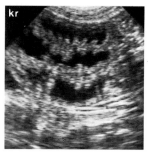
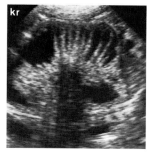

7.14a　　　　7.14b

7.14 Celiac disease in a 1-year-old girl with a 3-month history of bulky, pasty stool, no weight gain, whining. Sudden vomiting with marked abdominal distention. Plain abdominal radiograph showed small-bowel obstruction. Profuse stool followed contrast enema to exclude intussusception. **a, b.** Left flank longitudinal scans: fluid-filled loops of the small bowel with thickened wall and thickened Kerckring folds (cut tangentially in **b**). US findings with history and clinical presentation: celiac crisis, confirmed by biopsy. **DD** of thickened small bowel loops: hypoproteinemia (nephrotic syndrome, etc.), portal hypertension, gastroenteritis, celiac disease, cystic fibrosis, protein-losing enteropathy, regional enteritis (Crohn disease), giardiasis, eosinophilic gastroenteritis, intestinal lymphangiectasis, Zollinger–Ellison syndrome, constrictive pericarditis.

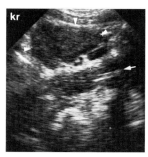
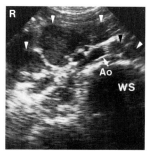
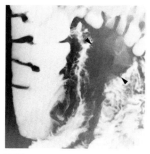

7.15a　　　　7.15b　　　　7.15c

7.15 Regional enteritis in a girl of 9 years, 3 months, 2 years after appendectomy. Had a 14-day history of abdominal pain, fever, diffuse abdominal tenderness and moderate muscular rigidity. No diarrhea. **a** Longitudinal scan of the right lower abdomen and **b** midabdominal transverse scan: multiple lymphomas (mesenteric; ▼), some lobulated, ranging up to 3.5 cm in size, located anterior to the psoas muscle (↓) and anterior and adjacent to the aorta (Ao). Little free intraperitoneal fluid. WS = spinal column. **DD:** malignant lymphoma, mesenteric lymphadenitis (large lymphomas especially characteristic of regional enteritis in *Yersinia* infection). Bone marrow aspiration: no malignancy. **c** Small-bowel series: spastic terminal ileum with irregular, partly nodular mucosa; separation of the bowel loops by the lymphoma (▼). Serology: *Yersinia enterocolitica*, serotype 3.

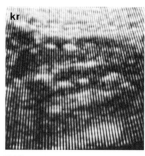
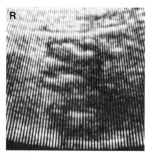
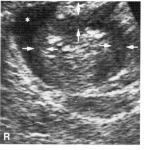
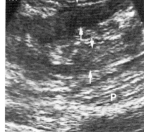

7.16a　　　　7.16b　　　　7.17a　　　　7.17b

7.16 Crohn disease in a 13-year-old boy with severe weight loss, abdominal pain, diarrhea, high ESR. Crohn disease suspected. **a** Longitudinal and **b** transverse scans of the right lower abdomen show "stacking" of three aperistaltic bowel loops with thickened walls (0.5 cm). Contrast enema: Crohn disease.

7.17 Crohn disease in a 23-year-old woman with clinical and radiographic signs of mechanical ileus. No previous gastrointestinal complaints. **a** Transverse and **b** longitudinal scans of the right midabdomen: considerable irregular, hypoechogenic bowel-wall thickening (↓) and free intraperitoneal fluid (★) consistent with seepage peritonitis. P = psoas muscle. Operation: cylindrical thickening of the terminal ileum with extension to the cecum and swollen mesenteric lymph nodes. Suspicion of Crohn disease confirmed histologically.

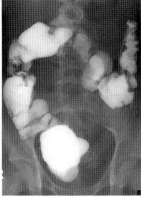

7.18a

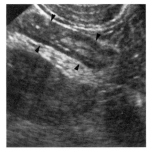

7.18b

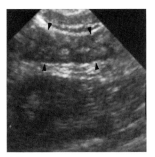

7.18c

7.18 Crohn disease in a 16-year-old girl with a 10-year history of the disease; presented with colicky pains during defecation and with a high ESR. **a** Contrast enema: luminal narrowing and rigidity of the left colic flexure, descending colon, and sigmoid colon with cobblestone pattern and pseudopolyps. **b, c** Left flank coronal scans: irregular wall thickening (hypoechogenic) of the descending colon (▼). Note the cobblestone appearance of the echogenic mucosa in **c**.

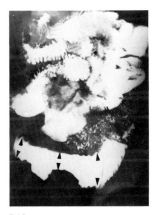

7.19a

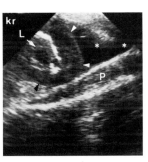

7.19b

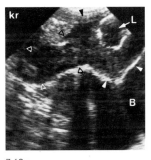

7.19c

7.19 Non-Hodgkin lymphoma of the small bowel in a 12-year-old boy with a 3-month history of lassitude and occasional upper abdominal pain. Palpable lower abdominal mass. Anemia (Hb 64 g/L), **a** Small-bowel series: rigid small bowel loop (▼) in the lower abdomen with a thickened wall and coarse mucosal folds. **b** Left longitudinal and **c** midsagittal scans of the lower abdomen: hypoechogenic thickening of the bowel wall (▼) and mesentery (▽; thickness 2 cm) and free intraperitoneal fluid (★). L = bowel lumen, B = bladder, P = psoas muscle. Liver, spleen, and kidneys appear normal. Suspicion of primary malignant lymphoma of small bowel. Histology: non-Hodgkin lymphoma, B-cell type.

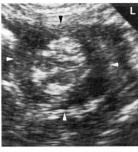

7.20a

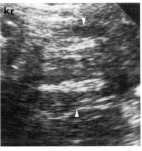

7.20b

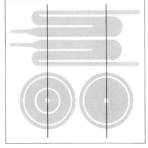

7.20c

7.20 Ileocolic intussusception in a 3½-month-old girl with a 1-day history of vomiting, refusal to eat, and one bloody stool. **a** Transverse and **b** longitudinal scans of the right lower abdomen: concentric layering of thickened (edematous), hypoechogenic walls (▼) of intussusceptum (see diagram **c**). Free intraperitoneal fluid. Ileocolic intussusception confirmed by contrast enema. Hydrostatic reduction not possible. **c** Diagram of intussusception: intussusceptum appears as concentric layers or as a wide hypoechogenic ring, depending on the scan plane.

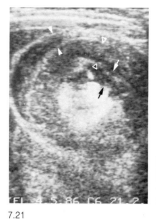

7.21

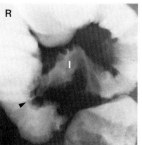

7.22a

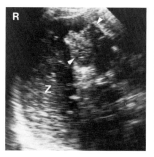

7.22b

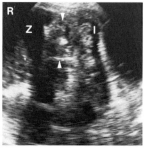

7.22c

7.21 Ileocecal double intussusception in a 9-month-old boy with a 4-day history of vomiting, thin stools, then colicky abdominal pain; finally, bloody stool, shocky, palpable rectal mass. Abdominal radiograph showed small-bowel obstruction. Transverse scan of the right lower abdomen: intussuscipiens (𝕏), outer (𝕏) and inner (⊹) layers of the intussusceptum (same findings in the left lower abdomen): ileocecal double intussusception extending to the rectum, confirmed at operation.

7.22 Intestinal intussusception in a 9-month-old boy with a 1-week history of fever and a 3-day history of diarrhea followed by sudden onset of vomiting, with some bile-stained vomitus. Plain abdominal radiograph showed bowel obstruction. US showed intussusception, reduced hydrostatically by nonionic contrast enema. **a** Contrast enema: swollen ileocecal valve (▼) and terminal ileum (I) following reduction. Coronal scans of the right lower abdomen show the thickened, hypoechogenic (edematous), projecting ileocecal valve (▼) in **b** longitudinal and **c** transverse section; thickened mucosal folds in the terminal ileum (I). Z = cecum.

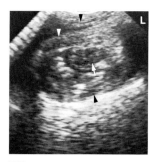

7.23a

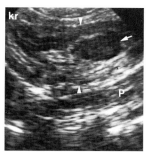

7.23b

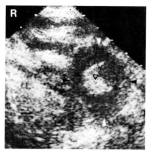

7.24

7.23 Intestinal intussusception due to lymphadenitis in a 6-year-old boy with colicky abdominal pain and vomiting 11 days before and on the day of admission; in the intervening period the patient was asymptomatic and had a normal stool. **a** Transverse and **b** longitudinal scans of the right lower abdomen: layered, thickened, hypoechogenic bowel walls (▼) with enclosed mesenteric lymph nodes (↓). P = psoas muscle.

7.24 Intestinal intussusception due to polyposis in a girl of 16 years, 9 months with known Pleutz-Jeghers syndrome; acute colicky abdominal pain with nausea, right periumbilical tenderness. US showed intussusception with polyps. Infraumbilical transverse scan: very thick, hypoechogenic bowel wall (▼) with polypoid projection (▽) into the bowel lumen. Operation disclosed two small-bowel intussusceptions, each in a region affected by polyps.

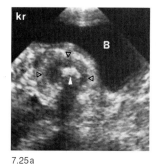

7.25a

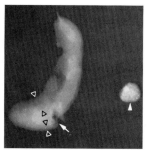

7.25b

7.25 Appendicitis and fecalith in a 3½-year-old boy with a 4-day history of abdominal pain, fever, diarrhea, and intermittent urinary retention; urine normal. **a** Right parasagittal scan of the lower abdomen: area of eccentric bowel wall thickening (▽) behind the bladder (B) with an intraluminal concretion casting an acoustic shadow (▼; no free fluid). Operation: appendix adherent to the bladder wall, intraoperative perforation. **b** Specimen radiograph: eccentric wall thickening (𝕏), perforation (↑), fecalith (▼).

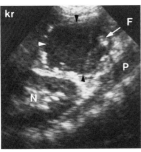
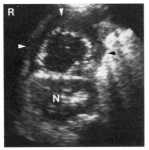

7.26a   7.26b

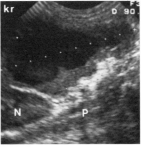
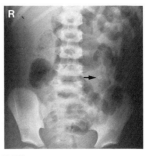

7.27a   7.27b

7.26 Perityphlitic abscess and fecalith in a 21-month-old boy with a 1-week history of anorexia and fever and a 1-day history of abdominal pain. **a** Longitudinal and **b** transverse right flank scans: hypoechogenic mass (▼) with a somewhat more echogenic rim bordering on the kidney (N) and psoas muscle (P). Concretion with acoustic shadow (F). Abdominal radiograph showed a fecalith and mass effect in the right midabdomen. Perityphlitic abscess with a fecalith confirmed at operation.

7.27 Perityphlitic abscess in a girl of 3 years, 9 months with a 1-week history of recurrent vomiting, abdominal pain, fever; admitted with diffuse peritonitis. **a** Right flank longitudinal scan: large abscess (+···+) bordering on the psoas muscle (P) and kidney (N; free intraperitoneal fluid). **b** Supine abdomen plain film: fecalith (arrow) in the left hemiabdomen. Operation: perityphlitic abscess ruptured into the free abdominal cavity (fecalith!), diffuse peritonitis.

7.28 Perforative appendicitis in a 13-month-old girl with a 4-day history of anorexia, repeated vomiting, mild diarrhea; 2-day history of high fever and abdominal pain. She presented with diffuse abdominal rigidity. Plain abdominal film showed intestinal obstruction. **a** Left flank coronal scan: strongly dilated fluid-filled small bowel loops (★) with antegrade and retrograde peristalsis. N = kidney (copious free fluid in cul-de-sac). **b** Longitudinal scan of the right lower abdomen: two wall-thickened bowel loops (in cross section; ▼) surrounded by a wide echogenic rim (▽). Echogenic structure with an acoustic shadow (fecalith, ←) posteriorly: perforative appendicitis with fibrinous adhesion of bowel loops leading to mechanical obstruction, peritonitis. Confirmed at operation.

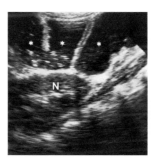
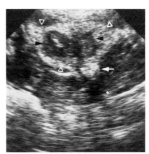

7.28a   7.28b

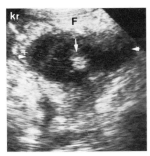
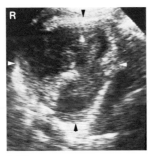

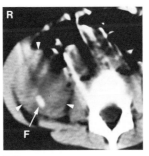
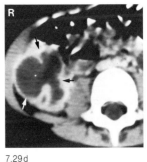

7.29a   7.29b   7.29c   7.29d

7.29 Perityphlitic abscess with fecalith, right renal agenesis in a boy 3 years, 9 months of age with initial vomiting, abdominal pain, and fever progressing in subsequent weeks to fever and anorexia with no abdominal pain. Firm, fist-size mass palpated in the right midabdomen. US: Wilms tumor suspected; patient hospitalized. **a** Longitudinal and **b** transverse scans of the right midabdomen: approximately 5-cm hypoechogenic mass with an echogenic border (▼) containing a hyperechogenic concretion (F →). Right kidney absent, left kidney very large with normal structure. CT scans of right midabdomen show **c** an abscess (▼) with fecalith (F) and **d** contrast enhancement of the abscess membrane (arrows).

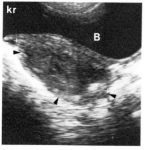 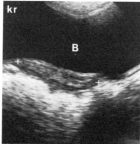

7.30a   7.30b

7.30 Cul-de-sac infiltrate in a 5-year-old girl who developed increased fever and leukocytosis 10 days after operation for perforative appendicitis. Palpable cul-de-sac infiltrate. **a** Longitudinal scan of the lower abdomen: 5-cm mass (▼) with a heterogeneous echo structure indenting the bladder (B) posteriorly and showing no change after defecation (indwelling intestinal tube visible posterior to the mass—cul-de-sac infiltrate). **b** Complete regression after a 6-day course of antibiotic therapy. ++ = uterus.

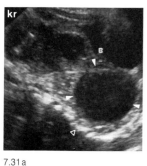 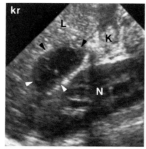   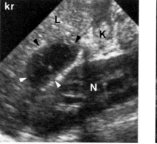 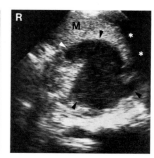

7.31a   7.31b   7.32a   7.32b

7.31 Intraperitoneal abscesses in a 3-year-old girl with intermittent fever 12 days after operation for perforative appendicitis with local peritonitis. **a** Longitudinal scan of the lower abdomen: spherical hypoechogenic mass (▼) between the bladder (B) and the sacrum (▽) and rectum: cul-de-sac abscess (was drained). **b** Longitudinal scan of the right upper abdomen: abscess (▼) between the liver (L), kidney (N), and colon (K; resolved with antibiotic treatment). Coexisting left-sided postoperative pleural effusion.

7.32 Intraperitoneal abscesses in a 12-year-old girl who became febrile 3 weeks after operation for a perforative appendicitis with diffuse peritonitis. Left subphrenic scans on **a** coronal and **b** transverse planes: hypoechogenic, indented mass (▼) with movable internal echoes and posterior acoustic enhancement below the spleen (M). Fluid between the spleen and diaphragm (★). Ao = aorta. US cannot differentiate a splenic abscess from an abscess in the splenic hilum. Radionuclide scans did not show splenic abscess. Operation: omentum-covered abscess at the lower splenic pole and subphrenic abscess on the left side. No splenic abscess (pyogenic splenic abscess is very rare!).

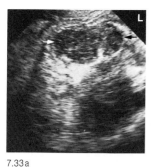 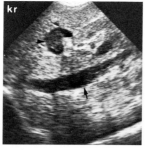   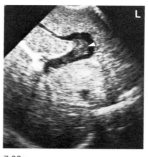 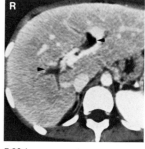

7.33a   7.33b   7.33c   7.33d

7.33 Perityphlitic abscess with subsequent pylephlebitis in a 10-year-old girl who developed septic fever, abdominal pain, jaundice, and hepatomegaly 1 week after a brief episode of diarrhea, vomiting, and fever. **a** Transverse scan of the right lower abdomen: hypoechogenic ovoid mass 4 × 2 cm in size: perityphlitic abscess, operatively confirmed. Free fluid in cul-de-sac, portal vein normal. Septic fever persisted after surgery. **b** Midsagittal and **c** oblique epigastric scans: dilatation of the portal vein with echogenic material in the lumen of the bifurcation and both side branches (▼). Portal vein trunk and superior mesenteric vein echo-free, hepatomegaly, no hepatic abscess. ↓ = inferior vena cava. Portal venous thrombosis associated with purulent endophlebitis of the portal vein. **d** CT: thrombus (▼) produces filling defect in the opacified portal vein. Purulent pylephlebitis may be associated with appendicitis, cholecystitis, pancreatitis, inflammatory small-bowel diseases, and other abdominal inflammations and tumors.

7.34 Necrotizing enterocolitis in a mature with bile-stained vomitus, bloody stool, and abdominal distention on the 3rd day of life. Plain abdominal radiograph showed intestinal pneumatosis, no air in the portal vein system. **a, b** Oblique scans through the liver hilum: intermittent (presumably due to respiratory variations of intra-/abdominal pressure) passage of very echogenic particles about 2 mm in size (↓; gas bubbles) from the mesenteric vein through the portal vein into the hepatic periphery. The embolized bubbles temporarily produce bright echoes in the hepatic parenchyma (▽; chiefly in the upper portions of the organ). Necrotizing enterocolitis is often manifested by visible gas in the portal vein and liver before radiographic signs appear.

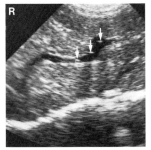
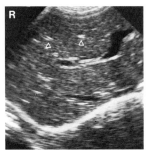

7.34a   7.34b

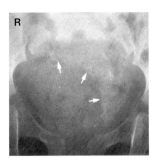
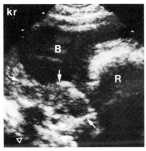
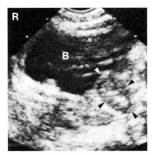
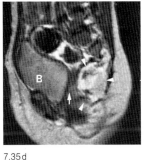

7.35a   7.35b   7.35c   7.35d

7.35 "Currarino triad" in a 6½-month-old girl. Three females on the paternal side had been operated for a presacral "cyst". Brother operated at the age of 6 months for an anorectal stenosis with suspected Hirschsprung disease (not histologically confirmed). Patient presented with difficult defecation and sacral asymmetry with increased pilosity. **a** Radiograph: right-sided sacral defect with a curved border (arrows): "scimitar sacrum." **b** Right longitudinal and **c** transverse pelvic scans: presacral mass with solid (↓) and cystic (▽) components. Rectum (R) is markedly dilated above a localized constriction with wall thickening (▼). B = urinary bladder. **d** Right parasagittal MR image of the pelvis: bladder (B), rectum (↑), and sacral mass (▼). Scimitar sacrum + anorectal stenosis + presacral mass (may consist of an anterior meningocele, lipoma, hamartoma or teratoma, dermoid cyst, or cystic enteric duplication) = "Currarino triad" (in at least 50%, autosomal dominant transmission).

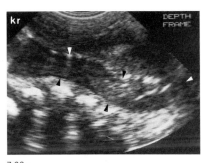
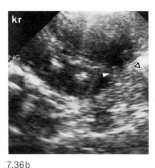

7.36a   7.36b

7.36 Low anal atresia in a newborn girl. Abdominal plain film on the 2nd day of life consistent with high anal atresia. Sacrum normal. **a** Longitudinal scan of the lower abdomen: meconium-filled rectal stump (▼; hence no bowel gas) extending distally past the coccyx. **b** Longitudinal transperineal scan: distance between the rectal stump (▼) and anal fissure (▽) is 0.8 cm. Low anal atresia confirmed at operation.

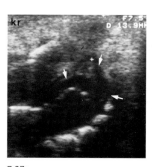
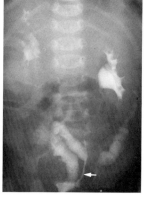

7.37a   7.37b

7.37 Anal atresia with rectovaginal fistula in a 1-day-old girl. **a** Transperineal longitudinal pelvic scan: fluid-filled rectal blind pouch (arrows) terminating 14 mm (+⋯+) above the anal fissure. **b** AP abdominal radiograph after angiocardiography (patent ductus, pulmonary sequestration) shows renally excreted contrast medium in the rectum and sigmoid colon due to a rectovaginal fistula. Arrow indicates the left ureter. Fluid in the blind pouch gives possible evidence of a fistula.

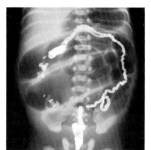
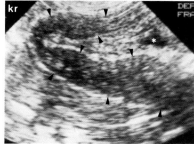

7.38a   7.38b

7.38 Meconium ileus in a preterm infant of 35 weeks' gestation, 2060 g; vomiting, abdominal distention, no meconium passage on the 2nd day of life. **a** Contrast enema: microcolon, greatly dilated loops of the small bowel. No meconium-containing bowel loops are visible. **b** Right flank coronal scan: greatly distended, meconium-filled small bowel loop (▼) and moderate free intraperitoneal fluid (★): meconium ileus with seepage peritonitis; operative treatment.

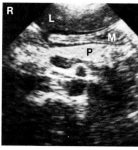
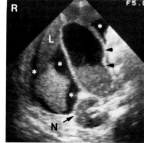

7.39   7.40

7.39 Cystic fibrosis in a 14-year-old boy. Epigastric transverse scan: markedly increased echogenicity of the pancreas. P = pancreas, M = stomach, L = liver.

7.40 Toxic hepatic failure with inspissation of bile in a 14-month-old boy with refractory status epilepticus and therapy-induced toxic hepatic failure with hypoproteinemic edema; parenteral nutrition. Right transverse epigastric scan: ascites (★), markedly distended gallbladder with thickened (edematous) wall and two layers of sludge (▼) of contrasting echogenicity. L = liver, N = kidney. Sludge (pigmentary granules and cholesterol crystals) forms with biliary stasis of any etiology (here, parenteral nutrition).

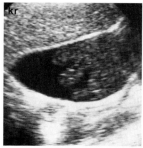
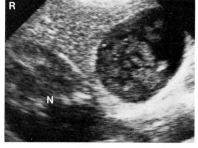
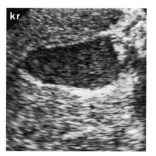

7.41a   7.41b   7.41c

7.14 Inspissation of bile in a 5½-year-old girl with microspherocytosis and right upper abdominal pain. **a** Longitudinal and **b** transverse scans of the right upper abdomen: moderately echogenic structures with no acoustic shadows in the well-filled gallbladder. **c** Longitudinal scan: incomplete contraction after a meal. N = kidney. Gallbladder sludge in a setting of hemolytic anemia (picture identical to that of biliary statis due, e.g., to parenteral nutrition). Complete resolution is possible.

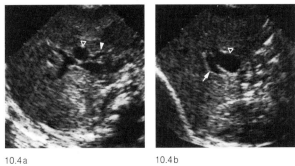
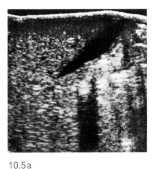
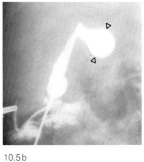

10.4a   10.4b   10.5a   10.5b

10.4   Choleductal atresia in a 3½-week-old boy with hyperbilirubinemia. Biliary obstruction. Suspected extrahepatic biliary
atresia. **a** Transverse and **b** longitudinal scans: cystic ectasia of
the common hepatic duct (△) and ectasia of the intrahepatic bile
ducts (▲); portal vein, →. Gallbladder not seen. Hepatoenterostomy (modification of Kasai type). Small gallbladder present;
atretic common dile duct.

10.5   Extrahepatic biliary atresia in a 2-month-old boy with
hyperbilirubinemia. **a** Longitudinal scan: full gallbladder, no visible bile ducts. **b** Intraoperative transvesicular cholecystography:
cystic ectasia of the cystic duct (△; not visible on sonogram).
Hepatoenterostomy (Kasai type).

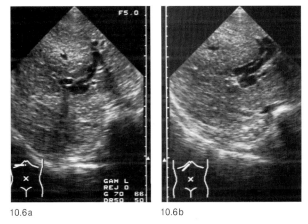
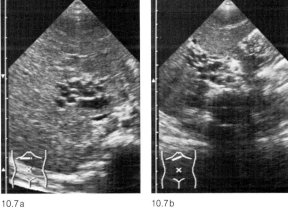

10.6a   10.6b   10.7a   10.7b

**10.6   Congenital hepatic fibrosis in the setting of polycys-
tic renal disease (recessive)** in a 10½-year-old girl with no
jaundice. **a, b** Sonograms show bile-duct ectasia (nonobstructive). Note general increase in echogenicity with an irregular
distribution, characteristic of hepatic fibrosis (same patient as in
Figs. 5.**41**, 14.**23**, and 14.**60**).

10.7   Venous malformation (portal? hepatic venous?) in an
11-month-old boy with **VATER association** (dextrocardia, spinal and rib anomalies, horseshoe kidney). **a, b** Sonograms
demonstrate "too many" vessels. All but the hepatic artery yield
a venous Doppler flow signal. No clinical or US evidence of portal
hypertension.

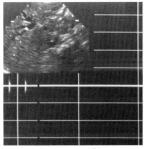
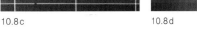
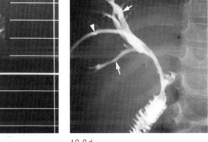

10.8a   10.8b   10.8c   10.8d

10.8   Liver transplant, abscess, biliary obstruction in a 3-
year-old girl who underwent a liver transplant following hepatic
failure associated with posthepatic fibrosis. **a** Transverse scan:
ill-defined hypoechogenic zone (arrows) suspicious for abscessation. Confirmed at reoperation; hepaticoduodenostomy followed by fever and progression of cholestasis. **b** Indeterminate,

large-caliber vascular structures in the right hepatic lobe
(arrows). **c** Duplex scan on the same plane: absence of flow
signal signifies ectatic bile ducts. **d** Radiographic correlate (→),
percutaneous contrast injected through the bile duct splint/drain
(▼).

11 Ascites

U. V. Willi

Free intraperitoneal fluid is a nonspecific symptom. A volume as small as several milliliters can be detected with ultrasound. In the clinical context and during the course of an illness, it is useful to grade the quantity of the fluid collection as small (mild), moderate, or massive (severe), and to note any changes that occur. Mild ascites may be physiologic (e.g., postovulatory) or may relate to a (local) inflammatory process.

An inflammatory process involving the peritoneum, mesentery, pancreas, hepatobiliary system, the urogenital and especially the gastrointestinal tract, or a subdiaphragmatic process, whether bacterial, viral, or parasitic, may be associated with a moderate or, at times, severe degree of ascites.

A large volume of free intraperitoneal fluid in a patient with no antecedent trauma and no severe or chronic disease of the heart, kidneys, liver, or gastrointestinal tract should raise suspicion of a malignant process (mesenteric, intestinal, peritoneal, pleural, or arising from an abdominal or retroperitoneal organ). The cytologic and bacteriologic examination of a percutaneously aspirated fluid sample is advised. For example, a lymphoma may be found to be causative.

Conversely, a massive fluid collection of relatively acute onset can present clinically as a large abdominal mass. Or ascites may displace a parenchymatous abdominal organ or accentuate its palpable contours, causing it to present (clinically) as a mass.

Impaired peritoneal fluid absorption is not uncommon in hydrocephalus patients with a ventriculoperitoneal shunt. A CSF pseudocyst of moderate size is not difficult to detect and in extreme cases is indistinguishable from massive ascites (see Fig. 5.**34**). Often the fluid is permeated by weblike echoes (proteinaceous substances).

While one can speculate as to the nature of free intraperitoneal fluid (exudate, transudate, chyle, urine, bile, pancreatic juice, blood), this cannot be reliably establishes with ultrasound. Corpuscular elements in the fluid can sometimes be made visible by the Gain manipulation. Ascitic fluid can be aspirated and subjected to bacteriologic, chemical, and/or cytologic analysis depending on the urgency fo the case and the nature of the inquiry.

Free fluid in the omental bursa can mimic an indeterminate cystic mass. Intraintestinal fluid can usually be identified as such even in the absence of intestinal peristalsis (signs of paralytic ileus).

It should not be difficult to distinguish between infra- and supradiaphragmatic fluid, although their combination cannot always be recognized. A chest radiograph taken in the proper position can be a useful adjunct. In many cases this film is already available and may itself provide the impetus for an abdominal ultrasound study.

References

Newman, B., R. Teele: Ascites in the fetus, neonate, and young child: emphasis on ultrasonographic evaluation. Semin. Ultrasound 5 (1984) 85–101

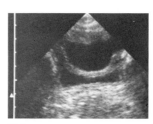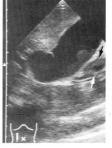

11.1a   11.1b

11.1 Salmonella typhosa infection in a boy 4 years, 9 months of age with fever, abdominal pain, and diarrhea. **a** Transverse scan: moderate ascites **b** Right longitudinal midabdominal scan: large gallbladder, sludge; local bowel wall thickening (arrows): presumably duodenal mucosa. Not shown: bile duct ectasia from biliary obstruction.

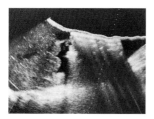

11.2 Constrictive pericarditis in a 15-year-old boy (from North Africa) with hepatosplenomegaly of unknown cause. Longitudinal scan: massive ascites. Chest radiograph showed calcified primary complex (TB); suspected pericardial calcification.

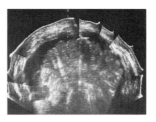

11.3 Global cardiac failure in a 14-year-old boy (from North Africa) with a "large abdominal mass." Radiograph showed cardiomegaly, Kerley B lines, massive pleural effusion. Transverse scan at about the level of the umbilicus: massive ascites and swelling of abdominal wall, both secondary to right-sided cardiac failure. Not shown: hepatomegaly. No tumor.

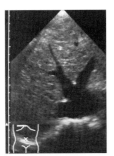 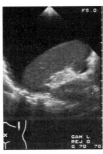 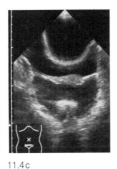 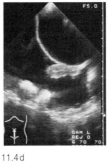 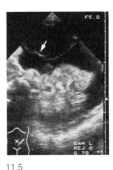

11.4a   11.4b   11.4c   11.4d   11.5

11.4 Endocardial fibrosis, tricuspid insufficiency in a 14-year-old girl. **a** Right transverse upper abdominal scan, **b** left flank longitudinal scan, **c** transverse pelvic and **d** longitudinal scans: massive ascites and severe ectasia of hepatic veins (right inflow stasis). Liver and spleen "float" in the ascites. Similar impression on the uterus and adnexa anteriorly and posteriorly by the fluid-distended peritoneal cavity.

11.5 Postenteritic syndrome with hypoproteinemia in a 2-month-old girl with a failure to grow, bloody stools, left flank mass. The first US 17 days before showed vigorous intestinal peristalsis (gastroenteritis?), no ascites. The second US, 9 days

before, showed mild splenomegaly, no ascites. Rapid subsequent weight gain. In this, the third examination, the longitudinal oblique scan of left hemiabdomen shows massive ascites and a thin, passively mobile, echogenic line (pseudocyst?), which later spontaneously disappeared. No evidence of tumor, adenopathy, or intussusception. **DD:** infection, tumor (e.g., lymphoma), malformation (e.g., a Meckel diverticulum), vascular lesion (e.g., intestinal or portal venous thrombosis), iatrogenic lesion (toxic effect from previous therapy). Laboratory: *Staphylococcus aureus* (aspirated ascitic fluid); hypoproteinemia. Good response to antibiotic treatment.

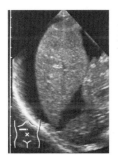 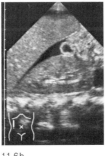 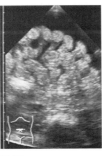 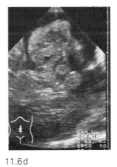 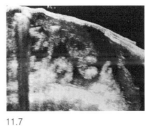

11.6a   11.6b   11.6c   11.6d   11.7

11.6 Multiple sulfatase deficiency in an 11-year-old girl with suspected bowel obstruction. **a** Right transverse upper abdominal scan, **b** right flank longitudinal scan, **c** umbilical transverse and **d** longitudinal scans: massive ascites: moderate hepatomegaly (and splenomegaly); renal swelling with increased cortical echogenicity. Scant intraintestinal fluid. Findings (including X-rays) did not arouse the suspicious of bowel obstruction. Not shown: the normal caliber of the hepatic veins.

11.7 Lymphoma in a 7-year-old boy with a suspected giant abdominal tumor. Longitudinal scan: massive ascites and extensive, diffuse bowel wall thickening suspicious for lymphoma. Chest radiograph showed massive bilateral pleural effusion. Laboratory/aspirate: confirmatory.

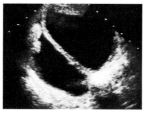 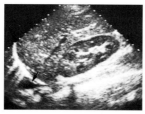

11.8a   11.8b

11.8 B-cell lymphoma in a 12-year-old boy with a 4-month history of fatigue (in retrospect). Respiratory tract infection 1 month before. Followed by pancreatitis? Referred for severe abdominal pain, fever, general malaise. Appendicitis suspected. **a** Longitudinal pelvic scan: massive ascites. Not shown: retroperitoneal lymph nodes (same patient as in Fig. 12.**17**).

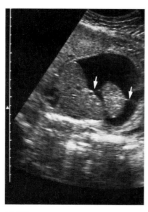 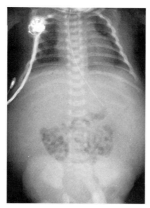

11.10a   11.10b

11.10 Gangliosidosis in a 32-week fetus. **a** US shows massive fetal ascites; free intestine fixed as a "mass" by cordlike structures (arrows) (ligaments and/or mesentery). Cranial to the "mass" is the liver, above that the heart. Not shown: normal sagittal diameter of the chest and kidneys, normal amniotic fluid volume. **DD:** ascites probably not of cardiac, urologic, or hepatobiliary origin; gastrointestinal cause (e.g., Meckel diverticulum); vascular disorder (e.g., mesenteric volvulus), etc. Infant delivered at term, showed similar postnatal US findings. **b** Radiographic correlate with fetal US; small bowel now contains air; laboratory investigation yields a diagnosis of gangliosidosis.

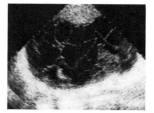 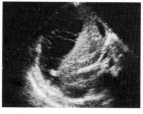

11.9a   11.9b

Appendectomy (normal-appearing appendix). **b** Right flank longitudinal scan 4 days later: mild pleural effusion (arrow). Progressive cachexia. Seven days later, cytologic diagnosis of B-cell lymphoma. The patient died the same day.

11.9 CSF pseudocyst in a 7-year-old girl with a myelomeningocele and a ventriculoperitoneal shunt. Abdominal pain, large abdomen. Abdominal tumor? **a** Right anterolateral longitudinal scan and **b** right transverse hemiabdominal scan: massive perihepatic fluid collection, presumably encapsulated and containing echogenic septations; intense acoustic enhancement: CSF pseudocyst with peritoneal malabsorption.

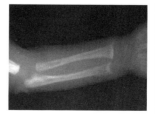 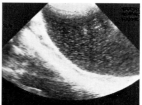

11.10c   11.11

c Radiograph 1 month later: rachitis-like change in the distal metaphyses of the forearm bones.

11.11 Hemolytic anemia in a 1-day-old male with ascites. Longitudinal abdominal scan: numerous fine echoes, accentuated by a high Gain setting. Chyle? Percutaneous aspiration: massive lymphocytes (fasted state) and erythroblasts. Later diagnosis: hemolytic anemia, unclassified (1 year, 5 months); spontaneous compensation.

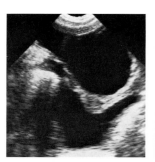 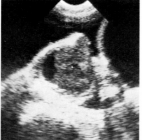

11.12a   11.12b

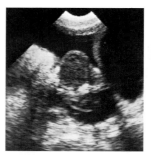 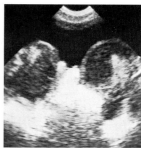

11.12c   11.12d

11.12 Tuberculous peritonitis/adnexitis in a girl of 12 years, 4 months with a 2–3 month history of general malaise, fatigability, pallor, anorexia. Abdominal distention and pain for several days prior to admission. Primary US and CT at the referring clinic showed massive ascites and bilateral adnexal masses; suspected malignant metastatic ovarian tumors with peritoneal carcinomatosis. **a** Midlongitudinal scan: the uterus is not adherent to the bladder, as is usual in ascites. **b** Right and **c** left longitudinal scans each show a supravesical adnexal mass with a capsule-like border, "solid"; the right mass has a fluid component. **d** Transverse scan shows both supravesical masses with ascites. **DD:** lymphoma. Laparoscopy: ascites yellow, turbid; ovaries small, normal; ovarian tubes strongly dilated, inflamed. Excellent, rapid response to antituberculosis drug therapy.

12 Lymphadenopathy

I. Forster

Enlarged peripheral lymph nodes usually present clinically as visible and palpable mass. Their size, shape, margins, echo structure, and spatial relationship to the muscles and blood vessels and, in the neck, to the trachea, esophagus, thyroid, and parotid gland can be evaluated with ultrasound. Nonpalpable lymph nodes also may be detected.

Enlarged infradiaphragmatic lymph nodes are rarely palpable. They may be associated clinically with nonspecific symptoms such as fever, abdominal and back pain, signs of intestinal and biliary obstruction, obstructive uropathy, or ascites. The most common indication for sonography is the suspicion of malignant disease.

The lymph nodes are sought at the following sites: *retroperitoneally* along the aorta, inferior vena cava, iliac vessels, peripancreatic area, renal hila, and perivesical area; *intra-abdominally* in the hepatic and splenic hilum, along the celiac trunk and its bifurcation, and the mesenteric vessels. The examiner should also be alert for abnormalities of the liver, spleen, pancreas, or kidneys and should watch for ascites or pleural effusion.

Sonographic Findings

Normal-sized peripheral lymph nodes appear sonographically as flat, oval, hypoechogenic structures. Normal-sized infradiaphragmatic nodes are rarely detectable with ultrasound, as they are virtually isoechogenic to surrounding tissues.

The echo structure of enlarged lymph nodes can range from hypoechogenic to hyperechogenic or heterogeneous (mixed). It is nonspecific and is not useful for differentiating benign from malignant disease. A single lymph node or a cluster of matted nodes cannot always be identified as such. Multiple well-defined hypoechogenic nodular masses can usually be diagnosed as lymhadenopathy by ultrasound, but differentiation between benign and malignant conditions is not possible.

Acute lymphadenitis often appears sonographically as an elliptical hypoechogenic mass or a heterogeneous mass with scalloped borders. Abscessed lymph nodes are cystic and usually cause acoustic enhancement. A similar pattern may be produced by tumor-infiltrated nodes that have undergone spontaneous degeneration or have been altered by chemotherapy or irradiation. Malignant lymphomas are typically hypoechogenic and can mimic cysts, but they do not cause enhancement phenomena. Lymph node metastases are usually more echogenic than malignant lymphomas or nodes affected by inflammatory change. Calcifications can be seen in association with chronic lymphadenitis and in metastatically involved nodes, appearing as intensely echogenic areas that may cast an acoustic shadow.

Intraperitoneal and retroperitoneal lymph nodes are often difficult to distinguish. Retroperitoneal lymph nodes lie behind the mesenteric vessels along the aorta and the inferior vena cava, whereas intraperitoneal nodes are located anterior to the mesenteric vessels or in the right mid- and lower abdomen, corresponding to the course of the mesentery. They may displace bowel loops, and bowel loops can mimic lymph nodes; usually these structures can be differentiated by noting the presence or absence of peristaltic motion. Peripancreatic lymph nodes are retroperitoneal and may be mistaken for a pancreatic tumor. Scalloped pancreatic margins are more consistent with lymphadenopathy than with a pancreatic tumor.

A knowledge of history and clinical findings is essential for the correct interpretation of sonographic findings. Acute lymphadenitis is painful, typically unilateral, and develops within 1−2 days. An infected lateral neck cyst can mimic lymphadenitis. If the inflammation is not definite, other lesions must be considered (dermoid cyst, hematoma, hemangiolymphangiomatous malformation, neoplasia); usually this necessitates a cytologic or histologic workup. The lymph nodes in acute lymphatic leukemia are frequently painful due to their rapid enlargement. Lymph nodes involved by malignant lymphoma generally are nonpainful and enlarge over a period of days to weeks. A Hodgkin lymphoma may be preceded by chronic, histologically nonspecific lymphadenopathy. Non-Hodgkin lymphomas frequently take a fulminating course and, when located intra-/abdominally, may present clinically as acute abdomen.

Computed tomography and magnetic resonance imaging can be useful adjuncts. Both are often superior to ultrasound in their ability to demonstrate mesenteric and iliac lymph nodes and the infiltration of adjacent structures in cases of extensive peripheral lymphadenopathy. Even computed tomography, however, cannot distinguish between benign and malignant causes of lymph node enlargement. Perhaps magnetic resonance imaging will occasionally advance diagnostic accuracy.

References

Beyer, D., P. E. Peters: Real-time ultrasonography – an efficient screening method for abdominal and pelvic lymphadenopathy. Lymphology 13 (1980) 142–149

Kraus, R., B. K. Han, D. S. Babcock, A. E. Oestreich: Sonography of neck masses in children. Amer. J. Roentgenol. 146 (1986) 609–613

Powell, R. W., A. L. Lightsey, W. J. Thomas, W. L. Marsh: Castleman's disease in children. J. pediat. Surg. 21 (1986) 678–682

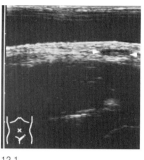 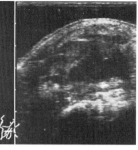

12.1   12.2

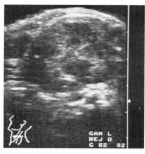 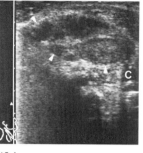

12.3   12.4

12.1 Normal lymph node (▲), of an 11-year old boy; left oblique inguinal scan.

12.2 Cervical lymphadenitis (clinical) in a 16-month-old boy with a firm, immobile swelling of acute onset on the left side of the neck. Swelling subsided rapidly with antibiotic treatment. Left transverse cervical scan: ill-defined mass of mixed echogenicity. US diagnosis: lymphadenopathy of unknown cause. **DD:** other mass lesion.

12.3 Malignant proliferating tumor in a 6-month-old boy with a left cervical swelling of acute onset. Left transverse cervical scan: mass of heterogeneous echogenicity composed of nodular elements. US diagnosis: lymphadenopathy, inflammatory or neoplastic. **DD:** other mass lesion. Histology: malignant, undifferentiated, highly proliferative tumor, nonclassifiable.

12.4 Cervical lymphadenitis (clinical) in a 4-year-old boy with a 4-day history of fever and neck swelling on the right side. Right oblique cervical scan: multiple nodular, partially confluent lesions with heterogeneous echo structure. C = Carotid artery, ▲ = lymph nodes. US diagnosis: lymphadenopathy of unknown cause. Possible lymphadenitis.

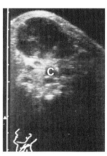 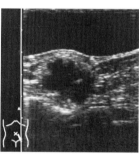

12.5   12.6

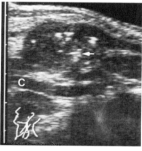

12.7

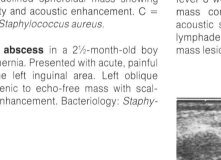

12.5 Lymphadenitis with abscess in a 6-month-old girl, HIV-positive, with a left-sided neck swelling of acute onset. Left oblique cervical scan: well-defined spheroidal mass showing very low internal echogenicity and acoustic enhancement. C = Carotid artery. Bacteriology: *Staphylococcus aureus*.

12.6 Lymphadenitis with abscess in a 2½-month-old boy with a history of left inguinal hernia. Presented with acute, painful swelling and redness in the left inguinal area. Left oblique inguinal scan: a hypoechogenic to echo-free mass with scalloped borders. No acoustic enhancement. Bacteriology: *Staphylococcus aureus*.

12.7 Lymphadenitis (clinical) in a 5½-year-old girl with a persistent swelling on the left side of the neck following scarlet fever 8 weeks before. Left longitudinal scan: well-defined solid mass containing some intensely echogenic elements with acoustic shadows (arrow). C = Carotid artery. US diagnosis: lymphadenopathy. Possibly chronic lymphadenitis. **DD:** other mass lesion.

12.8 Infectious mononucleosis (clinical) in a 13½-year-old girl with painful swelling of acute onset in the left submandibular, cervical, and supraclavicular areas, with subsequent involvement of the right side. **a** Left transverse and **b** longitudinal cervical scans: multiple nodular, solid, relatively hypoechogenic lesions. C = carotid artery, J = jugular vein. US diagnosis: lymphadenopathy of unknown cause. **DD:** inflammatory, neoplastic.

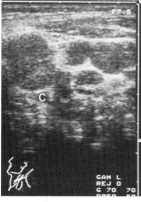 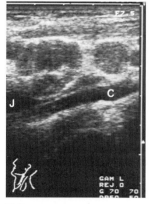

12.8a   12.8b

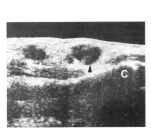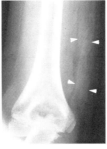

12.9a   12.9b

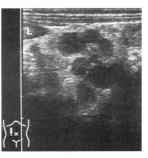

12.10

12.9 Cat-scratch disease in a 12½-year-old boy with nontender swelling on the right upper arm of 3 weeks' duration. **a** Longitudinal scan of the mediodistal portion of the right upper arm: 2 subcutaneous, hypoechogenic to anechogenic nodular lesions (▲). C = Medial condyle of the humerus. **b** AP radiograph of the right humerus shows 2 nodular soft-tissue densities (▲) corresponding to US findings. US diagnosis: lymphadenitis with abscess. Histology: cat-stratch disease.

12.10 Yersinia infection in a 5-year-old boy with unexplained appendicitis-like abdominal pain. Elevated ESR and white blood cell count. Longitudinal right midabdominal scan: multiple nodular, well-defined hypoechogenic lesions. L = Liver. US diagnosis: mesenteric lymphadenitis. Serology: *Yersinia* infection.

12.11 Benign lymphoma in a 12-year-old boy with a long history fo refractory iron deficiency anemia and a 2-month history of fatique and abdominal pain. Palpable nontender mass in the right midabdomen. **a** Transverse and **b** longitudinal scans: rounded, well-marginated, solid mass in the right midabdomen containing hypoechogenic areas with acoustic shadows (arrows). WS = Spinal column. US diagnosis: perityphlitic abscess. Histology: benign Castleman lymphoma.

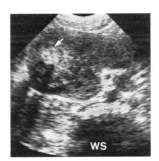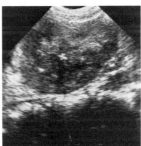

12.11a   12.11b

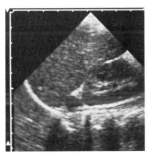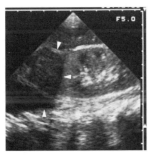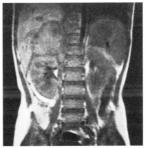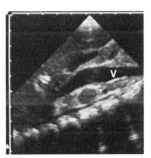

12.12a   12.12b   12.12c   12.12d

12.12 Suprarenal BCG abscess in a 2½-year-old girl (adopted from Sri Lanka). Lymphadenitis with abscess in the left supraclavicular area after BCG inoculation with subsequent right inguinal involvement. Right flank scan: **a** small hypoechogenic suprarenal mass, no lymphadenopathy; **b** 6 months later, a large heterogeneous, partly cystic suprarenal mass (▲) compressing

the upper pole of the right kidney. **c** T1-weighted MR image: right-sided suprarenal tumor. **d** Longitudinal scan of the right upper abdomen: retrocaval lymphadenopathy. V = Inferior vena cava. US diagnosis: suprarenal BCG abscess with retroperitoneal lymphadenopathy, confirmed operatively and by culture.

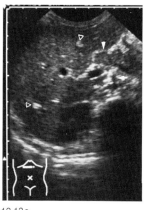
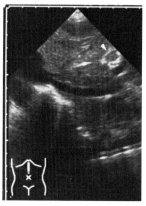

12.13a   12.13b

12.13 Septic granulomatosis in a 3-year-old boy with a history of hepatic abscesses. **a** Upper abdominal transverse and **b** midsagittal scans: lymph nodes (▲) anterior to the celiac trunk (←). △ = Hepatic granulomas.

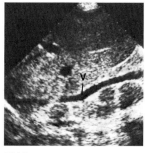
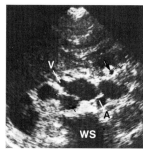
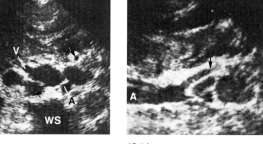
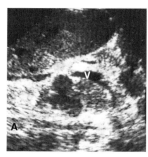

12.14a   12.14b   12.14c   12.14d

12.14 Hypo-IgA gammaglobulinemia in a 13-year-old boy with generalized peripheral lymphadenopathy, histologically nonspecific, benign. Acute, severe abdominal pain. Upper midabdominal US: **a** longitudinal scan: retrocaval lymph nodes. V = Inferior vena cava. **b** Transverse scan: lymph nodes between the inferior vena cava (V), aorta (A), and spine (WS).

The arrow points to the superior mesenteric artery (SMA). **c** Longitudinal scan shows elevation of the SMA by enlarged lymph nodes. **d** Coronal right flank scan shows interaortocaval nodes. US diagnosis: lymphadenopathy of unknown cause. Course with prednisone therapy: marked decrease in node size, no subjective complaints.

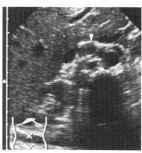
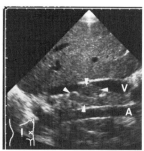
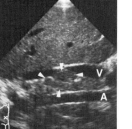

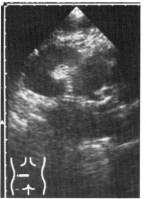
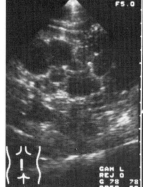

12.15a   12.15b   12.15c   12.15d

12.15 Follicular hyperplasia in a 13-year-old boy with immune deficiency of unknown etiology. **a** Transverse upper abdominal and **b** right coronal scans: retrocrural (←) and interaortocaval (▲)

lymph nodes. V = Inferior vena cava. **c** Transverse and **d** longitudinal left posterior paravertebral scans: retroperitoneal nodes projecting into the renal hilum.

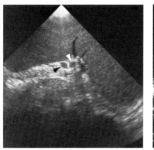
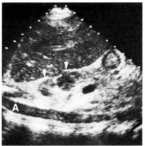

12.16   12.17a

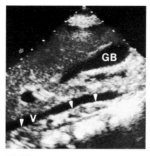
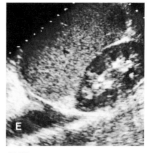

12.17b   12.17c

12.16 Acute lymphatic leukemia in a 15-year-old boy. Transverse left flank scan: massive splenomegaly with lymphadenopathy (▲) in the splenic hilum.

12.17 B lymphoma in a 12-year-old boy with acute abdominal pain, fever, general malaise. Laparotomy done for suspected perforative appendicitis; appendix appeared normal. Massive ascites. Lymph node biopsy: sinus histiocytosis. **a** Longitudinal

upper abdominal scan: lymph nodes (▲) between the aorta and the lower hepatic border. **b, c** Right flank scan: retrocaval lymph nodes (▲). V = Inferior vena cava, GB = gallbladder, E = pleural effusion. US diagnosis: lymphadenopathy of unknown cause, with massive ascites (see Fig. 11.**8**). Cytology of the pleural exudate 11 days after appendectomy: B lymphoma. Death occurred 9 hours later.

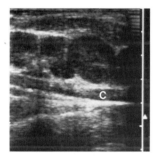
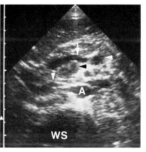

12.18   12.19a

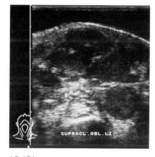
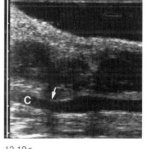

12.19b   12.19c

12.18 T-cell lymphoma in a 10½-year-old girl with progressive swelling on the left side of the neck for 1 week. Left longitudinal cervical scan: multiple nodular, solid, hypoechogenic lesions. C = Carotid artery. US diagnosis: malignant lymphoma suspected. Histology: T-cell lymphoma.

12.19 Malignant lymphoma in an 11½-year-old boy with intermittent fever and progressive lymph node swelling—first of the inguinal nodes, then of the axillary, cervical, and supraclavicular nodes on both sides. Three lymph node biopsies:

nonspecific. **a** Transverse upper abdominal scan: peripancreatic lymphadenopathy (▲). A = Aorta, WS = spinal column, arrow points to the splenic vein. **b** Left oblique supraclavicular scan: multiple hypoechogenic lymphomas. **c** Left longitudinal cervical scan: displacement (arrow) of the carotid artery (C) by the lymphomas. Rapid decrease in the node size with therapy, increase in the node echogenicity. US diagnosis: malignant lymphoma suspected. Histology: malignant lymphoma, probably T-cell (four lymph node biopsy, 3 months after the onset of the disease).

12.20 Hodgkin lymphoma in a 14-year-old boy with a 5-week history of progressive, nonpainful swelling on the left side of the neck. **a** Left longitudinal cervical scan: multiple nodular, hypoechogenic lesions arranged in a chainlike pattern. C = Carotid artery. **b** Transverse midcervical scan: lymph nodes (▲) impinge on the left thyroid lobe (T). C = Carotid artery. US diagnosis: malignant lymphoma suspected. Histology: Hodgkin lymphoma.

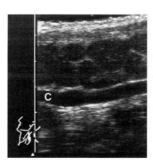
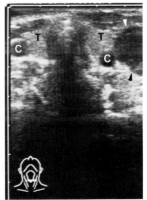

12.20a   12.20b

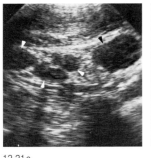
12.21a

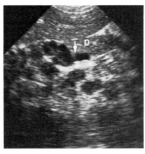
12.21b

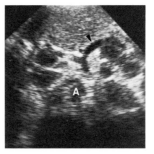
12.21c

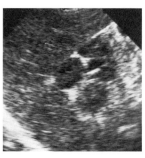
12.21d

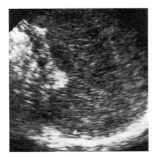
12.21e

12.21 Hodgkin lymphoma in a 13½-year-old boy with a 6-month history of progressive, nonpainful, bilateral swellings in the axillary, cervical and supraclavicular areas. **a** Right longitudinal axillary scan: lymphomas of varying size (▲). **b, c** Transverse upper abdominal scan: multiple lymph nodes of diverse size in the peripancreatic area and about the celiac trunk. Arrow points of the portal vein, P = pancreas, A = aorta. **d** Longitudinal left flank scan: lymphomas in the splenic hilum. **e** Transverse left flank scan: diffuse splenic infiltration (coarsening of the echo pattern). US diagnosis: malignant lymphoma. Histology: Hodgkin lymphoma.

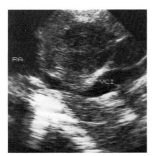
12.22a

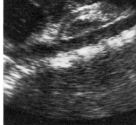
12.22b

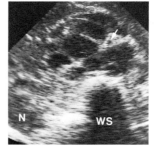
12.22c

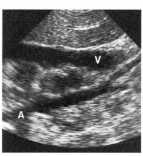
12.22d

12.22 Recurrence of a Hodgkin lymphoma in a 21-year-old man with increasing back pain 11 years after diagnosis. **a** Midsagittal upper abdominal scan: large precaval lymphomas compressing and displacing the inferior vena cava (VCI). RA = Right atrium. **b** Midsagittal and **c** transverse upper abdominal scans: lymphomas surrounding the superior mesenteric artery (arrow). WS = Spinal column, N = kidney. **d** Right coronal scan: interaortocaval lymphomas. A = Aorta, V = inferior vena cava. US diagnosis: recurrent Hodgkin lymphoma (confirmed).

13 Normal Kidney and Its Variants

R. D. Schulz

A special chapter is devoted to sonographic variants of renal anatomy, for the kidney may present more variations than any other parenchymatous organ (Table 13.1). The kidneys are subject to many disturbances during embryonic development which can affect their number, size, structure, position, and vascular supply. Approximately 10% of all kidneys exhibit some type of variation, so it is not uncommon to encounter such variants on sonograms. With the new high-resolution, real-time scanners and careful technique, almost all of these variants can be recognized. The less experienced examiner who is unfamiliar with the protean appearance of the normal kidney is apt to suspect an abnormality (e.g., mistake hypertrophic columns of Bertin for a tumor) and perhaps recommend unnecessary studies (intravenous urography, voiding cystourethrography, computed tomography, renal scintigraphy). As a rule, further radiologic studies are warranted only if the normal variant coexists with a truly pathologic finding (e.g, hydronephrosis of one pole in renal duplication or a duplex kidney with a ureterocele). This has led to the less frequent and more selective use of other imaging procedures.

Both kidneys can be sonographically examined from the flank or back; the right kidney can also be scanned transhepatically from the front. The flank scan is usually sufficient; a posterior scan may be needed if the lower renal pole is obscured by shadows from the overlying bowel. When the lesser pelvis is examined, the bladder should be moderately distended to provide an acoustic window so that a pelvic kidney can be recognized.

The renal sinus echo (central echo complex) is formed by the pyelocaliceal system and by peripelvic fibrofatty tissue. The sinus echo has a nonhomogeneous echo pattern and the shape of a flattened ellipse. In premature and young infants, there is not yet enough peripelvic fibrofatty tissue present to produce a visible sinus echo.

While the renal parenchyma is less echogenic than the hepatic parenchyma by about the 4th month of life, the kidney of the preterm infant is more echogenicity than the liver, and the neonatal kidney is approximately isoechogenic to the liver. The perirenal fat is not yet sufficiently developed in infants and small children to be sonographically visible. The renal fascia and fibrous capsule (Gerota fascia) are directly apposed, and the kidney is in very close proximity to the liver.

A hypermobile kidney is best examined in the upright patient by measuring the renal excursion during inspiration and expiration. Some of these normal variants have potential clinical significance due to associated complications such as urinary tract infection, urinary stasis, or lithiasis.

References

Carter, A. R., J. G. Horgan, T. A. Jennings, A. T. Rosenfield: Junctional parenchymal defect: sonographic variant of renal anatomy. Radiology 154 (1985) 499–502

Goodman, J. D., K. I. Norton, L. Carr, H. C. Yeh: Crossed fused renal ectopia: sonographic diagnosis. Urol. Radiol. 8 (1986) 13–16

Han, B. K., D. S. Babcock: Sonographic measurements and appearance of normal Kidneys in children. Amer. J. Radiol. 145 (1985) 611–616

Hayden, J. R., L. E. Swischuk: Pediatric Ultrasonography. Williams & Wilkins, Baltimore 1987

Hricak, H., T. L. Slovis, C. W. Callen, R. N. Romanski: Neonatal kidneys: sonographic-anatomic correlation. Radiology 147 (1983) 699–702

Kissane, J. M.: Congenital malformations. In Heptinstall, R. H.: Pathology of the Kidney. Little, Brown, Boston/Ma. 1974

Lafortune, M., A. Constantin, G. Breton, G. Vallee: Sonography of the hypertrophied column of Bertin. Amer. J. Radiol. 146 (1986) 53–56

Leekam, R. N., M. A. Matzinger, M. Brunelle, R. R. Gray, H. Grosman: Sonography of renal columnar hypertrophy. J. clin. Ultrasound 11 (1984) 491–494

McCarthy, S., A. T. Rosenfield: Ultrasonography in crossed renal ectopia. J. Ultrasound Med. 3 (1984) 107–112

Mildenberger, H.: Die Doppelniere im Kindesalter. Hippokrates, Stuttgart 1982

Trappe, B. O., L. von Rohden, F. Kleinhans, H. Handel, C. Nahrendorf, H. Koditz: Die Nierensonographie im Kindesalter. Normalbefunde. Z. Urol. Nephrol. 78 (1985) 641–647

Table 13.1 Normal variants of the kidney

Hyperechogenic kidney in preterm infant	Fetal lobation
Neonatal kidney with sinus echo	Neonatal kidney without sinus echo
Dendritic caliceal system	Ampullary caliceal system
Transition-form caliceal system	Splenic hump indenting left kidney
Cortical notch	Pseudotumor (hypertrophic columns of Bertin)
Renal hilum lip	Parenchymal nose
Incomplete duplication	Complete duplication
Triple kidney	Renal agenesis (aplasia)
Hypoplasia	Horseshoe kidney
Cake kidney	Intrathoracic kidney
Pelvic kidney	Crossed ectopia with fusion
Crossed ectopia without fusion	Ptotic or hypermobile kidney
Nonrotation (malrotation)	

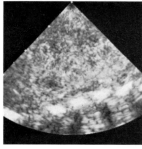
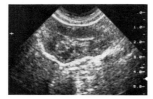

13.1

13.2

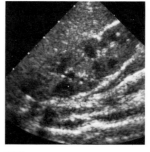
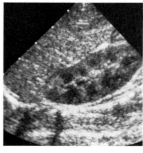

13.3

13.4

13.1 Kidney of a preterm infant of 27 weeks' gestation. Longitudinal right flank scan: hypoechogenic renal cortex and somewhat prominent, less echogenic medullary pyramids, which are approximately isoechogenic to the liver.

13.2 Infant kidney, aged 4 weeks. Posterior longitudinal scan of the right kidney: the renal cortex is isoechogenic to the adjacent liver parenchyma. The renal sinus is not visible.

13.3 Infant kidney with fetal lobation, aged 3 months. Right flank longitudinal scan shows a wavy renal contour: fetal lobation, with hypoechogenic medullary pyramids arranged concentrically about the renal sinus. Cortical echogenicity is decreased relative to the liver. Normal finding. Fetal lobation may persist into adulthood.

13.4 Infant kidney, aged 3 months. Right flank longitudinal scan: decreased echogenicity relative to the liver. Prominent hypoechogenic pyramids. *Caution:* no renal cysts, no fetal lobation.

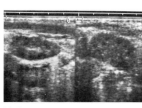
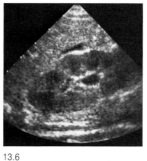

13.5

13.6

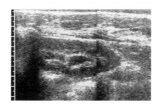

13.7

13.5 Infant kidney, aged 1 month. Right and left posterior longitudinal scans: a narrow, echogenic sinus is already visible on the right side. On the left there is no differentiation, between the parenchyma and sinus.

13.6 Infant kidney with fetal lobation, aged 4 months. Right flank longitudinal scan: marked lobation (scalloped renal contour) and a less echogenic renal cortex; normal sinus echo.

13.7 Infant kidney, 15-day-old girl. Posterior longitudinal scan: narrow anechogenic areas at the center of the sinus echo: ampullary collecting system. **DD:** vesicoureteral reflux, functional obstruction by a distended urinary bladder. Inspect urinary bladder.

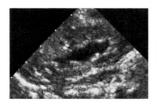
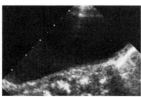

13.8a

13.8b

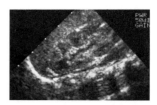

13.8c

13.8 Infant kidney, aged 4 days. **a** Right flank longitudinal scan: mildly distended, anechogenic renal pelvis: normal variant? **DD:** ampullary collecting system, distal ureteral stenosis, vesicoureteral reflux, functional obstruction by a distended bladder, increased postpartum diuresis. **b** Anterior longitudinal scan of the lower midabdomen: large urinary bladder whose fundus extends to the umbilicus; indicates widening of the renal pelvis due to a full bladder. **c** Right flank longitudinal scan at 10 days: no dilatation of the renal pelvis. The dilatation initially seen was most likely due to increased postpartum diuresis and bladder distention.

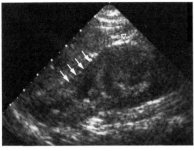

13.9

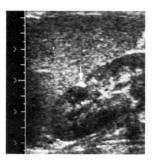

13.10

13.9 Splenic hump and renal indentation in a 6-year-old girl. Left flank longitudinal scan: curved indentation in the cranial part of the lateral border of the left kidney (←) with an associated bulging of parenchyma at the renal center (△): splenic hump impressing on the left kidney.

13.10 Renal notch in a 10-year-old boy. Right flank longitudinal scan: coarse, triangular echo at the lateral renal border at the junction of the upper and middle thirds (arrow): the renal notch, a common finding on the lateral margin is a vestige of incomplete fusion. Should not be confused with a pyelonephrotic scar.

13.11 Hypertrophic columns of Bertin in a 10-year-old boy. Posterior longitudinal scan: 1-cm, round, central "mass" arising from posterior side of the kidney (arrow) and projecting into the sinus.

13.12 Renal hilum lip in a 10-year-old boy. Transverse scan of the right upper abdomen: medial projection of parenchyma at the hilum: renal hilum lip (arrow). L = Liver, N = kidney, Ar = renal artery, WS = spinal column.

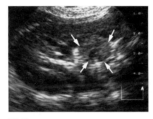
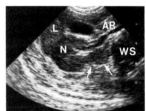

13.11   13.12

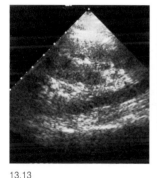
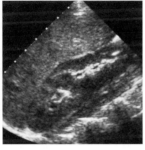

13.13   13.14a

13.13 Incomplete duplication in an 8-year-old girl. Posterior longitudinal paravertebral scan: "nose" of the parenchyma projects from the posterior side into the renal sinus: incomplete duplication of the collecting system.

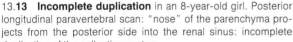

13.14b   13.14c

13.14 Duplex kidney in a 7-year-old boy. **a** Right flank longitudinal scan: parenchymal bridge completely divides the renal sinus: duplex kidney with a smaller upper and larger lower pole. **b** Transverse scan of the right upper abdomen: hypoechogenic subhepatic area at the site of the parenchymal bridge, where the echogenic renal hilum or renal sinus would normally occur. Second scan for suspected duplication: series of transverse sections proceeding from the anterior or posterior side. **c** Posterior longitudinal paravertebral scan (third scan for suspected duplication): continuous parenchymal bridge extends forward from the posterior side.

13.15 Suspected unilateral renal agenesis in a 9-year-old boy. **a** Posterior longitudinal left paravertebral scan: absence of renal tissue in the left fossa, consistent with agenesis. Examination had to be extended to check for a dystopic kidney or crossed ectopia; a second kidney was not found. Associated genital anomalies are present in 30% of cases. **b** Right posterior longitudinal scan: slightly enlarged, normal-appearing right kidney. Agenesis in newborns is signaled by the presence of large, prominent adrenals.

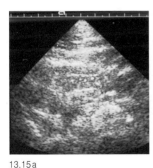
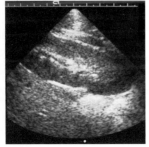

13.15a   13.15b

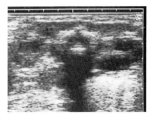
13.16a

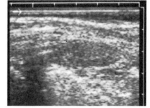
13.16b

13.16 Renal hypoplasia in a newborn boy. **a** Posterior transverse scan: small, echogenic left kidney and normal-sized, less echogenic right kidney: left-sided hypoplasia. **b** Left posterior longitudinal paravertebral scan: small, oval, echogenic left kidney without corticomedullary differentiation. Hypoplastic kidneys can be difficult to identify because they are often very echogenic. Congenital hypoplasia is probably secondary to an intrauterine vascular insult.

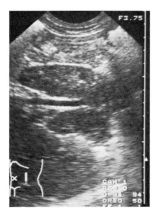
13.17

13.17 Horseshoe kidney in a 10-month-old boy. Left coronal scan: both hypoechogenic kidneys are imaged concurrently in the longitudinal view. The linear sonolucency between the kidneys is the aorta, covered caudally by a wide parenchymal isthmus connecting both lower poles: horseshoe kidney. The most common type of fusion anomaly, often associated with an atypical course of the vessels and ureters.

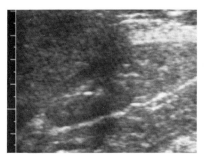
13.18a

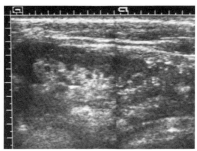
13.18b

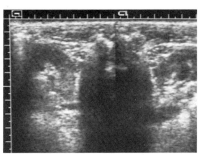
13.18c

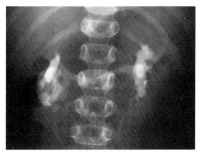
13.18d

13.18 Nonrotation and horseshoe kidney in an 8-year-old girl. **a** Right flank longitudinal scan on the standard plane: very narrow kidney with no sinus echo: nonrotation. Same on the left. **b** Posterior longitudinal left paravertebral scan: narrow kidney with no anterior parenchyma, "open sinus," renal axis almost parallel to the body surface: malrotation. Analogous scan on the right side showed the same finding. **c** Posterior transverse scan at the L3 level: renal hila point anteriorly instead of medially: bilateral nonrotation. Transverse scan from the front showed a parenchymal isthmus over the spine: horseshoe kidney. **d** EU: horseshoe kidney with bilateral malrotation; renal axes, normally divergent, are parallel to the spine. If the isthmus consists of fibrous tissue, it can seldom be directly visualized with US. An upper midabdominal scan will sometimes show a curved mass overlying the spine. An attempt should then be made to exclude horseshoe kidney before voicing suspicion of tumor.

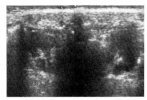
13.19a

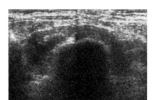
13.19b

13.19 Horseshoe kidney in an 8-year-old boy. **a** Posterior transverse scan shows rotation of both renal axes, with the hila anterior: nonrotation. Horseshoe kidney suspected. **b** Transverse midabdominal scan: uniform, hypoechogenic band curving from right to left in front of the spine: isthmus connecting the lower renal poles: horseshoe kidney.

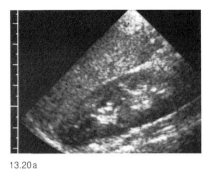

13.20a

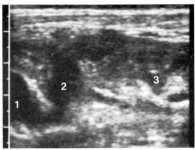

13.20b

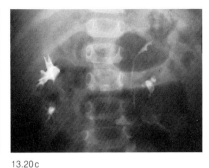

13.20c

13.20 Duplex and triple kidney in a 2½-year-old girl. **a** Left flank scan shows presence of a parenchymal bridge: left duplex kidney. **b** Right flank coronal scan: three separate, adjacent collection systems, each with a ureter: right triple kidney. Upper moiety shows hydronephrotic dilatation. Right ureterocele. **c** EU confirms duplex kidney on the left and triple kidney on the right. Upper pole on the right obstructed by a ureterocele, accounting for the faint opacification of the upper collecting system.

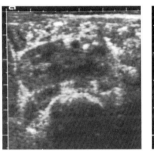

13.21

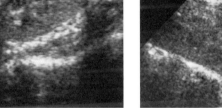

13.22a

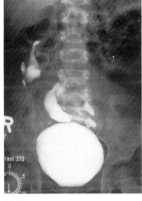

13.22b

13.22c

13.21 Lumbosacral dystopia in a 6-month-old boy. Transverse lower abdominal scan: right kidney anterior to the spine and great abdominal vessels. Normal corticomedullary differentiation, no obstruction.

13.22 Nonrotation in a 5-year-old girl. **a** Right flank longitudinal scan: malrotated right kidney lying against the psoas muscle.

A sinus echo is not visible on this section. Nonrotation of the right kidney. Left renal bed is empty. **b** Oblique lumbosacral scan through the lower midabdomen: hypoechogenic unobstructed left kidney, partly lumbar with the lower pole projecting into the lesser pelvis. Crossed ectopia. **c** 15-minute EU: nonrotated right kidney, lumbosacral left kidney with the collecting system directed craniolaterally.

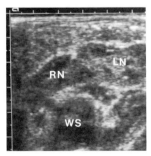

13.23

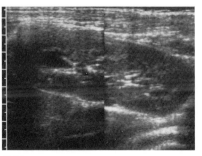

13.24

13.23 Renal dystopia in a 6-day-old neonate. Transverse upper abdominal scan: obliquely oriented right kidney (RN) in front of the spinal column (WS) and, directly adjacent, transversely oriented left kidney (LN). Renal dystopia, possibly with fusion. When malrotation is present, the renal hilum may lie anteriorly, laterally in rare cases, or even posteriorly in very rare cases.

13.24 Megacalix in an 11-year-old boy. Posterior longitudinal left paravertebral scan: normal left renal size and contour. Pear-shaped anechogenic area in the upper part of the sinus: large single calix. Confirmed by radiography.

14 Renal Abnormalities

I. Forster

Sonographic patterns

Alteration of size:
- Large kidney(s),
- Small kidney(s).

Alteration of echo structure:
- Increased echogenicity of the cortex (local/diffuse)
- Decreased echogenicity of the cortex (local/diffuse)
- Increased echogenicity of the renal pyramids
- Corticomedullary differentiation: accentuated, decreased, lost, reversed
- Cysts: number (solitary/multiple), size, location.

Large kidneys (Table 14.1) have a bulky appearance. The renal parenchyma is swollen. There is loss of definition of the central sinus echo complex.

Increased echogenicity of the renal pyramids (Table 14.2) is seen with medullary tubular ectasia, deposits of certain substances such as calcium, urates, or proteins. Increased echogenicity of the renal cortex (Table 14.3) if of heterogeneous origin and may affect any or all of the four constituents of the kidney: glomeruli, tubules, interstitium, and vessels. Compared with the diversity of possible histologic changes, the sonographic features are nonspecific and not indicative of the type of pathologic involvement nor do they correlate with the severity of the disease. Decreased renal cortical echogenicity is a less common finding (pyelonephritis, phlegmons, abscess; leukemia, lymphoma).

Key elements in the differential diagnosis are: the age of the child, the history, the clinical presentation, and a knowledge of the natural history of the various renal disorders.

Oligohydramnios can result from fetal obstructive uropathies, renal agenesis, renal hypoplasia, renal dysplasia, or polycystic renal disease. Renal disorders in neonates are most frequently secondary to renal vascular disease (renal vein thrombosis, acute tubular necrosis, acute cortical necrosis). Nephrosis, nephritis,

Table 14.1 Bilateral renal enlargement

Duplication
Obstruction
Nephritis
Nephrosis
Cystic abnormality
- polycystic kidney disease, autosomal recessive/dominant
- glomerulocystic kidney disease
- medullary sponge kidney
- other cystic changes
Tumor
- benign: hamartoma
- malignant: nephroblastoma (Wilms), other malignant tumors
Infiltration
- leukemia
- lymphoma
Volume overload
Mononucleosis
Toxic shock syndrome
Acquired immune deficiency syndrome (AIDS)
Kawasaki syndrome
Renal vein thrombosis
Schönlein–Henoch purpura
Biliary atresia
Fetal visceromegaly (Beckwith–Wiedemann)
Bartter syndrome
Lipoatrophic diabetes
Hereditary tyrosinosis
Type I glycogen storage disease (van Gierke)
Sickle cell glomerulopathy

Table 14.2 Increased echogenicity of the renal pyramids

Nephrocalcinosis: idiopathic, iatrogenic (Lasix [furosemid], vitamin D), immunobilization, hyperoxaluria, renal tubular acidosis, hyperparathyroidism, Cushing syndrome, Bartter syndrome
Cystic renal disease: polycystic kidneys, recessive; medullary sponge kidney
Tamm–Horsfall proteinuria
Congenital nephrotic syndrome (Finnish type)
Sickle cell anemia
Papillary necrosis

Table 14.3 Increased renal cortical echogenicity

Dysplasia
End-stage renal disease
Nephritis
Nephrosis
Polycystic kidney disease (recessive/dominant)
Glomerulocystic kidney disease
Nephronophthisis
Renal vein thrombosis
Acute tubular necrosis
Shock kidney
Hemolytic–uremic syndrome
Kawasaki's syndrome
Schönlein–Henoch purpura
Acquired immune deficiency syndrome (AIDS)
Type I glycogen storage disease (van Gierke)
Hereditary tyrosinosis
Amyloidosis
Nephrocalcinosis
Hyperoxaluria
Alport syndrome
Bartter syndrome
Fetal visceromegaly (Beckwith–Wiedemann)
Biliary atresia
Sickle cell glomerulopathy

Table 14.**4**   Polycystic kidney diseases in newborns (after Worthington)

	Unilateral	Bilateral	Size	Macro-cysts	Cortex	Cortico-medullary differentiation	Inheritance
Polycystic kidney disease autosomal recessive	−	+	Large	(+)	Hyper-echogenic	Lost or reversed	Recessive
Polycystic kidney disease autosomal dominant	+	+	Variable	+	hyper-echogenic	Lost	Dominant
Glomerulocystic kidney disease	−	+	Variable	+	hyper-echogenic	Lost	?

and hemolytic−uremic syndrome are predominantly diseases of preschool and school-age children.

Some disorders, such as polycystic renal disease and hemolytic−uremic syndrome, can present with different sonographic patterns (Tables 14.**4**, 14.**5**). In other conditions the sonographic features depend on the stage of the disease (Finnish-type congenital nephrotic syndrome, nephronophthisis; Table 14.**6**) or on the intensity and duration of the injurious process (shock kidney, renal vein thrombosis, nephrotoxic agents). Sonography may initially show normal kidneys in renal arterial thrombosis, in hemolytic−uremic syndrome of the arterial thrombotic microangiopathic type, and in lipoid nephrosis.

Medical renal disorders most frequently present with a nonspecific increased echogenicity of the renal cortex or pyramids. Exceptions are the terminal stage of nephronophthisis, the hemolytic−uremic syndrome of the glomerular thrombotic microangiopathic type, and in polycystic renal diseases, where a relatively characteristic pattern may be seen.

References

Avni, E. F., H. Szliwowski, M. Spehl, B. Lelong, P. Baudain, J. Struyven: L'atteinte rénale dans la sclérose tubéreuse de Bourneville. Ann. Radiol. 27 (1984) 207–214

Brenbridge, A. N., R. L. Chevalier, D. L. Kaiser: Increased renal cortical echogenicity in pediatric renal disease: histopathologic correlations. J. clin. Ultrasound 14 (1986) 595–600

Garel, L. A., R. Habib, C. Babin, D. Lallemand, J. Sauvegrain, M. Broyer: Syndrome hémolytique et urémique. Valeur diagnostique et prognostique de l'échographie. Ann. Radiol. 26 (1983) 169–174

Garel, L. A., R. Habib, D. Pariente, M. Broyer, J. Sauvegrain: Juvenile nephronophthisis: sonographic appearance in children with severe uremia. Radiology 151 (1984) 93–95

Gray, D. L., J. P. Crane: Prenatal diagnosis of urinary tract malformation. Pediat. Nephrol. 2 (1988) 326–333

Leumann, E. P.: Primary hyperoxaluria: an important cause of renal failure in infancy. Int. J. pediat. Nephrol. 6 (1985) 13–16

Worthington, J. L., G. D. Shackelford, B. R. Cole, E. D. Tack, J. M. Kissane: Sonographically detectable cysts in polycystic kidney disease in newborn and joung infants. Pediat. Radiol. 18 (1988) 287–293

Table 14.**5**   Variants of the hemolytic−uremic syndrome (after Garel and Habib)

	Morphology	Sonography
Type I	Glomerular Thrombotic Microangiopathy	Slightly enlarged kidneys Cortex hyperechogenic (compared to the liver) Corticomedullary differentiation preserved
Type II	Arterial Thrombotic Microangiopathy	Normal
Type III	Cortical necrosis (partial/complete)	Spectrum of shock kidney

Table 14.**6**   Nephronophthisis (terminal)

Relatively small kidneys
Sinus preserved
Cortex hyperechogenic
Corticomedullary differentiation lost
Corticomedullary cysts

Bilateral/Unilateral Renal Enlargement

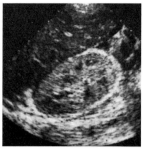 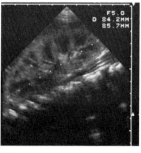 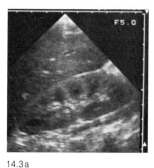 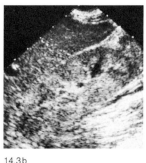

14.1   14.2   14.3a   14.3b

14.**1** **Meningococcal sepsis** in a 1-year-old boy. Right flank longitudinal scan: swollen kidney with a hypoechogenic cortex. The sinus is not visible. Accentuated corticomedullary differentiation. US: shock kidney.

14.**2** **Acute renal failure** after laparotomy for volvulus in malrotation, in a 5-year-old boy, status following omphalocele. **a** Right flank longitudinal scan: nephromegaly, increased cortical echogenicity, prominent renal pyramids, narrow sinus. **b** Scan 8 months later shows normal-sized kidneys with better sinus definition and less prominent papillae. Cortex still hypoechogenic. US: consistent with acute tubular necrosis.

14.**3** **Schönlein–Henoch purpura** in a 7-year-old boy with trisomy 21. Right flank longitudinal scan: nephromegaly, irregular increase of cortical echogenicity. US: glomerulonephritis. Renal biopsy: mesangial proliferative glomerulonephritis.

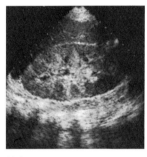 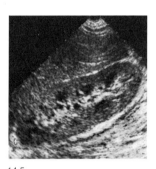 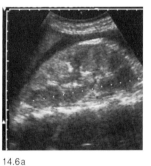 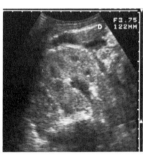

14.4   14.5   14.6a   14.6b

14.**4** **Acute renal failure** in a 10½-year-old boy. Right flank longitudinal scan: large kidney. Cortical hypoechogenicity is greater centrally than peripherally, giving increased corticomedullary contrast. Renal pyramids small due to cortical swelling. US: glomerulonephritis. Histology: membranoproliferative glomerulonephritis (same patient as in Fig. 14.**36**).

14.**5** **Poststreptococcal glomerulonephritis** with acute renal failure in a 12-year-old boy. Right flank longitudinal scan: moderately enlarged kidney with a hypoechogenic cortex. Corticomedullary differentiation is accentuated.

14.**6** **Disseminated lupus erythematosus** in an 11-year-old girl. Right flank **a** longitudinal and **b** transverse scans: large kidney with a hyperechogenic cortex, small renal pyramids, and reduced corticomedullary differentiation. Ascites. US: consistent with glomerulonephritis.

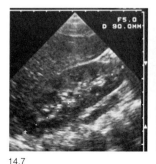 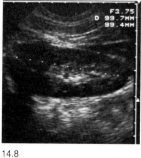

14.7   14.8

14.**7** **Lipoid nephrosis** in a 5-year-old girl. Right flank longitudinal scan: nephromegaly, small sinus. The renal pyramids are well defined. Irregular increase in cortical echogenicity.

14.**8** **Nephrotic syndrome** in a 9-year-old boy, recurrence after Endoxan (cyclophosphamide) therapy. Right posterior longitudinal scan: relatively large, bulky kidney(s) with normal cortical echogenicity. US: consistent with nephrotic syndrome.

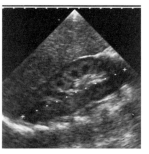 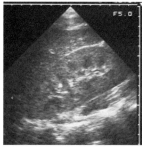

14.9   14.10

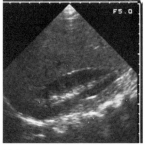 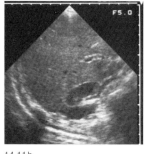

14.11a   14.11b

14.9 Nephrotic syndrome in hereditary spherocytosis in an 6-year-old boy. Right flank longitudinal scan: nephromegaly, cortex hypoechogenic at the periphery, hypoechogenic centrally (perimedullary region). Biopsy: "focal and segmental" glomerulosclerosis.

14.10 Cystinuria in a 19-year-old man with proteinuria and edema, on penicillamine therapy. Right flank longitudinal scan: nephromegaly with voluminous parenchyma and a very small sinus. Hyperechogenic cortex, decreased corticomedullary differentiation (same patient as in Fig. 14.**49**). US: consistent with nephrotic syndrome.

14.11 Type I glycogen storage disease in a 5-year-old boy. No hepatomas. Right flank **a** longitudinal and **b** transverse scans: large kidney, appears small in relation to the greatly enlarged liver. Increased attenuation of the beam by fatty infiltration of the liver makes cortical evaluation difficult; echogenicity presumably normal to slightly increased. The renal pyramids are less well defined.

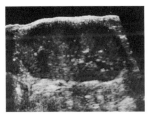 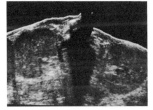

14.12a   14.12b

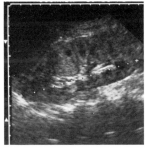 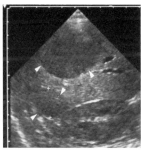

14.13a   14.13b

14.12 Hereditary tyrosinosis in a 4-month-old boy with a growth failure and suspected fructose intolerance. Left posterior **a** longitudinal and **b** transverse scans: large, voluminous kidneys with normal corticomedullary differentiation. **DD:** glycogen storage disease (?), hereditary tyrosinosis (subsequently confirmed; same patient as in Fig. 5.**50**, sister in Fig. 14.**14**).

14.13 Type I glycogen storage disease in a 15-year-old girl. **a** Left flank longitudinal scan: enlarged kidney with a narrow sinus and hyperechogenicity of the perimedullary region. **b** Transverse right upper abdominal scan shows two hypoechogenic hepatomas (▲).

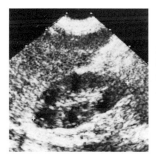 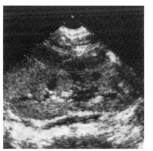

14.14a   14.14b

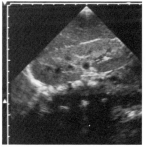 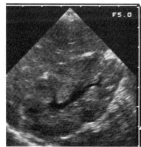

14.15   14.16

14.14 Hereditary tyrosinosis in an 11-day-old girl whose brother died of tyrosinosis (Fig. 14.**12**). Right flank longitudinal scan: **a** normal kidney. **b** Scan at 6 months: nephromegaly with a hypoechogenic renal cortex.

14.15 Lymphohistiocytosis in an 8-year-old girl with hepatosplenomegaly and suspected erythrophagocytosis. **DD:** immune defect. Left flank longitudinal scan: nephromegaly, narrow sinus, hyperechogenic cortex, very small renal pyramids. US: infiltrative process. **DD:** leukemia, lymphoma. Renal biopsy: tubulointerstitial nephritis with lymphocytic infiltration and partial destruction of the tubules.

14.16 Beckwith–Wiedemann syndrome in a 4-day-old girl. Right flank longitudinal scan: nephromegaly, voluminous parenchyma, reduced corticomedullary differentiation. Mild dilatation of the renal pelvis.

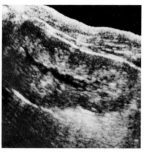
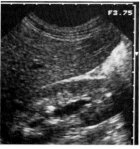
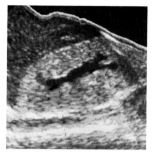
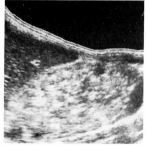

14.17a   14.17b   14.18   14.19

14.17 Bartter syndrome in an 8-year-old boy. **a** Right posterior longitudinal scan: nephromegaly, mild dilatation of the renal pelvis; medullary region hypoechogenic compared to the cortex: nephrocalcinosis? **b** Right flank longitudinal scan 6 years later: calcifications at the tips of some renal pyramids.

14.18 Unexplained dysmorphic syndrome in a 10-day-old boy. Right flank longitudinal scan: nephromegaly with intensely hypoechogenic renal parenchyma, loss of corticomedullary differentiation, mild hydronephrosis. US: polycystic kidney disease?

14.19 Polycystic kidney disease, recessive, in an 17-year-old girl. Right flank longitudinal scan: nephromegaly, intense hypoechogenicity, small peripheral macrocystic lesions.

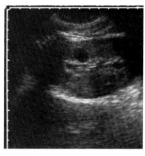
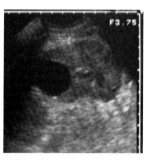

14.20a   14.20b

14.20 Polycystic kidney disease, recessive, in a 19-year-old man with a history of hepatosplenomegaly and esophageal varices at the age of 6. Multiple bilateral renal cysts and nephromegaly 3 years later. **a** Posterior right longitudinal and **b** left posterior transverse scan: voluminous parenchyma, hypoechogenic. There is no corticomedullary differentiation. Macrocysts.

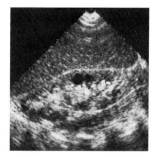
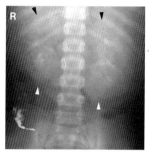
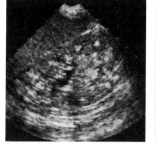
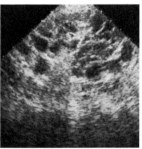

14.21a   14.21b   14.22   14.23

14.21 Polycystic kidney disease, recessive, and congenital hepatic fibrosis in a 10-year-old boy with esophageal varices. **a** Left flank longitudinal scan: nephromegaly, reversal of corticomedullary differentiation, several macrocysts. **b** EU: characteristic correlate. Appendix contrast-filled after gastrography.

14.22 Polycystic kidney disease, recessive, in a 9-month-old girl with recurrent urinary tract infections. Right flank longitudinal scan: massive nephromegaly. Increased echogenicity, accentuated in the medulla. EU showed characteristic tubular ectasia.

14.23 Polycystic kidney disease, recessive, and hepatic fibrosis in an 8-year-old girl (brother in Fig. 14.**24**). Parents: normal kidneys. Left flank longitudinal scan: moderately enlarged, poorly defined hyperechogenic kidney with multiple macrocysts (same patient as in Figs. 5.**41**, 10.**6**, and 14.**60**).

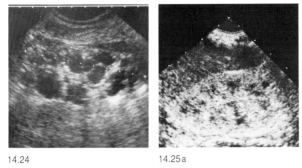

14.24   14.25a

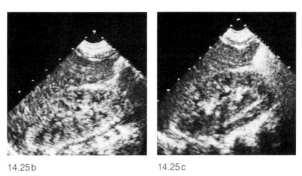

14.25b   14.25c

14.24   Polycystic kidney disease, recessive, in a 15-year-old boy with end-stage renal failure. Right posterior longitudinal scan: poorly defined kidney with multiple large cysts. Liver normal (sister in Figs. 14.**23** and 14.**60**).

14.25   Suspected polycystic kidney disease, dominant, in a 6-week-old boy (brother in Fig. 14.**35**). **a** Right flank longitudinal scan: large kidney. The renal cortex is significantly more echogenic than the adjacent liver parenchyma. **b** At 11 months: cortical hypoechogenicity has decreased. **c** At 18 months: regression of echogenicity and nephromegaly (related to age).

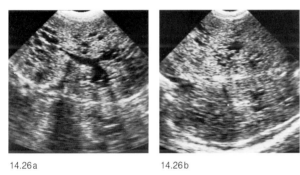

14.26a   14.26b

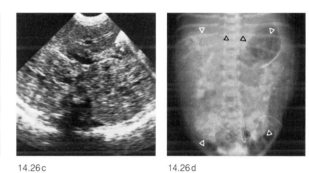

14.26c   14.26d

14.26   Polycystic kidney disease in a 3-day-old girl. **a** Left flank longitudinal, **b** right flank coronal, and **c** transverse upper abdominal scans: greatly enlarged, hyperechogenic kidneys with

numerous macrocysts. **d** EU: classic correlate. US: polycystic kidney disease, presumably dominant (mother: solitary renal cyst; grandmother: hepatic cyst).

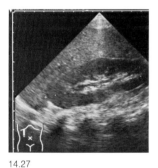

14.27

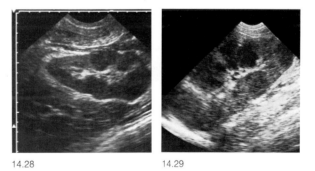

14.28   14.29

14.27   T-cell leukemia in a girl of 10 years, 4 months. Massive pleural effusion. Right flank longitudinal scan: nephromegaly, diffuse regular parenchymal proliferation (bilateral, also ascites and very large solid ovaries). Same patient as in Figs. 3.**28** and 18.**43**. **DD:** leukemia, lymphoma, ovarian tumor, Bone marrow: T-cell leukemia.

14.28   T-cell leukemia in a 14-year-old boy with fast-growing cervical lymphomas. Chest radiograph showed a mediastinal mass. Right posterior longitudinal scan: nephromegaly, irregular parenchymal involvement: knobby contour due to round hypoechogenic lesions. US: lymphoma suspected. Bone marrow: T-cell leukemia.

14.29   T-cell lymphoma in a 10-year-old girl with a mediastinal tumor and bony metastases. Right flank longitudinal scan: nephromegaly with multiple rounded, hypoechogenic lesions.

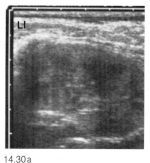
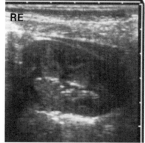

14.30a   14.30b

14.30 Febrile urinary tract infection. a Left posterior longitudinal scan: large, swollen kidney with a hypoechogenic cortex; sinus not defined. **b** Scan on the right shows a normal kidney. US: left pyelonephritis, confirmed.

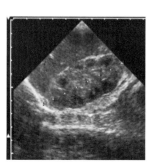
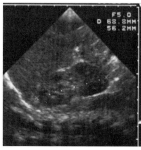
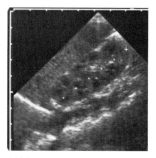

14.31a   14.31b   14.31c

14.31 Echerichia coli sepsis and right-sided nephritis. Right (left) flank longitudinal scan: **a** large kidney with a hyperechogenic cortex, corticomedullary differentiation visible. **b** Left kidney normal. **c** Later scan shows normalization with antibiotic therapy. Right vesicoureteral reflux diagnosed later.

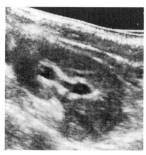
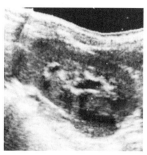
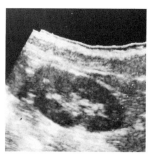

14.32a   14.32b   14.32c

14.32 Renal phlegmons with abscess in a 13-year-old boy with fever and left flank pain. Inflammation? Lithiasis? Posterior longitudinal scan: **a** diffuse renal swelling, anterioinferior parenchymal "tumor," mild hydronephrosis: renal phlegmon suspected. EU: ureteropelvic obstruction. **b** Four days later: abscess formation. Operation on the same day; 20 mL of pus drained from the lower pole parenchyma. **c** Two months later: local scar anteriorly. Remission of hydronephrosis. Normal EU.

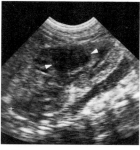
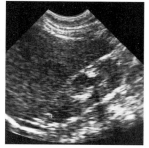

14.33a   14.33b

14.33 Urosepsis in a 4-week-old boy. **a** Right flank longitudinal scan: a relatively large, hyperechogenic kidney with hypoechogenic lesions anterolaterally (▲): pyelonephritis with abscess. **b** Six months later, the renal size is normal. Echogenic scar at the site of the former abscess. Vesicoureteral and massive intrarenal reflux were demonstrated later.

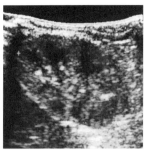 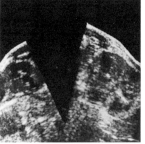

14.34a   14.34b

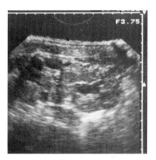

14.35

14.34 Renal vein thrombosis in a 4-day-old boy with gross hematuria and a "mass" in the right renal fossa. Posterior **a** right longitudinal and **b** bilateral transverse scans show a large kidney on the right side with increased cortical echogenicity.

14.35 Solitary left polycystic kidney (dominant) in a 7-year-old boy. Younger brother: bilateral renal enlargement (Fig. 14.**25**); father: left renal cyst. Left posterior longitudinal scan: nephromegaly, hypoechogenic cortex, and multiple macrocysts of varying size.

Bilateral/Unilateral Small Kidney(s)

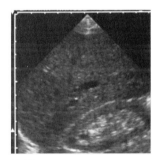

14.36

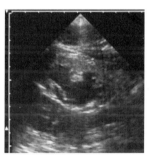 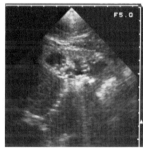

14.37a   14.37b

14.36 End-stage renal failure in chronic membrano-proliferative glomerulonephritis, 14-year-old boy (same patient as in Fig. 14.**4**). Right flank longitudinal scan: small kidney with a hyperechogenic cortex, reduced corticomedullary differentiation, a large sinus.

14.37 Bilateral reflux nephropathy. End-stage renal disease. **a** Left and **b** right posterior longitudinal scans: small kidneys with hyperechogenic cortex, loss of corticomedullary differentiation; moderate hydronephrosis.

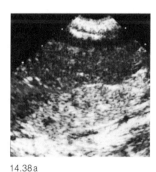 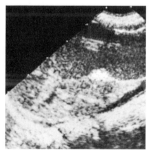

14.38a   14.38b

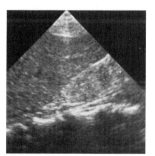

14.39

14.38 Recurrent urinary tract infections, hearing impairment, trisomy 21 in an 11-month-old boy. Creatinine high normal, calcium normal; hyperoxaluria excluded. **a** Right and **b** left flank longitudinal scans: small kidneys. Hyperechogenic cortex, partial reversal of corticomedullary differentiation. **DD:** reflux nephropathy, dysplastic kidneys, the Alport syndrome.

14.39 Suspected primary renal hypoplasia in a girl of 9 years, 4 months with end-stage renal failure. Right flank longitudinal scan: very small kidney(s). Cortex intensely echogenic, loss of corticomedullary differentiation.

Normal-Sized Kidneys

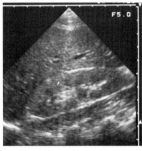 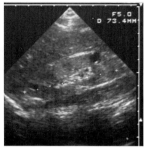 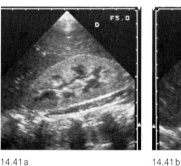 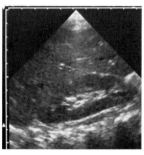

14.40a   14.40b   14.41a   14.41b

14.**40** **Nephronophthisis** in a girl of 11 years, 3 months with salt-losing syndrome and progressive renal failure. Three siblings with nephronophthisis. Right flank longitudinal scan: **a** normal-sized kidneys; hyperechogenic cortex, reduced corticomedullary differentiation, well-defined sinus. **b** One year later: end-stage renal disease. Renal size regressive, cysts in upper and lower poles (sister in Fig. 20.**1**).

14.**41** **Hemolytic—uremic syndrome** in a boy of 6 years, 10 months with acute renal failure following an upper respiratory infection. Right flank longitudinal scan: **a** mildly enlarged kidney with voluminous parenchyma, and a narrow sinus. The renal cortex is significantly more echogenic than the adjacent liver parenchyma. Accentuated corticomedullary differentiation. **b** Normal appearance at follow-up. Status post dialysis.

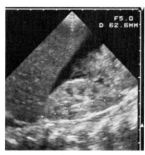 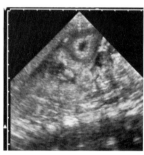 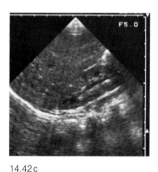

14.42a   14.42b   14.42c

14.**42** **Hemolytic—uremic syndrome** in a 16-month-old girl with fever and enterocilitis. **a** Right flank longitudinal scan: hyperechogenic cortex, ascites. **b** Left longitudinal upper

abdominal scan: thickening of the bowel wall. **c** Normal kidney 8 months later.

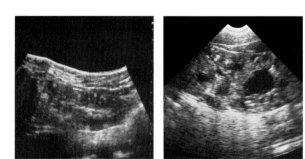 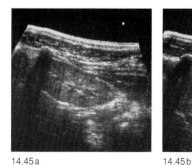 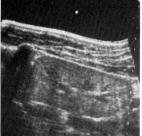

14.43   14.44   14.45a   14.45b

14.**43** **Tuberous sclerosis** in a 10½-year-old girl. Right longitudinal scan: normal-sized kidney with multiple small echogenic nodules in the cortex. US: angiomyolipomas (in both kidneys).

14.**44** **Tuberous sclerosis.** Left posterior longitudinal scan: multiple cysts of varying size, multiple small echogenic nodules consistent with angiomyolipomas.

14.**45** **Alport syndrome** in a girl of 14 years, 7 months with end-stage renal failure. **a** Right and **b** left posterior longitudinal scans: smaller right kidney with a hyperechogenic cortex and reduced corticomedullary differentiation.

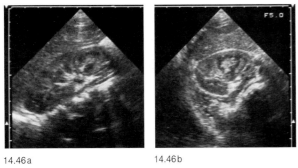
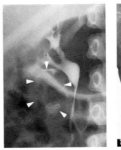
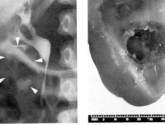

14.46a   14.46b   14.46c   14.46d

14.46 Multilocular renal cyst in a girl of 4 years, 4 months with acute, colicky abdominal pain and gross hematuria. **a** Longitudinal and **b** transverse right posterior scans: rounded lesion with a peripheral sonolucent rim and echogenic center with irregular margins. Normal renal contour. **c** EU: focal mass effect

in the lower renal pole with distortion of adjacent calices. **DD** (EU and US): most likely a malignant tumor (transitional cell carcinoma, nephroblastoma, rhabdoid tumor); benign tumor (hemangiomatous malformation). **d** Surgical specimen. Histology: multilocular renal cyst with an acute hemorrhage.

Nephrocalcinosis

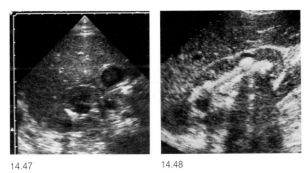
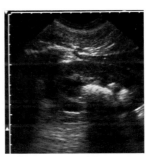

14.47   14.48   14.49

14.47 Nephrolithiasis in a 13½-year-old girl immobilized for 4 weeks because of multiple injuries including a tibial fracture and aortic rupture. Right flank transverse scan shows nephrolithiasis and sludge in the gallbladder.

14.48 Cystinuria in a 14-year-old boy with recurrent stone formation. Right flank longitudinal scan: massive stone formation in the pyelocaliceal system.

14.49 Cystinuria in a 19-year-old man. Left posterior longitudinal scan: nephrolithiasis with partial obstruction of upper-pole calices (same patient as in Fig. 14.**10**).

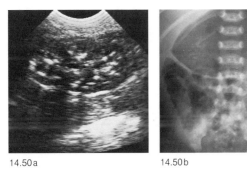
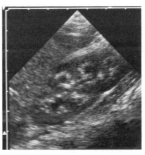
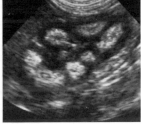

14.50a   14.50b   14.51   14.52

14.50 Previous renal vein thrombosis in a 5-month-old boy. **a** Right posterior longitudinal scan: multiple echogenic areas diffusely scattered throughout the right kidney (left kidney normal). **b** Radiograph at 4 weeks shows a branched, calcific pattern in the right kidney.

14.51 Medullary nephrocalcinosis in a 1-year-old boy with a urinary tract infection. Right flank longitudinal scan: echogenic outlining of renal pyramids at the periphery. Preserved echolucent center.

14.52 Medullary nephrocalcinosis in a 3-month-old boy showing reluctance to feed, dystrophy, and clinical signs fo idiopathic hypercalcemia. Right flank longitudinal scan: normal-sized kidney with intensely echogenic renal pyramids; the central area is less echogenic.

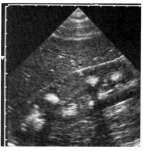
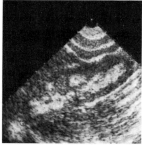
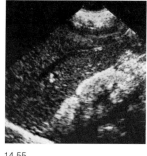
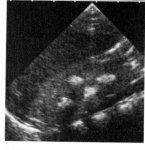

14.53   14.54   14.55   14.56

14.**53** **Renal tubular acidosis** in an 17-year-old male. Right flank longitudinal scan: the renal pyramids are intensely hyperechogenic, the cortex slightly so. Corticomedullary differentiation is reversed. US: cortical and medullary nephrocalcinosis.

14.**54** **Primary hyperparathyroidism, status following vitamin D intoxication,** 20-year-old male. Right flank longitudinal scan: cortex and medulla hyperechogenic; corticomedullary differentiation is reversed. US cortical and medullary nephrocalcinosis.

14.**55** **Primary hyperoxaluria** in an 11-month-old boy with a failure to grow and renal failure. Right flank longitudinal scan: intensely echogenic parenchyma with partial acoustic shadowing. No corticomedullary differentiation. US: nephrocalcinosis, hyperoxaluria (confirmed; sister in Fig. 14.**56**).

14.**56** **Primary hyperoxaluria** in a 4-month-old girl. Her brother (Fig. 14.**55**) died at the age of 2 years with hyperoxaluria and end-stage renal disease. Right flank longitudinal scan: medullary and cortical nephrocalcinosis. Reversal of corticomedullary differentiation (renal pyramids already intensely echogenic at 3 weeks).

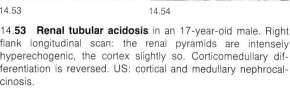
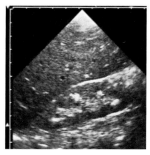

14.57   14.58

14.**57** **Primary hyperoxaluria** in a boy of 13 years, 10 months with a long history of fatigue and overweight; suspected developmental retardation. Hematuria, proteinuria, glucosuria; anemia; end-stage renal disease. Right flank longitudinal scan: relatively small kidney, intensely echogenic, especially in the region of the renal pyramids. US: massive nephrocalcinosis. **DD:** hyperoxaluria (confirmed; brother in Fig. 14.**58**).

14.**58** **Primary hyperoxaluria** in a boy of 9 years, 10 months. His brother (Fig. 14.**57**) has end-stage renal disease in hyperoxaluria. Right flank longitudinal scan: hyperechogenicity of the cortex (mild) and renal pyramids (intense). Reversal of corticomedullary differentiation.

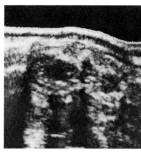
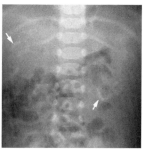
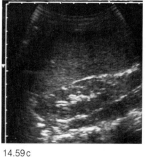

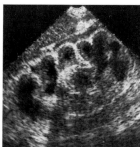

14.59a   14.59b   14.59c   14.60

14.**59** **Renal cortical necrosis** in a 3-month-old boy who underwent 3 previous operations for coarctation of the aorta. Microhematuria. **a** Left posterior longitudinal scan: marked thinning of the intensely echogenic, garlandlike cortex. **b** Radiograph: calcification of the renal cortex (arrow). US: cortical necrosis secondary to shock or renal vein thrombosis. **c** Left flank longitudinal scan 7 years later: small kidney with a partially sonodense border; mild renal insufficiency.

14.**60** **Renal cortical necrosis** (US) in an 8½-year-old girl 4 weeks after renal transplantation (end-stage renal disease) in the setting of recessive polycystic kidney disease and hepatic fibrosis. From the beginning, a nonfunctioning graft. Right flank longitudinal scan: graft enlargement. Cortex hypoechogenic peripherally and very hyperechogenic centrally; prominent medullary papillae. Scintigraphy: no perfusion. Subsequent nephrectomy (same patient as in Figs. 10.**6**, 14.**23**, and 5.**41**; brother in Fig. 14.**24**).

15 Urinary Tract Infection

U. V. Willi

Urinary tract infection, after "abdominal pain," is the second most common abdominal indication for ultrasound scanning. Sonography in these cases will disclose an abnormality with some frequency: unilateral or bilateral ectasia of the ureter or pyelocaliceal system; a related or independet abnormality in the size, shape, echo structure, or position of one or both kidneys; evidence of a unilateral or bilateral urinary-tract duplication anomaly, possibly combined with a ureterocele; regular or irregular bladder wall thickening; an intravesical lesion, possibly with an associated foreign body; or even a lesion extrinsic to the kidney and urinary tract which secondarily incites a urinary tract infection by obstructing urinary drainage.

Urinary tract infection, by its *direct or indirect effects on the urinary organs*, can initiate a variety of complex morphologic and functional changes in the kidney and urinary tract. This means that the findings of a given ultrasound examination are relative, and that the timing of the subsequent uroradiologic study is important. Once the infection is clinically controlled (almost always) and emergency intervention is unnecessary, it is prudent to delay definitive evaluation for 4−6 weeks after the institution of effective anti-infectious treatment. This allows sufficient time for the regression of most *bladder wall changes*, which can mask the presence of vesicoureteral reflux in two ways: (1) a reduced bladder capacity due to inflammatory irritation prohibits adequate stressing of the ureterovesical junction, and (2) inflammatory swelling of the bladder mucosa in this area may cause an inherently incompetent ureterovesical junction to appear competent.

Urinary tract infection can have direct or indirect *effects on the upper urinary tract and kidneys:* toxic infectious paralysis in (usually small) children with urosepsis can lead to a potentially severe dilatation of the ureter and pyelocaliceal system. Acute pyelonephritis can produce a local, tumorlike swelling of the parenchyma or a more generalized swelling leading to a variable, possibly severe degree of renal function impairment. This situation can precipitate an acute compensatory enlargement of the unaffected kidney or, if the latter is not fully functional, progress to acute renal failure. Again, this underscores the need for caution in interpreting sonographic findings (renal size, shape, echo structure) and the questionable value of excretory urography in the stage of acute infection.

"Recurrent" or chronic bladder inflammations are not uncommon in small girls about 4−7 years of age. Sonograms in these patients often reveal significant bladder wall thickening, usually no ectasia of the upper urinary tract, and normal-appearing kidneys. There seems to be little rationale at present (or in general) for a uroradiologic workup of these cases or for prolonged anti-infectious therapy. However, a urodynamic evaluation (uroflowmetry and pelvic floor electromyography) is sometimes useful and will occasionally permit the diagnosis of urinary dysfunction.

Some sonographic findings are characteristic of the condition diagnosed by that modality ar secondarily by uroradiography, but many are nonspecific. It is not unusual to find complex abnormalities (ureterovesical obstruction with concomitant reflux, e.g., in patients with posterior urethral valves and bladder wall hypertrophy) that have a relatively simple morphologic presentation. In cases where a morphologic abnormality is identified (e.g., ectasia of the upper urinary tract), the functional status of the affected system remains unclear or at best speculative until function testing (voiding cystourethrography, excretory urography or radionuclide alternatives) is done to complete the evaluation.

On the other hand, sonography gives us a reasonably accurate picture of the possible differential diagnoses. This "prejudical" information sets the stage for an accurate and expeditious diagnosis, which generally can be made using simple, conventional radiographic methods.

The typical morphologic features of renal and urinary tract abnormalities are illustrated in chapter 16 (Hydronephrosis and Hydroureter), chapter 17 (Bladder Wall Changes), and chapter 14 (Renal Abnormalities).

References

Ben-Ami, T.: The sonographic evaluation of urinary tract infections in children. Semin. Ultrasound 5 (1984) 19–34

Gross, G., R. L. Lebowitz: Infection does not cause reflux. Amer. J. Roentgenol. 137 (1981) 929–932

Kangarloo, H., R. H. Gold, R. N. Fine, M. J. Diament, M. I. Boechat: Urinary tract infection in infants and children evaluated by ultrasound. Radiology 154 (1985) 367–373

Lebowitz, R. L.: The detection of vesicoureteral reflux in the child. Invest. Radiology 21 (1986) 519–531

Lebowitz, R. L., J. Mandell: Urinary tract infection in children: putting radiology in its place. Radiology 165 (1987) 1–9

16 Hydronephrosis and Hydroureter

U. V. Willi

While some authors use the terms "hydronephrosis" and "hydroureter" in reference to obstructive uropathy, there these terms are *synonymous with ectasia of the pyelocaliceal system or ureter*. This avoids any etiologic implications, for a severe *vesicoureteral reflux* can mimic an obstruction morphologically or may coexist with one (e. g., refluxing, primary obstructive megaureter). A *full urinary bladder* can cause a unilateral or bilateral reduction of urinary drainage through the ureterovesical junction, creating a temporary "functional obstruction." Whether this condition is physiologic or is based on a pathologic process (e. g., an infravesical obstruction) cannot always be ascertained by sonography.

Some *complex situations with variable urodynamic parameters* (urine flow; urinary drainage; renal size; distensibility of calices, pelvis, and ureter; ureterovesical passage; functional bladder or urethral change) lead to a more or less pronounced dilatation of the upper urinary tract. Pure *morphologic variants*, whether physiologic or pathologic (e. g., megacalices), compound the diversity of the phenomenon of hydronephrosis/hydroureter. *Acute urinary tract infection* is a relatively frequent cause of significant morphologic changes in the urinary tract and can influence the parameters cited above.

More and more frequently the *presentation* of hydronephrosis, with or without hydroureter, is being recognized antenatally (often described sonographically as a fairly nonspecific "cystic renal change"). It may also present in urinary tract infection, as an abdominal mass, as an incidental finding, in association with another abnormality (e. g., myelomeningocele; cloacal anomaly; duplication of the upper urinary tract, possibly combined with a ureterocele) or as part of a syndrome.

The most common form of *obstructive uropathy* is a proximal stenosis of the ureter at the ureteropelvic junction: *ureteropelvic junction obstruction*. A "relative" ureteropelvic stenosis exists in patients with a large or very distensible extrarenal pelvis once the ureteral capacity has been exhausted (e. g., due to ureterovesical obstruction) or in patients with massive vesicoureteral reflux. Once the ureterovesical obstruction is cleared or reflux has resolved, the ureteropelvic junction is found to be abnormal. An unusual form of proximal "ureteral obstruction" exists in conjunction with *pelvoinfundibular hypoplasia*, i. e., absence of the renal pelvis. The extreme form of ureteropelvic junction stenosis is proximal ureteral atresia. This lesion is regarded as an early-fetal pathogenetic process along the lines of the classic *multicystic dysplastic kidney*. The complete or nearly complete ureteral obstruction that develops later in the fetal period leads to "microcystic renal dysplasia," appearing sonographically as a relatively thick renal parenchyma with increased echogenicity.

Obstructions can occur at various levels of the ureter and can have various etiologies. A familiar intrinsic form is *fibrotic ureteral stenosis*, while a common extrinsic form is due to *vascular ureteral compression* (e. g., proximally by an accessory renal artery or a renal artery taking an anomalous course, in the midureter by a preureteric vena cava: "retrocaval ureter"). More common than both forms is intraluminal ureteral obstruction by a *calculus*. A ureteral calculus is easier to diagnosis in the proximal or distal segment than in the midureter. With acute obstruction of the ureter by a calculus, no ectasia of the collecting system proximal to the obstruction is seen initially, perhaps for a period of days.

A relatively common lesion compromising drainage at the ureterovesical junction is the *"primary obstructive megaureter,"* which occasionally is detected by its hyperperistaltic activity. It may be associated with vesicoureteral reflux, because its distal, functionally abnormal segment has a normal caliber. Not infrequently, primary obstructive megaureter as well as primary refluxing megaureter present with wall thickening due to hypertrophy. Renal pelvic wall thickening, on the other hand, is more likely to have a (chronic) inflammatory pathogenesis.

Complex forms of ureterovesical obstructive uropathy, possibly with reflux, can arise in conjunction with *posterior urethral valves* (in boys). The potential for ureterovesical obstruction despite massive ipsilateral reflux is noteworthy and may be one reason for the inadequacy of diagnosis based on morphologic ultrasound criteria.

The primary task of sonography is to define the *morphology of upper urinary tract ectasis:* unilateral or bilateral; affecting the calices, pelvis, and/or ureter; belonging to a solitary system or segmental; with or without an associated nephrourologic or other malformation; constant or intermittent. Other important criteria for the presumptive evaluation of the kidneys and urinary tract are *renal size* (may be increased due, say, to the successful compensation of an obstruction by the well-functioning kidney), *renal shape* (may be very abnormal due, say, to multicystic dysplasia), and the *thickness and echogenicity of the renal parenchyma*. In the setting of prenatal diagnosis, a normal amniotic fluid volume provides strong evidence of normal global renal function.

It should be stressed that the *(morpho)dynamic examination* of the urinary tract by voiding cystourethrography (VCUG) and excretory urography (EU) or by alternative or complementary radionuclide scanning is essential for the adequate evaluation of a dilated upper urinary tract.

Several points should be noted in this context:
- Massive dilatation of the upper urinary tract may not be amenable to further sonographic differentiation (obstruction, vesicoureteral reflux, or both combined).
- Even with massive vesicoureteral reflux, urinary tract ectasia may be missed, and the reflux undiagnosed, in the absence of an acute event during the ultrasound examination.
- Inadequate urinary drainage due to obstructive or malformative uropathy predisposes both to infection and to lithiasis; it is likely that each of these conditions can be the cause or the effect of the other.
- Megacalices are not easily distinguished from an obstructive hydronephrosis by ultrasound. In itself, the condition does not require surgical treatment. However, it may be associated with an obstructive uropathy, which in turn may require correction. Generally the diagnostic criteria for megacalices are well demonstrated by EU, although the picture may be less clear when there is associated obstructive uropathy.
- Despite the frequently massive degree of hydronephrosis with a very thin parenchyma (especially with ureteropelvic stenosis), the finding of normal parenchymal echogenicity with the preservation of renal shape implies a good prognosis in terms of the preservation of renal function. However, this does not remove the obligation to complete the evaluation with appropriate radiographic and/or radionuclide procedures (as described above).

References

Brown, T., J. Mandell, R. L. Lebowitz: Neonatal hydronephrosis in the era of sonography. Amer. J. Roentgenol. 148 (1987) 959–963

Caldamone, A. A.: Duplication anomalies of the upper tract in infants and children. Urol. Clin. N. Amer. 12 (1985) 75–91

Chopra, A., R. L. Teele: Hydronephrosis in children: narrowing the differential diagnosis with ultrasound. J. clin. Ultrasound 8 (1980) 473–478

Holthusen, W., B. Lundius: Megapolycalicosis with ureteric obstruction: a retrospective analysis of ten childhood cases. Ann. Radiol. 27 (1984) 191–198

Kenawi, M. M., D. I. Williams: Circumcaval ureter: a report of four cases in children with review of the literature and a new classification. Brit. J. Urol. 48 (1976) 183–192

Nussbaum, A., J. P. Dorst, R. D. Jeffs, J. P. Gearhart, R. C. Sanders: Ectopic ureter and ureterocele: their varied sonographic manifestations. Radiology 159 (1986) 227–235

Paltiel, H. J., R. L. Lebowitz: Neonatal hydronephrosis due to primary vesicoureteral reflux: trends in diagnosis and treatment. Radiology 170 (1989) 787–789

Williams, D. I., J. H. Johnston: Paediatric Urology, 2nd ed. Butterworths, London 1982

Young, D. W., R. L. Lebowitz: Congenital abnormalities of the ureter. Semin. Roentgenol. 21 (1986) 172–187

Ureteropelvic Junction Obstruction

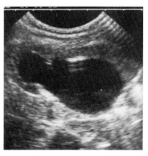 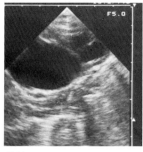 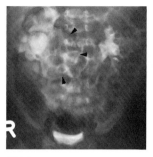 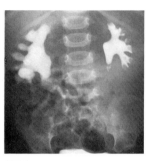

16.1a   16.1b   16.1c   16.1d

16.1 **Unilateral ureteropelvic junction obstruction** in a 5½-week-old boy with a prenatal US diagnosis of a "cystic structur" in the right renal area. No urinary tract infection. Posterior **a** longitudinal and **b** transverse scan: massive hydronephrosis and large extrarenal pelvis, consistent with UPJO. Large kidney, well-preserved parenchyma with normal echogenicity. **c** EU 2 hours postcontrast: relatively dense opacification. Wide extrarenal pelvis (▲). **d** 15-minute EU 5 months after an Anderson−Hynes pyeloplasty: normal function. *Note:* US and EU suggested a good functional prognosis.

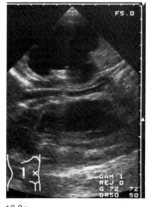 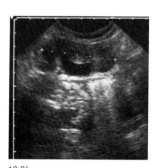 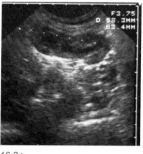

16.2a   16.2b   16.2c

16.2 **Bilateral ureteropelvic junction obstruction** in a 6-day-old girl with a prenatal diagnosis of bilateral hydronephrosis. No urinary tract infection. **a** Right flank coronal scan: massive bilateral hydronephrosis; parenchyma appears more prominent on the left than on the right. Urography showed a higher-grade obstruction on the right side. Anderson−Hynes pyeloplasty performed on the right kidney at the age of 19 days. **b** Left and **c** right posterior longitudinal scans 2 weeks later: residual caliceal ectasia on the right; complete, transient remission of the hydronephrosis on the left (secondary operation on the left kidney for recurrence of massive hydronephrosis). Result satisfactory on both sides.

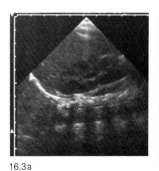 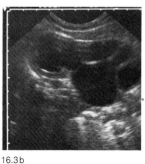

16.3a   16.3b

16.3 **Unilateral ureteropelvic junction obstruction** (incidental finding) in a 3½-month-old boy with suspected hypertrophic pyloric stenosis. No urinary tract infection. **a** Right and **b** left flank coronal scans: normal right kidney. Massive dilation of the left pyelocaliceal system; kidney very large; parenchyma appears relatively prominent, especially in the upper pole. Radioisotope assessment of renal function: 52% on the right, 48% on the left. Anderson−Hynes pyeloplasty. *Note:* the diagnosis was made possible by a routine evaluation of the kidneys and urinary tract in the case of pyloric stenosis.

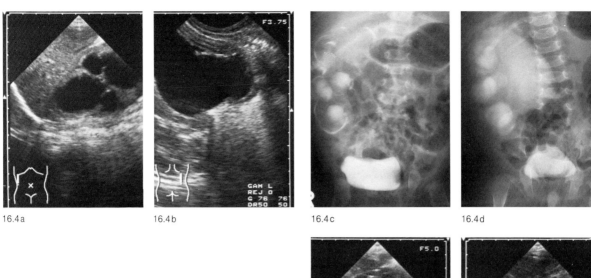

16.4a   16.4b   16.4c   16.4d

16.4 Ureteropelvic junction obstruction with a solitary right kidney in a 3½-year-old boy with a right-sided abdominal mass; suspected Wilms tumor. a Anterior and **b** posterior longitudinal scans: massive hydronephrosis; large pelvis; very large kidney; relatively prominent parenchyma with normal echogenicity. EU at **c** 15 and **d** 120 minutes postcontrast: early, strong opacification of the excretory channels of the medulla (crescent sign) and dependent calices: good function. Longitudinal right flank scans at **e** 9 days and **f** 5 months after an Anderson–Hynes pyeloplasty: remarkable, progressive reversal of caliceal ectasia with corresponding normalization of parenchymal morphology. Creatinine consistently normal.

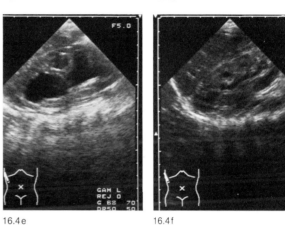

16.4e   16.4f

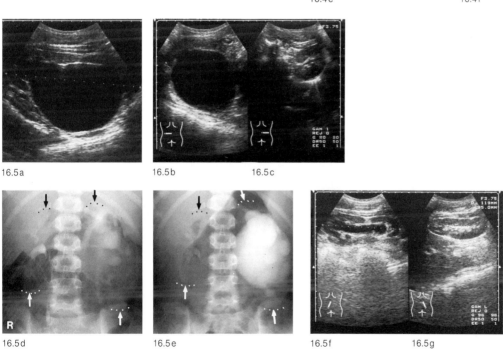

16.5a   16.5b   16.5c

16.5d   16.5e   16.5f   16.5g

16.5 Unilateral ureteropelvic junction obstruction in a boy of 8 years, 8 months with a "stitch" in the left side for 1½ years; firm "tumor mass" in the left hemiabdomen. **a** Longitudinal and **b, c** transverse posterior scans: massive left-sided hydronephrosis with a large pelvis; left kidney greatly enlarged, but parenchyma still generally prominent. EU at **d** 15 minutes and **e** 3 hours postcontrast: fairly early, dense opacification of the caliceal

system, wide parenchymal rim, pronounced renal enlargement (poles marked with arrows): all signs consistent with good renal function. **f** Left and **g** right posterior longitudinal scans 3 months after an Anderson–Hynes pyeloplasty: moderate residual pyelocaliceal ectasia; relative and absolute regression of the left renal size. EU showed normal function.

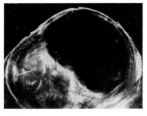
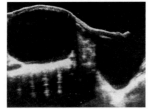

16.6a   16.6b

16.6 Unilateral ureteropelvic junction obstruction, complete (silent kidney) in a 12-year-old boy who sustained a minor flank trauma followed by pain and a very large, firm mass in the left hemiabdomen. EU showed a solitary functioning right kidney with compensatory enlargement. **a** Transverse and **b** longitudinal scans: very large, sharply marginated cystic mass—hydronephrotic sac suspected. Operative removal (confirmed). In retrospect, mass had probably been present for some time.

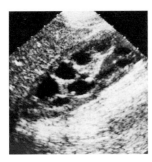
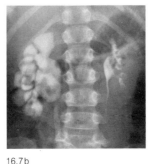
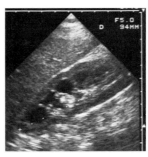
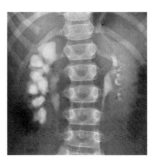

16.7a   16.7b   16.7c   16.7d

16.7 Ureteropelvic junction obstruction associated with unilateral megacalices in a 5½-year-old girl with recurrent urinary tract infections. Right flank longitudinal scans **a** before and **c** after the operation; 30-minutes EU **b** before and **d** after the operation (Anderson–Hynes pyeloplasty). Both modalities demonstrate a regression of the caliceal dilation following the correction of the stenosis. Megacalices diagnosed by urography.

Multicystic Dysplasia

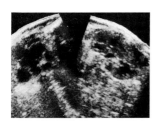
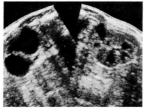
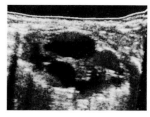

16.8a   16.8b   16.8c   16.8d

16.8 Multicystic dysplastic kidney in a 8-week-old female with suspected galactosemia. Posterior transverse scans at the **a** cranial, **b** middle, and **c** caudal levels and **d** a longitudinal scan show multiple cystic elements of varying size forming a grapelike cluster with no identifiable parenchyma; renal shape very abnormal: characteristic of multicystic dysplastic kidney.

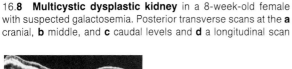
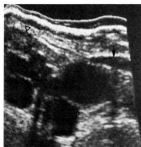
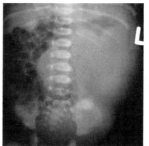
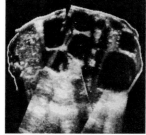

16.9   16.10a   16.10b

16.9 Multicystic dysplastic kidney in a 13-month-old girl with orofaciodigital syndrome. Left posterior longitudinal scan: multiple cystic elements of varying size; abnormal renal shape. Posterosuperior P ($\triangledown$): spleen; posteroinferiorly ($\rightarrow$): quadratus lumborum muscle.

16.10 Multicystic dysplastic kidney in a 6-day-old boy with an abdominal mass. **b** Radiograph: large mass in the left hemiabdomen with extension to the right, displacing the bowel. **b** Transverse sonogram: multiple cystic elements of varying size; extensive structure lacking a characteristic renal shape: typical of multicystic dysplastic kidney.

16.11 Microcystic renal dysplasia in a 3-day-old premature male (31 weeks' gestation) with respiratory distress syndrome. US elsewhere raised suspicion of posterior urethral valves. **a** Left flank coronal scan: massive hydronephrosis on the left side, moderate on right. Suspicion of bilateral ureteropelvic junction stenosis. Urography: silent left kidney. Scintigraphy: reduced parenchymal uptake. Nephrostomy with contrast injection: no drainage on the left side. Nephrectomy: renal surface studded with tiny nodules, consistent with microcystic changes (**b**); two discrete sites of ureteral atresia (arrows). P = renal pelvis. *Note:* it is reasonable to assume that a complete upper urinary tract obstruction would have developed in the late fetal period with this type of microcystic dysplasia (see also Fig. 16.**28**).

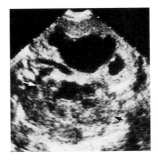
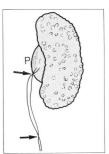

16.11a   16.11b

Ureteral Stenosis Distal to the Ureteropelvic Junction

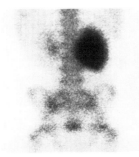
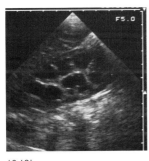
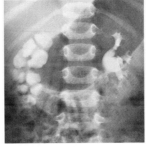
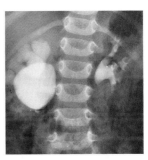

16.12a   16.12b   16.12c   16.12d

16.12 Proximal stenosing ureteral compression by a vessel, associated megacalices (incidental finding) in a boy of 3 years, 10 months with Schönlein–Henoch purpura and gonarthritis. **a** Posterior radionuclide bone scan: hydronephrosis on the right, ureteropelvic junction obstruction suspected. **b** Right flank coronal sonogram: massive caliceal ectasia, consistent with ureteropelvic junction obstruction. **c** EU 15 minutes postcontrast: megacalices; **d** 45 minutes postcontrast: proximal ureteral loop; (in retrospect) evidence of vascular effect, confirmed at operation: Anderson–Hynes pyeloplasty with transposition of the ureter in front of the compressing vessel.

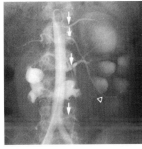
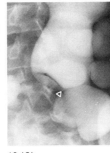
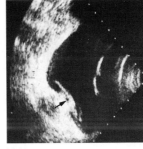

16.13a   16.13b   16.13c

16.13 Horseshoe kidney, proximal unilateral obstructive ureteral compression by an aberrant artery in a 12-year-old boy with a urinary tract infection. US showed horseshoe kidney and left-sided hydronephrosis with moderate proximal ureteral ectasia. **a** Angiography: four renal arteries on the left side (→), one taking a downward oblique aberrant course (△). **b** Postangiographic EU: proximal ureteral compression suspected (△). **c** US: pulsating vessels subsequently identified (arrow). Operation: ureter divided and reimplanted anterior to the compressing vessel. *Note:* US is specific when combined with angiography, otherwise it is nondiagnostic. Also: there is a frequent association of horseshoe kidney with aberrant vessels.

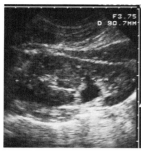

16.14a   16.14b

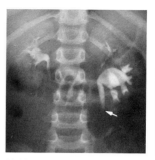

16.14c   16.14d

16.**14   Proximal ureteral stenosis** in a 6-year-old boy with recurrent urinary tract infections. **a** Longitudinal and **b** oblique posterior scans: duplex system; moderate ectasia of the lower pole moiety with the ureteral segment. **c** EU 45 minutes postcon-

trast: correlates with US; ureteral stenosis (arrow). **d** Retrograde ureteropyelography confirms the stenosis (arrow). Resection of the stenosis, end-to-end anastomosis.

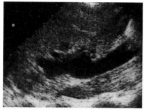

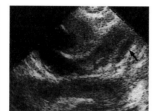

16.15a   16.15b

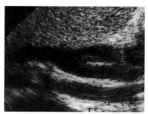

16.15c

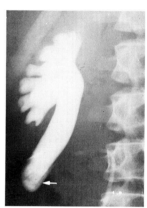

16.15d

16.**15   Retrocaval ureter (preureteric vena cava) with partial duplication of the inferior vena cava** in a 15-year-old male with hematuria. Right flank coronal scan: **a** moderate ectasia of the pyelocaliceal system, massive ureteral ectasia. **b** Loop in midureter (arrow). **c** Duplication of the lower inferior vena cava. **d** EU: broad ureteral loop through the duplicated vena cava; the distal part fo the ureteral loop has a normal caliber (arrows; corresponds to the part marked in **b**); massive ureteral ectasia proximal to the loop, with hydronephrosis. Good renal function. *Note:* relatively early diagnosis for this type of lesion.

Stenosis at the Ureterovesical Junction ("Primary Megaureter")

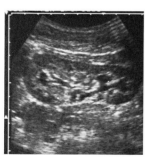

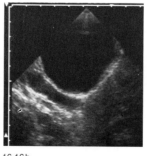

16.16a   16.16b

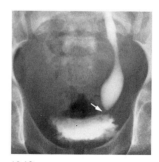

16.16c

16.**16   Primary obstructive megaureter** in a 7-year-old boy with a single episode of gross hematuria. No trauma or urinary tract infection. **a** Left posterior longitudinal scan: mild ectasia of the caliceal system. **b** Anterior scan: moderate distal ureteral

ectasia. **c** EU 20 minutes postcontrast, postvoiding: characteristic "tight" (normal-caliber) distal ureteral segment (arrow; aperistaltic and functionally obstructed; here the obstructive effect was mild, so primary surgical correction was withheld).

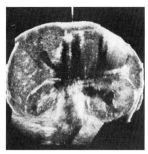 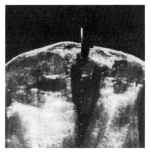 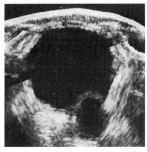 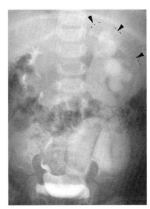

16.17a   16.17b   16.17c

16.**17 Primary obstructive megaureter** in a 3½-month-old
boy with pyelonephritis. **a** Anterior and **b** posterior transverse
scans: moderate left hydronephrosis; swollen left kidney. **c**
Anterior pelvic scan: massive left hydroureter impressing on the
bladder wall. **d** Two hour EU 6 weeks after antibiotic therapy:
massive ectasia of the left upper urinary tract. *Note:* persistence
fo the nephrogram (▼) and reduction of parenchymal thickness

16.17d

due to obstruction. Regression of parenchymal swelling after
treatment of the infection. Surgical correction.

16.**18 Solitary left kidney with a primary obstructive
megaureter and renal failure** in a 7-month-old boy with a
urinary tract infection. **a** Left flank coronal scan: massive hydronephrosis, parenchyma relatively prominent laterally (arrows). **b**
Anterior longitudinal scan: massive ureteral ectasia; normal-
caliber, aperistaltic distal ureteral segment (arrow). Primary
transcutaneous nephrostomy; antibiotic treatment. Normalization
of renal function. Subsequent surgical correction.

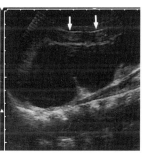 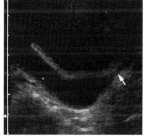

16.18a   16.18b

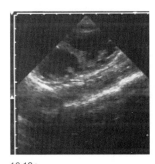 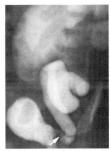 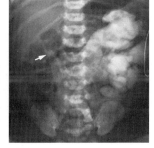

16.19a   16.19b   16.19c

16.**19 Solitary left kidney with primary obstructive and
refluxing megaureter** in a 1-day-old boy with a prenatal diagnosis of a solitay hydronephrotic left kidney. No renal failure. **a**
Left flank coronal scan: massive hydronephrosis; duplex system? **b** VCUG: massive reflux; normal-caliber, aperistaltic distal

ureteral segment (arrow). **c** 1 hour postvoiding: persistence of
opacity in a partial duplex system, consistent with ureterovesical
obstruction. Umbilical clamp (arrow). Surgical correction. *Note:*
the urologic aspect of the upper urinary tract evaluated by
VCUG; EU is unnecessary.

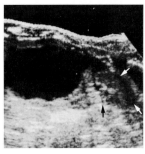
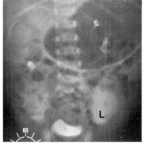
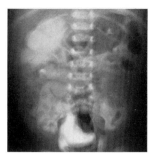

16.20a   16.20b   16.20c

16.**20 Unilateral primary obstructive megaureter with a bilateral duplex system** in a 17-day-old boy diagnosed prenatally with right hydronephrosis. **a** Posterior longitudinal scan: duplex system on the right side; upper-pole hydronephrosis; relatively well-preserved parenchyma; normal lower pole

(arrows). **b** 10-minutes EU: prominent crescent sign as evidence of good function. **c** 4-hour urogram. Despite adequate renal function, upper-pole nephroureterectomy was performed on the right side.

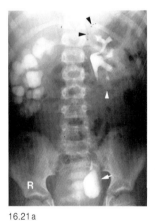
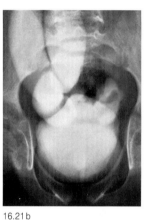
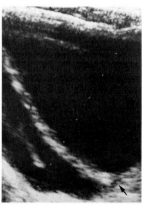

16.21a   16.21b   16.21c   16.21d

16.**21 Primary obstructive megaureter on the right with incomplete duplication and megacalices, (para)ureteral diverticulum on the left with left-sided reflux nephropathy** in a boy 8 years, 9 months of age with recurrent urinary tract infections. **a** Thirty-minute EU elsewhere: megacalices and delayed excretion on the right side; parenchymal reduction (▲) and diverticulum (→) on the left side. **b** Three-hour urogram,

postvoiding: duplex megaureter on the right; diverticulum on the left. Anterior longitudinal scan **c** on the left: diverticulum with ureteral orifice (arrow) draining into the diverticulum; **d** on the right: common distal portion of megaureters; normal-caliber aperistaltic distal ureteral segment (arrow). Surgically corrected by bilateral ureteral reimplantation, en bloc reimplant on the right following resection of the adynamic segment.

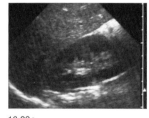
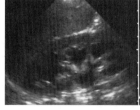
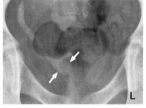
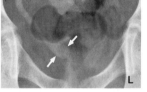

16.22a   16.22b   16.22c   16.22d

16.**22 Bilateral ureteroceles with nonduplex systems** in a 7-year-old boy with the Kawasaki syndrome. Incidental urologic finding. **a** Right and **b** left flank coronal scans: normal-appearing right kidney, moderately hydronephrotic left kidney. **c** EU 3 minutes postcontrast: right ureterocele (arrows) already opacified, delayed excretion on the left; **d** 23 minutes postcontrast, postvoid: both ureteroceles opacified (arrows), ectatic left ureter. Obstruction moderate on the left, minimal (if any) on the right. Bilateral surgical correction (same patient as in Fig. 17.**23**).

16.**25 Complete duplication on the right, obstructive ▶ upper-pole pyoureterocele** in a 4-week-old boy with an acute urinary tract infection, sepsis. **a** Right longitudinal pelvic scan: thick-walled pyoureterocele; associated ureter is redundant and ectatic. Following bladder catheterization, progressive bilateral ureterovesical obstruction by a ureterocele. **b, c** Right and left flank coronal scans: massive bilateral hydronephrosis. Emergency incision of the pyoureterocele. **d** Subsequent right flank coronal scan: significant regression of hydronephrosis in both poles. Secondary en bloc reimplantation of the right ureters.

Duplex Systems with Obstruction (and Reflux)

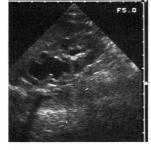

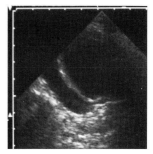

16.23a

16.23b

16.23 Complex duplication on the right, ureterovesical obstruction of the upper pole system (primary megaureter?) in a 5-month-old boy with a urinary tract infection. **a** Right flank coronal scan: massive upper-pole hydronephrosis; moderately thick parenchyma with normal echogenicity. **b** Right longitudinal pelvic scan: ectatic upper pole ureter; normal-caliber distal segment. **c, d** EU at 3 and 120 minutes postcontrast: crescent sign; adequate nephrogram; later, relatively dense opacification of the right upper pole ureter (arrows). En bloc reimplantation of the right ureters. 15-minute EU **e** 9 days and **f** 1 year after surgery: progressive improvement of right upper pole drainage.

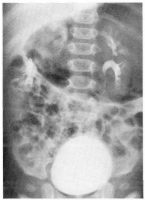

16.23c

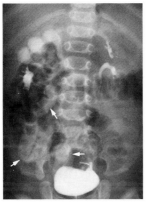

16.23d

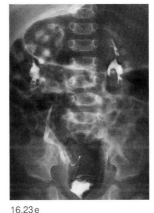

16.23e

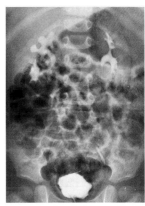

16.23f

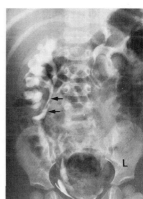

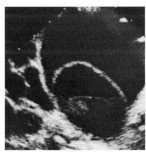

16.24a

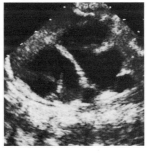

16.24b

16.24c

16.24d

16.24 Complete duplication on the right, obstructive upper pole ureterocele, lower pole reflux in a 4-month-old girl with a urinary tract infection. **a, b** Right flank coronal scans: massive hydronephrosis and hydroureters (arrows). **c** 2-hour EU: good opacification of the upper pole system (lower pole has adequate function despite reflux); ureterocele (▼). (On original,

the contrast-filled ureterocele was visible within the contrast-filled bladder.) Upper-to-lower-pole ureteroureterostomy (**d**, arrows). **d** 15-minute EU 1 year postoperatively: satisfactory result. Secondary reimplantation of the right ureter due to persistent reflux.

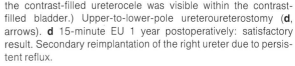

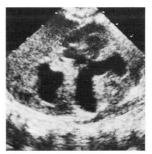

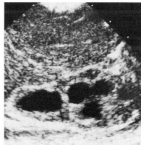

16.25a

16.25b

16.25c

16.25d

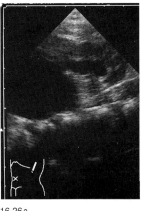 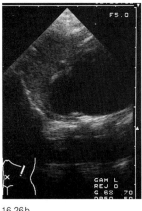 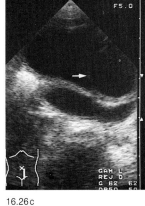 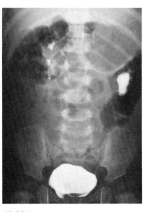

16.26a   16.26b   16.26c   16.26d

16.26 Complete duplication on the left and obstructive upper pole ureterocele in a 1-year-old girl with a urinary tract infection. **a, b** Left flank coronal scans: massive upper pole hydronephrosis; apparently intact parenchyma; moderate lower pole ectasia. **c** Right longitudinal pelvic scan: massive ureteral ectasia; ureterocele (arrow). **d** 1-hour EU: marked displacement of the normal left lower pole moiety by a poorly functioning

hydronephrotic upper pole moiety. Upper pole nephroureterectomy on the left side. Histology: severe chronic pyelonephritis with focal renal dysplasia. *Note:* weak or absent contrast excretion in urography is a poor prognostic sign. In this case, with normal parenchymal echogenicity and relatively severe ectasia, there was renal dysfunction, possibly caused (in part) by transient infection.

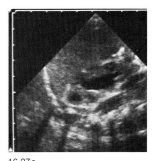 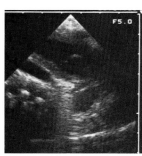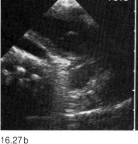

16.27a   16.27b

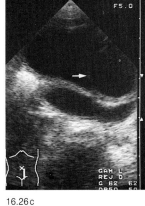

16.27c

16.27 Complete duplication on the right with obstructive upper pole ureterocele in a 5-week-old boy referred for right-sided hydroureteronephrosis diagnosed elsewhere. **a** Right flank coronal scan: moderate hydronephrosis of both poles, upper pole less extensive; upper pole parenchyma shows a diffuse increase of echogenicity. **b** Right longitudinal pelvic scan: moderate ureteral ectasia; ureterocele. **c** 15-minute EU: displacement of the lower pole system by an upper pole hydroureter;

mild lower pole hydronephrosis from the obstructive effect of the ureterocele on the lower pole orifice. Treated by a right upper pole nephroureterectomy, leaving behind the evacuated ureterocele. Histology: dysplatic renal tissue. Subsequent reflux into the right lower pole system (initially prevented by the ureterocele). *Note:* increased parenchymal echogenicity, mild dilatation of the collecting system, and nonopacification on urogram are consistent with inadequate function.

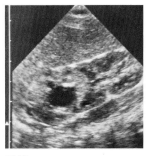 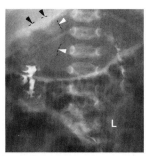

16.28a   16.28b

16.28 Complete duplication on the right with ureterovesical obstruction of the upper pole system in a 7-week-old girl diagnosed prenatally with right-sided hydronephrosis. **a** Right flank coronal scan: moderate ectasia of the upper pole collecting system (including the ureter); subtle caliceal ectasia; relatively thick parenchyma, hyperechogenic (resembles the case in Fig. 16.**11**). **b** EU, 15 minutes: displacement of the normal lower pole by an upper pole hydroureter; faint nephrogram (▼; no subsequent increase in contrast excretion). Treated by an upper pole nephroureterectomy. Histology: renal dysplasia, medullary fibrosis (see also Fig. 16.**11**).

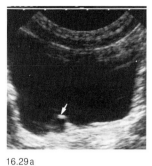
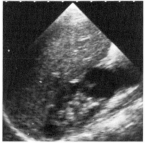

16.29a   16.29b

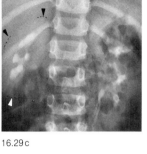

16.29c

16.**29** **Complete duplication on the right, nonobstructive upper pole ureterocele, lower pole reflux with massive reflux nephropathy** in a 4½-year-old boy with recurrent urinary tract infections. **a** Transverse pelvic scan: small ureterocele on the right (arrow). **b** Right flank coronal scan: normal upper pole; massive lower pole hydronephrosis. EU at **c** 3 minutes and **d** 3½ hours postcontrast: normal function of the upper pole (▼); reflux into the lower pole system (confirmed by VCUG); both ureters

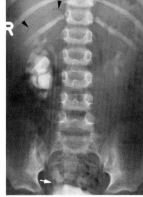

16.29d

distinguishable distally (upper pole ureter thin: →). Treated by lower pole nephroureterectomy. Histology: atrophic dysplastic kidney.

16.**30** **Complete duplication on the right, obstructive upper pole ureterocele, massive lower pole reflux with severe reflux nephropathy** in a 3½-year-old boy with recurrent urinary tract infections. **a, b** Right flank coronal scans: upper pole hydronephrosis with a very thin hyperechogenic parenchymal rim; variable reflux-induced lower pole hydronephrosis. EU: no appreciable renal function; massive lower pole reflux. Treated by a complete nephroureterectomy on the right, leaving behind the evacuated ureterocele. Histology: atrophic kidney with dysplasia in both moieties.

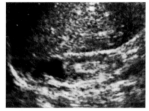
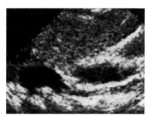

16.30a   16.30b

16.**31** **Complete duplication on the left with a ureterovesical upper pole obstruction leading to compressive obstruction of the lower pole system** in a 1-day-old girl with a prenatal differential diagnosis of a urogenital vs. gastrointestinal lesion. **a–c** Pelvic and left flank scans: massive ectasia and redundancy of the left upper urinary tract; hyperechogenic parenchyma. **DD:** solitary vs. duplex system. **d** Renal scintigraphy (dimercaptosuccinylic acid) at 2 days: unexpectedly good "function"; unusual renal shape. **e** Antegrade ureteropyelography of the upper pole system at 2 months, 1 day later transcutaneous catheter insertion into the lower pole system; abdominal film 1 day later: obstructive upper pole system still contrast-filled; catheter in the lower pole system. Unnecessary cutaneous upper pole ureterostomy; splinting of the lower pole ureter. **f** One week later, 45-minute EU: moderate statis of the lower pole system. Managed by upper pole nephroureterectomy. Histology: chronic pyeloureteritis, medullary fibrosis, dysplasia. *Note:* diagnosis not possible without interventional radiology.

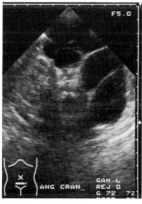
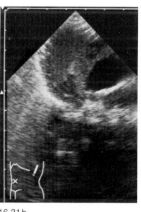

16.31a   16.31b

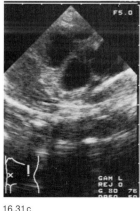
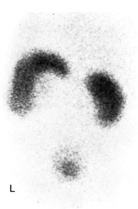
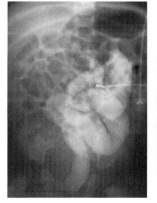
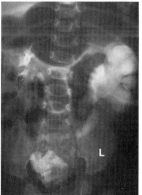

16.31c   16.31d   16.31e   16.31f

Posterior Urethral Valves

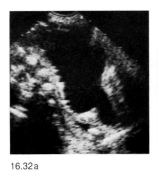 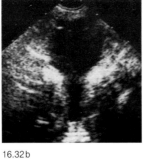 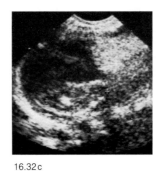 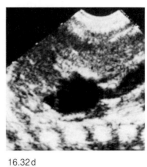

16.32a   16.32b   16.32c   16.32d

16.32 Posterior urethral valves in a 12-day-old boy. Oligohydramnios, neonatal asphyxia, bilateral pneumothorax, pulmonary hypoplasia; progressive renal failure. Referred at 12 days. Umbilical US scan angled toward the perineum: **a** longitudinal, **b** transverse: micturition induced by slight transducer pressure; characteristic dilatation and elongation of the prostatic urethral segment. Left flank coronal scans **c** before and **d** during micturition: reflux-induced dilatation of the upper urinary tract (**d**). Similar on the right. The infant died the following day.

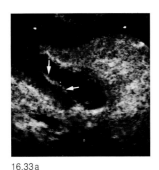 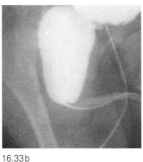

16.33a   16.33b

16.33 Posterior urethral valves in a 7-week-old boy with urosepsis and a weak urine stream. **a** Longitudinal pelvic scan: greatly elongated and dilated prostatic urethral segment; visible portion of the valve (arrows). **b** VCUG: classic radiographic correlate to US. Also massive right-sided reflux with diffuse intrarenal reflux. No renal failure. Surgical correction. Normal renal function at the age of 6 years.

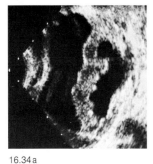 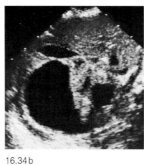 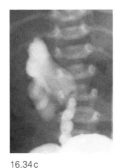 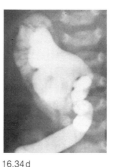

16.34a   16.34b   16.34c   16.34d

16.34 Posterior urethral valves and perirenal urinoma in an 11-day-old boy with a recent prenatal diagnosis of a cystic lesion in the right renal area. Right flank **a** coronal and **b** transverse scans: large perirenal cystic mass consistent with urinoma; moderate hydronephrosis. VCUG **c** before and **d** during micturition: massive reflux on the right; massive intrarenal reflux during micturition (higher pressure); no current evidence of renal rupture. Spontaneous resolution of the urinoma. Surgical correction of the valves; temporary cutaneous right ureterostomy; later reconstruction. Right kidney became very small and athropic, with compensatory hypertrophy of the left kidney. Normal renal function at the age of 5 years.

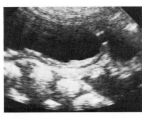 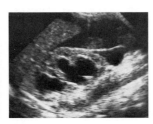 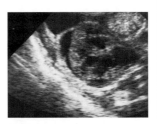 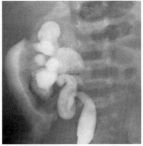

16.35a   16.35b   16.35c   16.35d

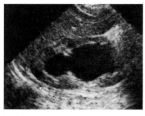
16.36a

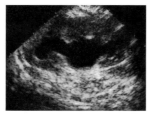
16.36b

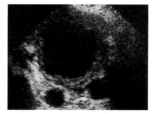
16.36c

16.36 Posterior urethral valves, massive left-sided reflux combined with ureterovesical obstruction in a 6-month-old boy with a urinary tract infection, and a weak urine stream; presumptive diagnosis by a pediatrician. **a** Right and **b** left flank coronal scans show massive hydronephrosis on each side. **c** Transverse pelvic scan: bilateral hydroureter; bladder wall thickening. Findings consistent with the preliminary diagnosis. VCUG: confirmed diagnosis; massive reflux on the left side. **d** Ten-minute and **e** 120-minute postvoiding films: massive ureterovesical obstruction. *Note:* exhaustion of the ureteral capacity leads to functional ureteropelvic obstruction. Continuous catheter drainage of the bladder provides only gradual resolution, but without this treatment the condition will persist more or less unchanged.

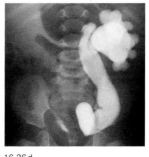
16.36d

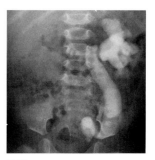
16.36e

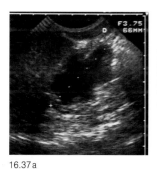
16.37a

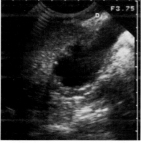
16.37b

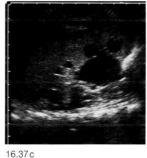
16.37c

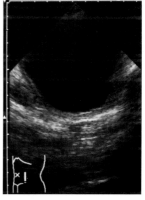
16.37d

16.37 Prune-belly syndrome in a 10½-year-old boy. Diagnosis known since early childhood. The patient had previously had the Boari procedure elsewhere. Renal failure. **a, b** Right and **c** left flank coronal scans: massive bilateral hydronephrosis with more severe dilatation and thinner parenchyma on the right; left renal parenchyma hyperechogenic; massive hydroureter on the right. **d** Anterior cornal pelvic scan: bladder wall thickening (hypertrophy due to an infravesical "valvelike" obstruction). *Note:* the bladder wall is usually thin in prune-belly syndrome.

Vesicoureteral Reflux

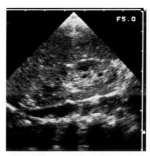
16.38a

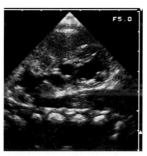
16.38b

◀ **16.35 Posterior urethral valves, reflux-induced right renal rupture, perirenal urinoma, urinary ascites** in a 9-day-old boy with sepsis. **a** Longitudinal pelvic scan: characteristic dilatation and elongation of the prostatic urethral segment; bladder wall thickening, Right flank **b** coronal and **c** transverse scans: moderate perirenal fluid, copious intraperitoneal fluid: urine. **d** VCUG: massive right-sides reflux with perirenal and intraperitoneal contrast accumulation.

16.38 Massive bilateral vesicoureteral reflux in a 4-week-old boy with diarrhea and a urinary tract infection. Right flank coronal scan **a** before and **b** after voiding: progressive hydronephrosis, suggestive of reflux. Confirmed by VCUG (same patient as in Fig. 17.**16**: bladder wall thickening! **DD:** posterior urethral valves). *Note:* massive primary vesicoureteral reflux leads to the compensatory hyperthrophy of the detrusor muscle.

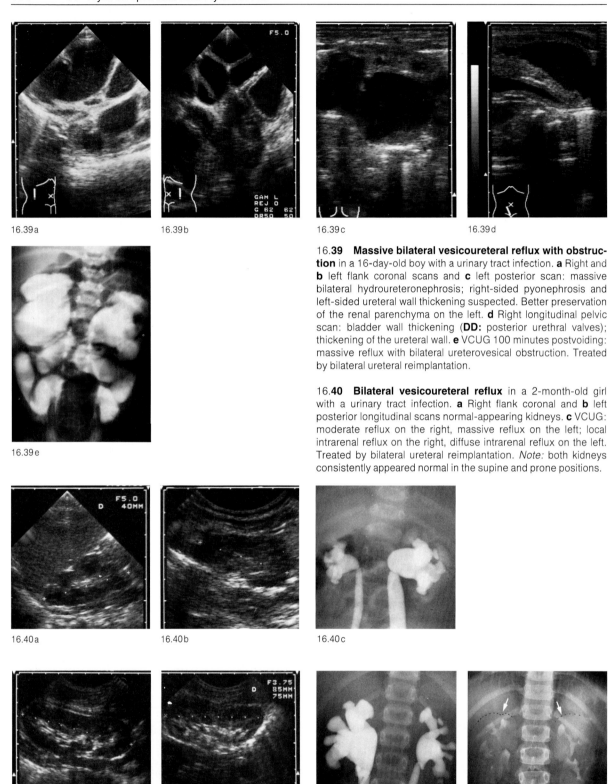

16.39a   16.39b   16.39c   16.39d

16.39e

16.40a   16.40b   16.40c

16.41a   16.41b   16.41c   16.41d

16.**39** **Massive bilateral vesicoureteral reflux with obstruction** in a 16-day-old boy with a urinary tract infection. **a** Right and **b** left flank coronal scans and **c** left posterior scan: massive bilateral hydroureteronephrosis; right-sided pyonephrosis and left-sided ureteral wall thickening suspected. Better preservation of the renal parenchyma on the left. **d** Right longitudinal pelvic scan: bladder wall thickening (**DD:** posterior urethral valves); thickening of the ureteral wall. **e** VCUG 100 minutes postvoiding: massive reflux with bilateral ureterovesical obstruction. Treated by bilateral ureteral reimplantation.

16.**40** **Bilateral vesicoureteral reflux** in a 2-month-old girl with a urinary tract infection. **a** Right flank coronal and **b** left posterior longitudinal scans normal-appearing kidneys. **c** VCUG: moderate reflux on the right, massive reflux on the left; local intrarenal reflux on the right, diffuse intrarenal reflux on the left. Treated by bilateral ureteral reimplantation. *Note:* both kidneys consistently appeared normal in the supine and prone positions.

16.**41** **Massive bilateral vesicoureteral reflux with reflux nephropathy** in a girl of 6 years, 10 months with recurrent urinary tract infections. **a** Left and **b** right posterior longitudinal scans: normal-appearing left kidney, apparent parenchymal reduction at the upper and lower poles of the right kidney. **c** VCUG: massive bilateral reflux, more severe on the right. **d** Three-minute EU: moderate bilateral reflux nephropathy, with severe involvement of the upper poles (arrows). *Note:* "normal" US findings do not exclude reflux or reflux nephropathy.

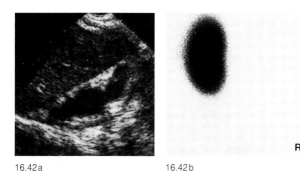
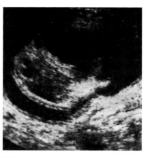

16.42a   16.42b

16.43

16.42 Massive vesicoureteral reflux on the right, anterior urethral valve in a 14-month-old boy referred for right-sided hydronephrosis and urethral stenosis. **a** Right flank coronal scan: massive hydronephrosis; parenchyma intensely echogenic and irregularly thinned, consistent with diffuse fibrosis. **b** Renal scintigram (dimercaptosuccinylic acid), posterior view: nonfunctioning right kidney. Nephroureterectomy performed after a previous urethroplasty. *Note:* intense echogenicity of renal parenchyma implies a poor prognosis in terms of renal function. Function test indicated prior to operation.

16.43 Myelomeningocele with neurogenic bladder and massive bilateral vesicoureteral reflux in a 10-year-old girl. Right pelvic longitudinal scan: hydroureter with a greatly thickened wall. Compensatory hyperthrophy due to massive reflux (bilateral findings); irregular bladder wall contour ("trabeculated bladder"). Partial regression of reflux achieved by intermittent catheterization.

Urolithiasis

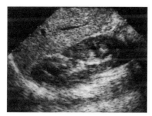
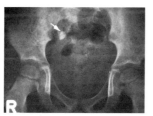
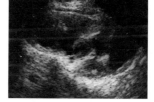
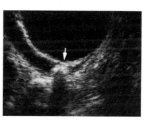

16.44a   16.44b   16.44c   16.44d

16.44 Ureterolithiasis (without malformation) in a boy of 5 years, 8 months with a history of leukocyturia for about 6 months. No urinary tract infection. Normal US scans 3 weeks and 1 week before. **a** Third right flank coronal scan: normal. Questionable distal ureteral calculus (not shown). **b** Radiograph: calcification on the right side (arrow). **c** Right posterior longitudinal scan 3 weeks later: massive hydronephrosis. **d** Right longitudinal pelvic scan: hydroureter; prevesical stone (arrow), "acoustic shadow."

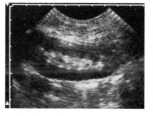
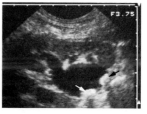

16.45a   16.45b

16.45 Proximal urolithiasis with ureteropelvic stenosis in a girl of 4 years, 5 months with a 3-month history of "abdominal pain." Erythrocyturia, leukocyturia, proteinuria. **a** Left and **b** right posterior longitudinal scans: left side unremarkable, moderate hydronephrosis on the right; relatively large extrarenal pelvis; 2 stones (arrows) with acoustic shadows.

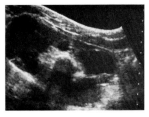
16.46a

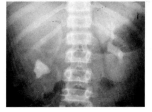
16.46b

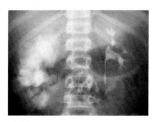
16.46c

16.46   Unilateral urolithiasis, megacalices, and ureteropelvic stenosis in an 11-year-old boy with colicky right flank pain, nocturnal enuresis, and "pyuria." **a** Right posterior longitudinal scan: massive ectasia of the caliceal system; central sonodensity with an acoustic shadow. EU **b** 3 minutes and **c** 45 minutes postcontrast: large "staghorn calculus" in the renal pelvis,

obstructive; megacalices. *Note:* megacalices in themselves do not require surgical treatment; here, associated with ureteropelvic stenosis, there is a true obstruction with calculus formation. Cause/effect relationship unclear. Megacalices predispose to lithiasis.

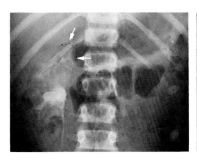
16.47a

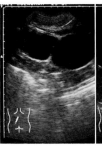
16.47b

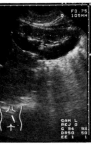
16.47c

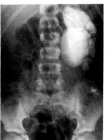
16.47d

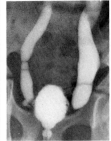
16.47e

16.47   Unilateral urolithiasis and megacalices associated with ipsilateral ureteropelvic stenosis and bilateral reflux in a 12-year-old boy with a urinary tract infection. Abdominal radiograph showed calcifications on the left side. **a** Three-minute EU shows 2 relatively large calcifications laterally, no nephrogram (now or later); parenchymal loss superomedially in the upper pole of the right kidney (arrows). Posterior scans: **b** massive hydronephrosis on left, **c** normal-appearing right kidney. **d**

VCUG: bilateral vesicoureteral reflux, more severe on the left. **e** 3 hours postvoiding: persistent dense opacification of the greatly dilated left pyelocaliceal system. Radionuclide scan showed absence of left renal function. *Note:* ureteropelvic stenosis may be primary, secondary to reflux, or exacerbated by reflux. Prolonged persistence of opacification after reflux suggests absence of "vis a tergo," i.e., a nonfunctioning kidney.

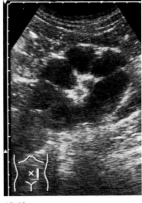
16.48a

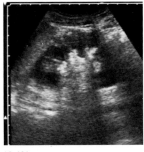
16.48b

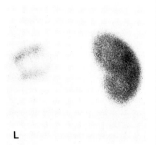
L
16.48c

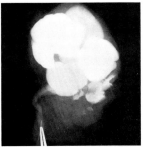
16.48d

16.48   Uro(nephro)lithiasis with pelvoinfundibular hypoplasia in a boy of 14 years, 10 months with a urinary tract infection. **a** Anterior scan: massive hydronephrosis with a "flower" configuration. **b** Left flank coronal scan: numerous central calculi; no pelvis. **c** Renal scintigram (dimercaptosuccinyl-

ic acid): minimal residual "function" with unusual distribution. Nephrectomy. **d** Surgical specimen: contrast filling corresponds to the US pattern. Small pelvis with stenoses at the junction of the calices (infundibulae) and pelvis. Histology: severe chronic pyelonephritis.

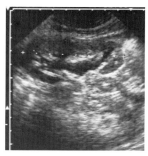

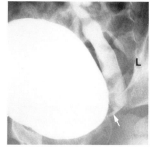

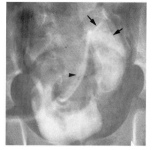

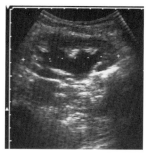

16.49a   16.49b   16.49c   16.49d

16.49 Missed urolithiasis with primary obstructive megaureter in a 19-month-old boy with a recurrent *Proteus mirabilis* urinary tract infection. **a** Left posterior longitudinal scan: mild to moderate hydronephrosis. VCUG (not shown) interpreted as reflux into the distal segment of the megaureter. **b** EU, 30 minutes: characteristic of primary megaureter; normal-caliber distal segment (arrow). Surgical correction: mobilization of the ureter, distal resection, and reimplantation by the Cohen technique. **c** Early postoperative 70-minute EU: evidence of residual ureteral ectasia; ureteral stone surrounded by contrast (→), missed; suprapubic catheter (▼). Four months later: **d** left posterior longitudinal scan: progressive hydronephrosis. **e** Transverse pelvic scan: left ureteral calculus (arrow). **f** Abdominal radiograph (detail): confirms missed left ureteral calculus. Secondary operative removal. *Note:* stone misinterpreted as reflux on VCUG; preliminary abdominal radiograph not obtained.

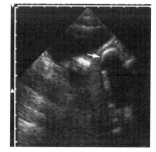

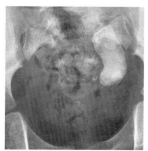

16.49e   16.49f

17 Bladder Wall Changes

U. V. Willi

Bladder wall changes, aside from certain diverticular formations, are demonstrated far better with ultrasound than with conventional radiographic techniques. As a general rule, sonography should be the initial procedure for evaluating the urinary bladder. Bladder wall thickening are *often morphologically nonspecific*, in which case their interpretation remains speculative. However, ultrasound will sometimes permit the morphologic differentiation of the mucosa and detrusor muscle, especially when newer instruments are used. The history and clinical picture (age; pollakiuria, dysuria, possibly hematuria; usually no fever) in patients with general bladder wall thickening are suggestive of (chronic) cystitis, and this is often confirmed by response to long-term antibiotic treatment or perhaps by cystoscopy, which generally is not indicated. But even with chronic cystitis, bladder wall thickening may have a *complex etiology* in which mucosal swelling results from the inflammation itself while muscular thickening represents detrusor hypertrophy due perhaps to a coexisting dyssynergia between the detrusor and external sphincter muscles. In other cases there may be an infravesical obstruction (posterior uretheral valves in males) leading to detrusor hypertrophy with an associated cystitis that results in mucosal swelling.

The highly chronic nature of some cystitides is frequently associated with chronic constipation (generally in girls about 4–8 years of age). When bladder wall thickening is noted in these cases, we recommend temporarily withholding uroradiologic procedures (voiding cystourethrography, VCUG). If the kidneys appear normal, as they usually do, a uroradiologic study after normalization of the bladder wall is usually negative or unnecessary.

Bladder wall thickening tends to be general and regular but may occasionally be local or irregular, depending on the cause.

As in other areas of pediatric radiology, the presence of bladder wall changes (thickening) raises differential diagnostic issues of inflammation/infection, infiltration/tumor, malformation, metabolic process, trauma/iatrogenesis, or anatomic/functional variant. The response to *inflammatory mucosal processes* can vary greatly and is occasionally extreme. The causative agents may be infectious (bacterial, viral, fungal, parasitic) as well as chemical (toxic) or physical (mechanical).

Hypertrophy of the detrusor muscle is usually the result of increased muscular effort, which my in turn result from an anatomic (posterior urethral valves in males) or functional infravesical obstruction (neurogenic bladder) or from abnormally frequent ("aberrant") micturition associated with primary vesicoureteral reflux or a large-volume bladder diverticulum.

Infiltrative bladder wall changes may be inflammatory or neoplastic in nature (eosinophilic cystitis, TB, septic granulomatosis; leukemia, lymphoma; neurofibromatosis, etc.).

Local bladder wall changes include primary (possibly associated), secondary, and iatrogenic diverticula, ureteroceles, urachal remnants, and polypoid lesions.

The normal range of variation of bladder wall thickness is thought to be quite large. Redundant mucosa after voiding in a previously overdistended bladder is apt to create the impression of "wall thickening" and should be distinguished from a pathologic process. Marked variability of bladder wall thickness can also be seen in abnormal conditions (e. g., cystitis, Fig. 17.**7**; hypertrophy, Fig. 17.**24**). The accentuation of bladder wall tickness in the presence of free intraperitoneal or retroperitoneal fluid, especially blood resulting from abdominal trauma, is not well understood. Is the phenomenon a normal finding due to simultaneous intravesical and extravesical delineation of the bladder wall, or does it represent a true morphologic correlate of pathophysiologic change, possibly relating to differences in intravesical and extravesical osmolarity?

The difficulty of *evaluating the quality and thickness of the bladder wall* varies with the degree of bladder distention. Hence the evaluation relies more on diagnostic circumspection (assessing the situation at the time of examination in the light of the history and clinical presentation) and the personal experience of the examiner than on a straightforward comparison of bladder wall thickness with a scale. An overdistended bladder can make diagnosis impossible; this pertains both to the bladder wall itself and to any abnormality in close proximity to the urinary bladder (see, for example, Fig. 5.**30**).

The "double chambered bladder" is a typical finding in smaller children and should not be mistaken for a urachal remnant (Fig. 17.**9b**).

The simple urodynamic workup (uroflowmetry and pelvic floor electromyography using painless perineal surface electrodes) is an easily performed adjunctive study in cooperative children (generally older than 4–5 years of age). A urodynamic study is recommended in some patients with "refractory chronic cystitis" and may disclose a functional correlate for the morphologic bladder wall thickening (Fig. 17.**10c**).

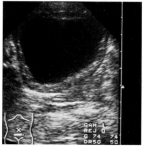

17.1

17.1 Cystitis in a 7½-year-old girl with recurrent urinary tract infections, no fever. Transverse scan: thickened bladder mucosa (4–6 mm) within a normal-appearing, less echogenic muscular layer. Bladder volume approximately 55 mL. Normal kidney duplex renal system on the left. Due to bladder wall thickening, VCUG was not performed. Findings 3 months later were unchanged, implying chronic cystitis. Suggestion of external sphincter acivity during micturition (dysfunctional).

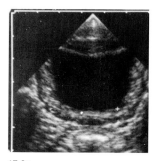
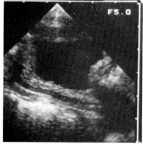

17.2a   17.2b

17.2 Cystitis in a girl of 6 years, 2 months with celiac disease in remission. Recurrent urinary tract infections, no fever. **a** Transverse and **b** longitudinal scans: thickening of the mucosa (approximately 5 mm), normal-appearing muscular layer (1–2 mm). Bladder volume approximately 15 mL. Kidneys appear normal. Findings consistent with cystitis. Urodynamic tests normal. VCUG at 5 years, 11 months showed small bladder diverticulum, no reflux, and slight bladder wall thickening.

17.3 Cystitis in a girl of 6 years, 7 months. Recurrent urinary tract infections, no fever; pollakiuria; secondary enuresis. **a, b** Transverse and longitudinal scans: thickened mucosa (5–7 mm) with the bladder almost empty (approximately 9 mL); muscular layer appears normal. **c, d** Repeat scans 5 months later: similar findings, relatively less acute due to moderate bladder distention (approximately 27 mL). Kidneys still normal. Findings consistent with cystitis.

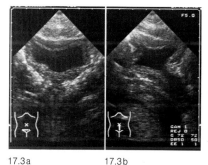

17.3a   17.3b   17.3c   17.3d

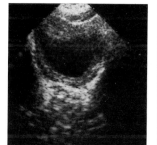
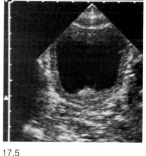

17.4   17.5

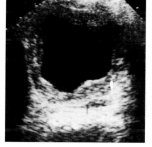
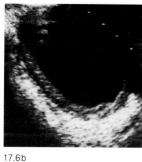

17.6a   17.6b

17.4 Hemorrhagic cystitis in an 8-year-old boy with a urinary tract infection and repeated episodes of acute, gross terminal hematuria; dysuria. Vague suspicion of a urethral polyp. Transverse scan: moderate bladder wall thickening, presumably mucosal. Bladder volume approximately 10 mL. Kidneys normal. Subsequent VCUG showed a small bladder diverticulum on the right and a normal-appearing urethra. Remission of cystitis achieved with antibiotic treatment.

17.5 Hemorrhagic cystitis in a boy of 4 years, 9 months with a 1-day history of pollakiuria, dysuria, and hematuria (small amount of blood at the end of micturition). Acute urinary tract infection, no fever. Transverse scan: diffuse bladder wall thickening; mucosa and muscularis not clearly distinguishable. Local "tumorous" lesion centrally above the trigone: polyp? Bladder volume approximately 40 mL. Kidneys normal. Symptoms and bladder changes regressed with antibiotic treatment. No further uroradiologic evaluation.

17.6 Hemorrhagic cystitis in an 8½-year-old girl who underwent nephrectomy at the age of 6 years, 4 months for a Wilms tumor with concomitant excision of a solitary hepatic metastasis. Vincristine-induced polyneuropathy, transient. Admitted with dysuria and hematuria. **a** Transverse and **b** longitudinal scans: diffuse bladder wall thickening; mucosa and muscularis not clearly distinguishable. Bladder volume approximately 70 mL. Solitary right kidney with compensatory enlargement. Findings and course consistent with hemorrhagic cystitis.

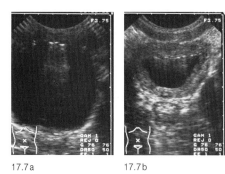

17.7a   17.7b

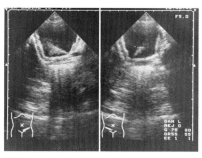

17.8

17.7 Cystitis in a 9-year-old girl with recurrent urinary tract infections apparently unrelated to earlier constipation. Secondary enuresis (psychogenic?). US at 8 years, 8 months showed bladder wall thickening. Reexamined now following 3 months' antibiotic treatment. US after VCUG (no reflux) **a** with approximately 135 mL bladder volume: bladder wall thickening poorly demonstrated, intravesical air (anterior); **b** with approximately 7 mL bladder volume after voiding: mucosa about 1 cm thick, persistence of intravesical air. Kidneys normal. Findings consistent with cystitis. Catheter specimen obtained at VCUG showed an active urinary tract infection. *Note* the marked variability of mucosal swelling with different degrees of bladder filling.

17.8 Cystitis in a girl of 9 years, 4 months with recurrent urinary tract infections. **a, b** Slightly oblique transverse scans on the left and right: diffuse mucosal thickening to approximately 5 mm. Prominent urine jet from the left and right ureterovesical orifices, presumably reflecting increased outflow resistance due to active ureteral peristalsis. Not shown: bilateral intermittent ureteral ectasia with no caliceal dilation; normal kidneys. Bladder volume approximately 60 mL. Findings consistent with cystitis.

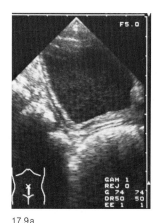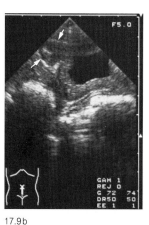

17.9a   17.9b

17.9 Cystitis in a 4½-year-old girl with recurrent febrile urinary tract infections. **a** Longitudinal scan with approximately 50 mL bladder volume: mucosal thickness approximately 3−4 mm (intravesical echoes probably artifacts). **b** Repeat scan 5 weeks later with a bladder volume of 4mL: mucosal thickness approximately 6−7 mm. Each presentation consistent with cystitis. Kidneys unremarkable. VCUG at the age of 4 years, 9 months showed mild bilateral reflux. *Note:* empty, collapsed bladder fundus in **b** (arrows; "double chambered" pediatric bladder).

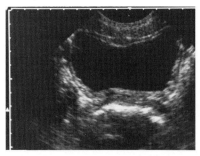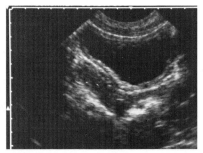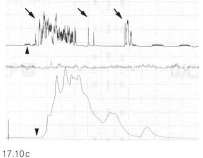

17.10a   17.10b   17.10c

17.10 Chronic cystitis with voiding dysfunction in a 12½-year-old girl. Primary enuresis at the age of 4 years, secondary enuresis later on. Presented with a 3-year history of recurrent urinary tract infections, no fever, intermittent dysuria. **a** Transverse and **b** longitudinal scan: mucosal thickening of approximately 3−5 mm consistent with cystitis. Bladder volume approximately 70 mL. Kidneys normal. **c** Urodynamic study shows abnormal pelvic floor (external sphincteric) activity (→) during voiding (▼ start of voiding): classic pattern with detrusor-external sphincter dyssynergia. Successfully managed by micturition training (instruction), diazepam, and antibiotics. **c** Upper trace: pelvic floor activity; middle trace: no abdominal wall activity; lower trace: flow rate. 1 unit of the abscissa = 2.5 seconds; 1 unit on the ordinate = 5 mL/s (relative shift of 2.5 seconds between the upper and lower traces).

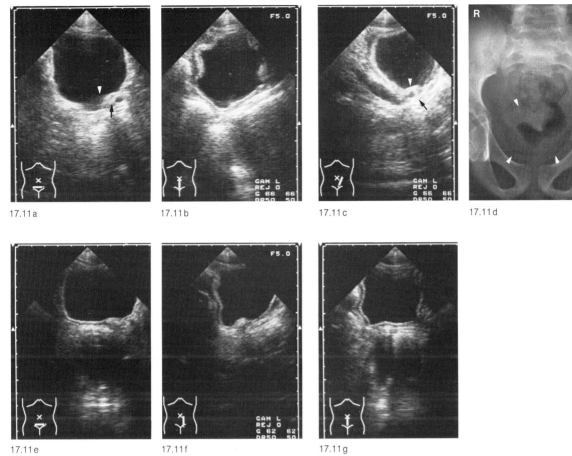

17.11a 17.11b 17.11c 17.11d

17.11e 17.11f 17.11g

17.11 Schistosomiasis of the urinary tract (*Schistosoma haematobium*) in a boy of 9 years, 2 months who lived in South Africa until the age of 9. Gross hematuria, slight pollakiuria, no dysuria. **a–c** Scans show irregular thickening of hyperechogenic bladder mucosa (▼); similar wall change may involve the prevesical and/or intramural part of the left ureter (→) with an obstructive effect; left hydroureter and hydronephrosis (not shown). Bladder shape distorted; volume approximately 55 mL. **d** Plain radiograph: mucosal calcification (▼). **e–g** Repeat scans 3½ months later: persistent, probably calcified mucosal change, regressive in thickness. Granulomatous residue about the left ureteral orifice, now without obstruction. Bladder shape still irregular; volume approximately 40 mL. Clinically asymptomatic.

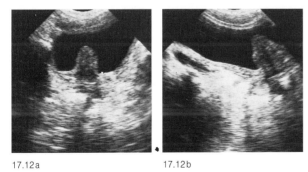

17.12a 17.12b

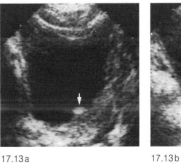
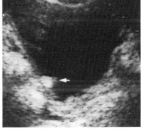

17.13a 17.13b

17.12 Tumorous eosinophilic cystitis in a 1-year-old girl with an interlabial mass. Prolapsing ureterocele? **a** Transverse and **b** longitudinal scans show a solid mass projecting into the bladder from the trigone, with a loss of clear differentiation of the bladder wall layers; possible involvement of the bladder margin. VCUG showed an intravesical mass, consistent with US findings, prolapsed into the urethra on voiding. No reflux. **DD:** rhabdomyosarcoma, leiomyosarcoma, etc. Biopsy: tumor-forming eosinophilic cystitis. Gradual resolution with Bactrim (co-trimoxazole) therapy.

17.13 Suture granuloma in a girl 6 years, 9 months of age, 3 months after bilateral ureteral reimplantation (Cohen) for reflux. Uncomplicated course. **a** Transverse and **b** longitudinal scans: suture granuloma (arrow) at the newly constructed orifice of the right ureter (transposed to the left).

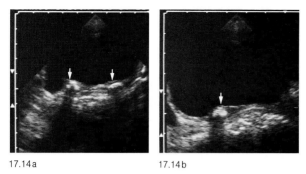

17.14a   17.14b

17.14   Bilateral submucous Teflon deposits in a girl 6 years, 5 months of age, 1 day after bilateral submucous Teflon (polytetrafluoroethylene) injections for bilateral vesicoureteral reflux. **a** Transverse and **b** right longitudinal scans: submucous Teflon deposits (arrows) with acoustic shadows, more prominent on the right. Deposits have a tendency to contract and form granulomatous residue.

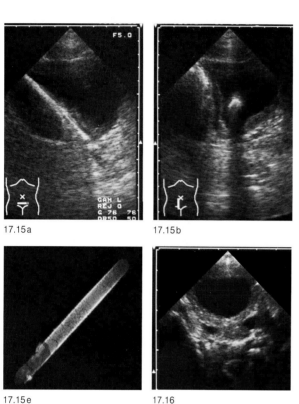

17.15a   17.15b

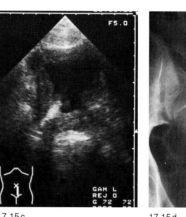

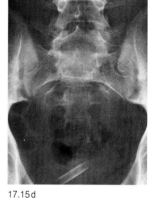

17.15c   17.15d

17.15e   17.16

17.15   Cystitis due to a foreign body (intravesical calcified plastic rod inserted transurethrally) in a 15-year-old boy with about a 5-month history of occasional burning on micturition. Pollakiuria. Later, episodes of gross hematuria. Antibiotics given for a presumed urinary tract infection. Referred for US due to recurrence. **a** Transverse and **b, c** longitudinal scans (right, left): hyperechogenic, rod-shaped foreign body with an acoustic shadow; irregular thickening of the bladder wall, possibly involving the mucosa and muscular layer, more pronounced on the left due presumably to greater irritation on the left side. **d** Radiograph: cylindrical calcific density. Operatively removed by the transvesical route. **e** Specimen radiograph: calcium shell damaged with forceps at the operation.

17.16   Compensatory bladder wall hypertrophy with massive bilateral reflux (associated with cystitis?) in a 4-week-old boy with a urinary tract infection and fever. Transverse sonogram (postvoid): thickening of the bladder wall (approximately 4 mm with a volume of about 12 mL), wall layers not separately defined; bilateral hydroureter. Massive bilateral hydronephrosis (not shown). **DD:** posterior urethral valves with or without unilateral or bilateral reflux; possible obstruction of ureterovesical drainage. VCUG showed massive bilateral reflux with a normal urethra. *Note:* especially in patients with massive primary reflux, the constant recirculation of urine can lead both to detrusor hypertrophy and to its dilatation with secondary bladder enlargement (same patient as in Fig. 16.**38**).

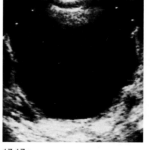

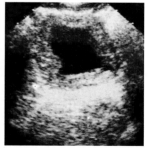

17.17a   17.17b

17.17   Persistent detrusor hypertrophy following reflux in a boy of 5 years, 7 months who at 3 years, 4 months underwent a left nephrectomy for extreme reflux nephropathy with no residual renal function and right ureteral reimplantation (Cohen) for presumed primary megaureter. Known detrusor hypertrophy. Transverse scans with **a** approximately 110 mL bladder volume and **b** approximately 6 mL volume: wall of distended bladder appears normal; mild bilateral ureteral ectasia (residual ureteral stump on the left); postvoid scan shows diffuse bladder wall thickening (approximately 9 mm).

17.18 Posterior urethral valves, bilateral reflux, left-sided infrarenal urinoma. Fetal sonograms taken at 17 weeks were normal. Oligohydramnios. "Cystic change in the left kidney" noted 1 day before birth (premature) at 34 weeks. **a** Left flank coronal scan on the 1st day of life: moderately full urinary bladder with a thickened wall (▼); large cystic lesion in the left hemiabdomen: infrarenal or pararenal urinoma; hydronephrotic left upper pole (→). **b** VCUG at 6 days: trabeculated bladder; bilateral reflux, on the left massive and diffuse intrarenal; left ureter displaced to the right by a left infrarenal urinoma. Posterior urethral valves (poorly shown here). Urography showed unsatisfactory left renal function; radionuclide scan at 13 months showed no function on the left side. Creatinine variable in the 1st month of life, 70–185 mmol/L, later becoming high normal: 58 mmol/L at 4 years.

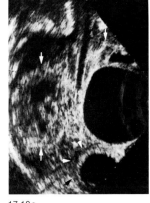 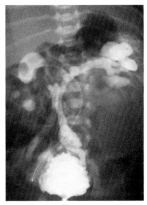

17.18a   17.18b

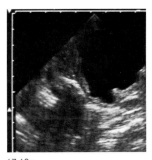 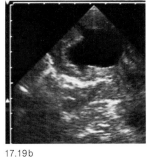

17.19a   17.19b

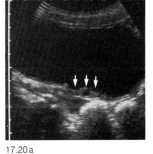 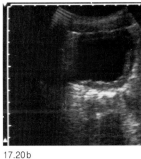

17.20a   17.20b

17.19 Status following posterior urethral valves complicated by right-sided reflux in a boy of 16 years, 3 months who previously underwent a left nephrectomy. Moderate, stable renal failure (creatinine 200 mmol/L). Longitudinal scan **a** with approximately 60 mL bladder volume: irregular inner bladder contour, similar mucosal and muscular thickness (each about 2 mm); **b** with approximately 20 mL bladder volume: mucosal thickness a similar, muscular layer now about 8–9 mm = hypertrophy (residual and/or compensatory hypertrophy due to reflux?).

17.20 Neurogenic bladder in a boy of 8 years, 7 months misdiagnosed elsewhere with "bladder neck stenosis," prompting two unnecessary transurethral resections; absence of S4 and S5 segments not noted in 7 uroradiologic examinations. **a** Longitudinal scan with approximately 150 mL bladder volume: trabeculation of the bladder wall with pseudodiverticula (arrows); **b** transverse scan with approximately 25 mL volume: muscular layer 5–8 mm thick = hypertrophy (pseudodiverticula not visible on contraction). Neurogenic dysfunction with an anatomic cause diagnosed at the age of 8 years, 7 months. Micturition improved greatly with medical treatment.

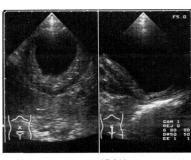 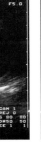 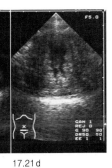 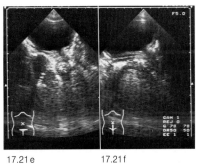

17.21a   17.21b   17.21c   17.21d   17.21e   17.21f

17.21 Suspected physical cystitis. Enuresis. Suspected intermittent overflow incontinence. Mildly stenosing concentric stricture of the posterior urethra. Endoscopic dilation to 14 Fr restored normal micturition. Transverse and longitudinal follow-up scans **a, b** with approximately 30 mL bladder volume and **c, d** with 0 or 1–2 mL volume: massive thickening of the mucosa. No hematuria, no dysuria! Effect of the irrigating fluid during cystoscopy? Malfunction of "cold" fiberoptic light during cystoscopy? Etiology remains unclear. **e, f** Scans 3½ weeks later with a bladder volume of approximately 25–30 mL: significant regression of mucosal change. Clinically symptomatic.

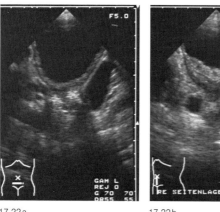
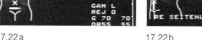
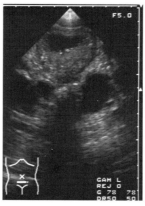
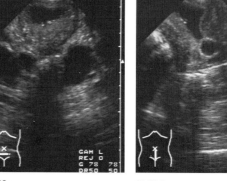

17.22a   17.22b   17.22c   17.22d

17.22 Suspected physical (and chemical?) cystitis in an 8-year-old boy with posterior urethral valves diagnosed at age 7. Massive reflux, severe left-sided reflux nephropathy. Right kidney very small, supicious for reflux nephropathy/dysplasia. Urethral stricture following the resection of valves. **a** Transverse scan: moderate bladder wall thickening; massive ureteral ectasia on the left, mild on the right. Five days after the second valve resection: dysuria, hematuria, right flank pain. **b** Longitudinal scan: extreme mucosal swelling in the trigone region (constant in the right lateral decubitus); massive hydroureters (each with hydronephrosis), presumably obstructive. **c** Transverse and **d** longitudinal scans 3 days later: progression of mucosal swelling, diffuse; balloon catheter. Suspected electrocauterization of the mucosa by increased conductivity of the bladder irrigating fluid (antiseptic agent).

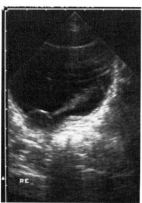
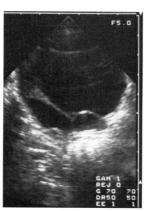

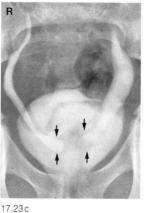
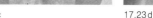
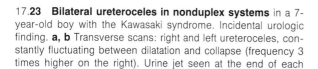

17.23a   17.23b   17.23c   17.23d

17.23 Bilateral ureteroceles in nonduplex systems in a 7-year-old boy with the Kawasaki syndrome. Incidental urologic finding. **a, b** Transverse scans: right and left ureteroceles, constantly fluctuating between dilatation and collapse (frequency 3 times higher on the right). Urine jet seen at the end of each dilatation phase, followed by an emptying of the sac. EU 15 minutes after i.v. contrast injection: **c** ureteroceles (arrows); **d** upper urinary tract, mild ureteral dilation on the right, moderate hydronephrosis/hydroureter on the left (same patient as in Fig. 16.**22**).

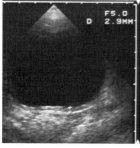
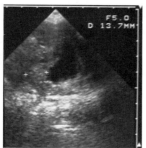

17.24a   17.24b

17.24 Dynamics of bladder wall thickening in a boy of 6 years, 10 months, diagnosed at the age of 4 with embryonic prostatic rhabdomyosarcoma, who presented with acute urinary retention. Subtotal resection, chemotherapy; good course. **a** Transverse follow-up scan with approximately 120 mL bladder volume: moderate bladder wall thickening. **b** Londitudinal post-voiding scan with approximately 3–4 mL bladder volume gives the impression of a massive bladder wall thickening: residual hypertrophy, possibly complex with mucosal involvement? (same patient as in Fig. 5.**30**).

References

Berger, R. M., M. Maizels, G. C. Moran, J. J. Conway, C. F. Firlit: Bladder capacity (ounces) equals age (years) plus 2 predicts normal bladder capacity and aids in diagnosis of abnormal voiding patterns. J. Urol. 129 (1983) 347–349

Hernanz-Schulman, M., R. L. Lebowitz: The elusiveness and importance of bladder diverticula in children. Pediat. Radiol. 15 (1985) 399–402

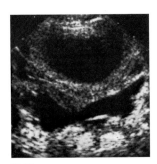

17.25

17.25 Acute lymphatic leukemia in a girl 8 years, 7 months of age. Abdominal evaluation. Transverse scan: moderate amount of free intraperitoneal fluid. Moderate bladder wall thickening, diffuse; leukemic bladder wall infiltrate suspected. Also hepatomegaly and mild nephromegaly. All findings normalized with chemotherapy.

18 Pediatric Gynecologic Problems

U. V. Willi

Information on the patient's *history* (family, growth, menstruation, diseases), on the *clinical manifestations* (general findings, secondary sexual characteristics, findings of the gynecologic examination), and often on the *laboratory results* (vaginal cytology, possibly hormonal and chromosome studies and hand X-ray) is necessary for a meaningful interpretation of ultrasound findings. Sonograms can demonstrate the presence, size, shape, and structure of the uterus and ovaries, confirm gestation as early as 2–3 weeks, and reveal genital and extragenital abnormalities. Moderate (not massive) distention of the urinary bladder is an essential technical prerequisite for a successful examination. The neonatal uterus is often relatively large (3.5–5 cm long) and has a prominent endometrial echo due to the influence of maternal hormones. During the first months of life the neonatal uterus assumes the infantile shape and size, retaining them until the age of 7–8 years (thin, 2.5–3 cm long). The cervix and isthmus at this stage make up more than half the organ. The uterine volume gradually increases 2–3 years before the onset of puberty, and this growth accelerates during puberty. Thus, uterine growth appears to be strictly age-dependent in the prepubertal period but becomes both age- and hormone-dependent during puberty. The greatest growth occurs in the fundus and corpus, imparting the characteristic pear shape to the postpubescent organ (length 6–8 cm). The endometrial echo becomes prominent, acquiring a thickness of several millimeters during the secretory (premenstrual) phase. Growth (maturation) of the ovaries appears to proceed at a continuous rate from the first years of life, showing a dependence on age but not on hormonal stimulation. Average ovarian volumes of 1 mL have been measured at 2 years, and 2 mL at 12 years. The average volume of a mature ovary is 3–6 mL. The small cystic elements in the ovaries of small children and the larger cysts that occur with some requency at puberty may result from low-level intermittent secretions of gonadotropins, perhaps before other signs of puberty are observed. While "functional" cysts of this kind can easily lead to overestimation of ovarian size, they should not be interpreted as an expression of ovarian "dysfunction." Often their clinical significance remains unclear despite hormonal tests.

Indications for "gynecologic" sonography in girls are:

Disturbances of puberty (unusual or abnormal pubertal development). *Precocious puberty* (premature appearance of secondary sexual characteristics and menarche) may be partial or complete, isosexual or heterosexual. True precocious puberty is isosexual, while precocious pseudopuberty may be either isosexual or heterosexual. The true form is usually idiopathic and is less commonly caused by neoplastic, malformative, postinflammatory, or posttraumatic (usually intracranial) processes, endocrinologic disorders, or phakomatoses. Isosexual precocious puberty may be provoked by exposure to exogenous or endogenous estrogens, the heterosexual form by virilizing tumors of the ovary or adrenal cortex or by congenital adrenal hyperplasia (AGS). Appreciable uterine growth signifies a hormonal effect and is the hallmark of true precocious puberty. *Delayed puberty* is often constitutional or may result from systemic disease. Hypo- or hypergonadotropic (Turner syndrome: infantile uterus, rudimentary ovaries) hypogonadism are potential causes.

Disturbances of menstruation. In patients with *primary amenorrhea* and well-developed secondary sexual characteristics, an organic lesion must be excluded: hymenal atresia, various grades of vaginal and/or uterine atresia (even if the vagina appears normal externally). Hematocolpos and hematometrocolpos are possible with partial vaginal atresia, vaginal septum, hymenal atresia/septum, or simple labial adherence. Potential causes of primary amenorrhea include Rokitansky–Küster–Mayer syndrome (absence of the uterus with variable vaginal hypoplasia) and peripheral androgen resistance ("testicular feminization"). Primary and *secondary amenorrhea* can result from anorexia. Uterine size and volume appear to change with body weight (relative smallness/thinness of uterus). Clinical rule of thumb: in patients with secondary amenorrhea due to anorexia with weight loss, menstruation usually does not resume until the patient has reached the body weight she had while still menstruating. The most important condition to be excluded in secondary amenorrhea is intrauterine or ectopic pregnancy (with or without a pelvic mass and/or abdominopelvic pain).

Other disturbances of menstruation are: *menorrhagia* or hypermenorrhea (excessive bleeding), *polymenorrhea* (too frequent bleeding), *oligomenorrhea* (too infrequent bleeding), and *metrorrhagia* (bleeding between menstrual periods). Episodes of "functional" menorrhagia or metrorrhagia occur in approximately 5% of girls during the first 2 years after menarche. Rare organic causes of these conditions are infectious or neoplastic processes involving the vagina, uterus or ovaries, bleeding anomalies (von Willebrand's disease), or pregnancy. In the rare cases of primary (first 6–12 months after menarche) *dysmenorrhea* (painful menstruation), an organic cause must be excluded.

Possible causes of later (secondary) dysmenorrhea are genital tract infections or endometriosis. Psychological factors are frequency involved in these cases.

Genital anomalies (frequently undiagnosed in newborn girls). More often than hydrocolpos/hydrometrocolpos in neonates, hematocolpos/hematometrocolpos in postmenarchal females is manifested by pain, pelvic mass, abnormal vaginal discharge, and possibly meno-/metrorrhagia in the presence of uterine duplication. Rokitansky−Küster−Mayer syndrome and peripheral androgen resistance are counted among the genital anomalies. Some malformations are discovered in the course of a uro(radio)logic evaluation. Duplication anomalies of the uterus, with or without vaginal duplication, result from failure of normal fusion of the müllerian ducts (paramesonephric duct). This may be primary (with normal development of the cloaca, abdominal wall and urinary tract) or secondary (with persistence of the cloaca and/or bladder exstrophy, possibly with cloacal exstrophy, or ureteral ectopy; each of these structures appears able to interfere with fusion of the müllerian ducts). Unilateral occlusion in a duplex uterus (with possible vaginal duplication) is consistently associated with an abnormal ipsilateral upper urinary tract, usually with renal agenesis, and less frequently with ipsilateral ureteral ectopy. An even less common differential diagnosis is ectopic ureteral insertion into a Gartner (wolffian) duct, associated with renal hypoplasia. This condition can mimic hydrocolpos or unilateral vaginal obstruction in a duplication anomaly (as described above) on sonograms.

Interlabial masses often can be differentiated by clinical observation. An ectopic ureter protruding into the vagina must be distinguished from a ureterocele protruding into the urethra. In acute cases the latter is pink or light red in color, whereas a chronic ureterocele is dark and livid due to impaired perfusion; it may be similar in form to a closed hymenal septum, which has a more whitish color due to retention of mucoid fluid. Paraurethral and vulvar cysts are eccentrically located and tend to be smaller in size. A prolapsed urethra is identifiable by its central meatus. Rhabdomyosarcoma (sarcoma botryoides) may arise vaginally or vesicourethrally and has a glass-bead or grape-like appearance.

Pelvic masses can be classified in various ways: genital or extragenital, cystic or solid, neonatal or postneonatal, etc. Only mass lesions of the *ovaries, uterus,* and *vagina* or prerectal masses specific to the female pelvis are illustrated here (see chapter 5: Abdominal Masses). On the list of possible *cystic* abdominopelvic masses, including a large urinary bladder, ovarian cysts (with or without hemorrhage), hydro(metro)colpos, and hemato(metro)colpos are relatively common. Even more common are cystic changes of follicles or a corpus luteum, although these do not often present as a mass. Ovarian teratomas may be cystic or solid but are usually mixed (cystic−solid). Though usually benign, a teratoma in a young girl is more likely to be malignant than one in an adult female (benign dermoid cyst). *Solid ovarian tumors* are less common in girls, are usually malignant, and many can be curatively treated. They are either *germ cell tumors*—seminoma (dysgerminoma), teratoma (differentiated and/or malignant, yolk sac tumor)—or *non−germ cell tumors*—stromal tumor (granulosa theca cell tumor, Sertoli cell tumor, etc.), tumor of unknown origin (possibly endocrine). A cystic mass in the adnexal region may respresent a paraovarian cyst,

a fimbrial cyst, or a hydrosalpinx (occasionally bilateral). The possibility of an ectopic pregnancy should also be considered. Gonadal tumors associated with peripheral androgen resistance generally develop after adolescence and are initially benign (e. g., Sertoli cell tumor). A rhabdomyosarcoma may arise from the uterus, vagina, or bladder. A fast-growing solid tumor can be difficult to assign sonographically to a specific organ because of its proximity to surrounding structures. With a sacrococcygeal (retrorectal) teratoma or neuroblastoma, direct or indirect involvement of the genital organs is occasionally seen. Due to the potential for urinary tract involvement by a pelvic tumor, excretory urography (EU) is often indicated as a simple and reliable routine investigation (after exclusion of pregnancy). A plain abdominal survey radiograph should be obtained whenever there is a question of a pelvic mass (see the introduction to chapter 5).

Vaginal bleeding (prepubertal) is relatively uncommon, and about half of cases are caused by a vaginal infection with or without a foreign body within the vagina. Vaginal bleeding clearly illustrates the importance of the clinical examination (including inspection of the vulva and urethral metaus, rectal examination, and vaginoscopy with a smear for cytology and bacteriology). Other possible etiologies are: vaginal trauma, urethral prolapse, cervical polyp, vaginal tumor (rhabdomyosarcoma), the rare adenocarcinoma of the cervix or vagina (prenatal exposure to diethylstilbestrol), increased exposure to endogenous or exogenous estrogen (isolated menstruation; precocious puberty; idiopathic or in the McCune−Albright syndrome). An ovarian tumor with vaginal bleeding is thought to be extremely rare.

Abdominopelvic pain, pelvic inflammatory disease. Inflammatory, posttraumatic, postoperative, neoplastic, and malformative processes and dysfunctions of the gastrointestinal or urogenital tract are potential causes of abdominopelvic pain. Cystic or solid neoplastic changes of the ovaries or adnexa and lesions of the uterus can cause varying degrees of *pain* regardless of their etiology (functional, inflammatory, malformative, neoplastic, posttraumatic). An ordinary ovarian cyst with torsion or hemorrhage (chocolate cyst); follicular, corpus luteum, paraovarian or fimbrial cysts; hydro-, pyo-, and hematosalpinx; as well as intrauterine or ectopic pregnancy may be causative. Torsion of the adnexa and/or ovary is usually very painful and is signaled by adnexal or ovarian enlargement (venous stasis) or an unusual position of these structures. Ovaries with chronic torsion may additonally manifest cysts of varying size, especially at the organ periphery. The term "pelvic inflammatory disease" (PID) is used by some to denote venereal disease; however, gonorrhea frequently produces nonspecific sonographic changes: hypoechogenic uterine or adnexal structures with ill-defined margins, adnexal mass (hydrosalpinx or pyosalpinx), pelvic abscess, or "disorganized pelvic structures" with (unilateral) abdominal wall swelling. Endometriosis and uterine myoma appear to be very infrequent causes of pain in girls.

References

Gilsanz, V., R. H. Cleveland: Duplication of the Muellerian ducts and genitourinary malformations, Part I. Radiology 144 (1982) 793–796

Gilsanz, V., R. H. Cleveland, B. S. Reid: Duplication of the Muellerian ducts and genitourinary malformations, Part II. Radiology 144 (1982) 797–801

Hall, D. A., L. E. Hann, J. T. Ferrucci, E. B. Black, B. S. Braitman, W. F. Crowley, N. Nikrui, J. A. Kelley: Sonographic morphology of the normal menstrual cycle. Radiology 133 (1979) 185–188

Hays, D. M., H. Shimada, R. B. Raney, M. Tefft, W. Newton, W. M. Crist, W. Lawrence, A. Ragab, H. M. Maurer: Sarcomas of the vagina and uterus: the intergroup rhabdomyosarcoma study. J. pediat. Surg. 20 (1985) 718–724

Lucraft, H. H.: Ovarian tumors in children – a review of 40 cases. Clin. Radiol. 30 (1979) 279–285

Nussbaum, A., R. L. Lebowitz: Interlabial masses in little girls: review and imaging recommendations. Amer. J. Roentgenol. 141 (1983) 65–71

Nussbaum, A. R., R. C. Sanders, M. D. Jones: Neonatal uterine morphology as seen on real-time US. Radiology 160 (1986) 641–643

Nussbaum, A. R., R. C. Sanders, D. S. Hartman, D. L. Dudgeon, T. H. Parmley: Neonatal ovarian cysts: sonographic-pathologic correlation. Radiology 168 (1988) 817–821

Paniel, B. J., J. B. Truc, J. M. Beuzit, C. Pelissier, Ph. Poitout: Diagnostic des malformations congénitales de la vulve et du vagin. Ann. pédiat. 34 (1987) 11–25

Salardi, S., L. F. Orsini, E. Cacciari, L. Bovicelli, P. Tassoni, A. Reggiani: Pelvic ultrasonography in premenarcheal girls: relation to puberty and sex hormone concentrations. Arch. Dis. Childh. 60 (1985) 120–125

Stanhope, R., J. Adams, H. S. Jacobs, C. G. D. Brook: Ovarian ultrasound assessment in normal children, idiopathic precocious puberty, and during low dose pulsatile gonadotropin releasing hormone treatment of hypogonadotrophic hypogonadism. Arch. Dis. Childh. 60 (1985) 116–119

Yeh, H.-C., W. Futterweit, J. C. Thornton: Polycystic ovarian disease: US features in 104 patients. Radiology 163 (1987) 111–116

Introduction

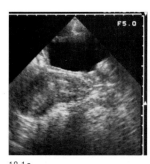
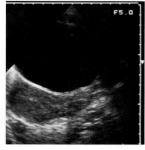
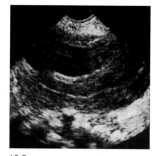

18.1a   18.1b   18.2

18.1 Normal postpubertal uterus in a 12-year-old girl with menorrhagia. Longitudinal scan: **a** inadequate bladder distention, partial visualization of the uterus plus the bowel mimics "retroflexed uterus." **b** Adequate bladder distention: normal postpubertal uterus!

18.2 Normal neonatal uterus in 3-day-old infant with low anal atresia. Longitudinal scan: relatively large uterus, approximately 5 cm, with prominent endometrial echo, physiologic (maternal estrogen effect).

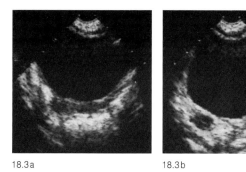
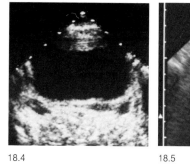
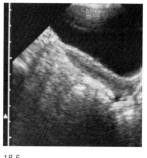

18.3a   18.3b   18.4   18.5

18.3 Normal infantile uterus, physiologic ovaries in a girl of 3 years, 8 months who underwent left nephrectomy for a stage I Wilms tumor at the age of 9 months. Healthy. **a** Longitudinal scan: infantile uterus, 3.1 cm. **b** Transverse scan: left ovary approximately 1.3 mL, right approximately 0.9 mL, each with cystic elements.

18.4 Physiologic findings in a healthy girl 4 years, 10 months of age. Transverse scan: ovaries approximately 0.7–0.8 mL, relatively hypoechogenic. Uterus appears medial to the left ovary.

18.5 Normal pubescent uterus in a girl of 10 years, 8 months. Longitudinal scan: uterus, 5 cm, narrow.

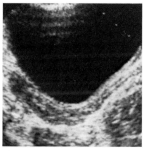
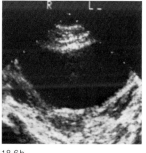
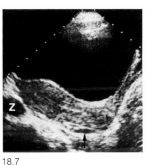
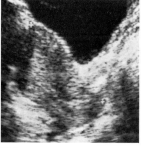

18.6a   18.6b   18.7   18.8

18.6 Normal pubescent uterus, physiologic ovaries in a girl of 12 years, 9 months beginning to develop secondary sexual characteristics. **a** Longitudinal scan: pubescent uterus, approximately 5.5 cm. Longitudinal growth apparent; still no increase in fundal thickness. Visible endometrial echo. **b** Transverse scan: right ovary approximately 1.5 mL with a cystic follicle; left ovary approximately 1.2 mL.

18.7 Normal postpubertal uterus in a 12-year-old with heavy menarche, anemia. Longitudinal scan 2 weeks postmenstruation: uterus, approximately 8 cm. Proliferative-phase endometrial echo. Follicular cyst (Z) of the right ovary; small amount of free fluid (arrow) in the cul-de-sac (may be postovulatory).

18.8 Normal postpubertal uterus in a 12½-year-old girl. Menstruation. Longitudinal scan: uterus during secretory/menstrual phase; very prominent endometrial echo; "full" uterus, often less well delineated than in the proliferative phase. Length 6.7 cm.

Disturbance of Puberty

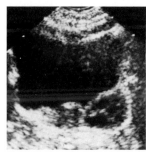
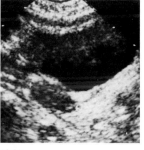
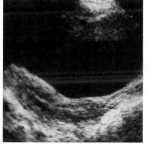
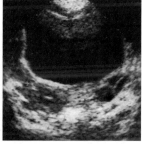

18.9a   18.9b   18.10a   18.10b

18.9 Isolated thelarche at 20 months. Vaginal cytology and cranial CT normal. FSH and osseous maturity in the high normal range. **a** Transverse scan: left ovary approximately 1.1 mL, contains multiple cystic elements; normal infantile uterus (cross section). **b** Longitudinal: right ovary approximately 0.9 mL. Idiopathic precocious puberty unlikely. Review clinical and US findings.

18.10 Progressive precocious puberty in a 4-year-old girl with accelerated growth and osseous maturity. Elevated estradiol. **a** Longitudinal scan: uterus enlarged for her age, approximately 4.4 cm; prominence of the fundus and an endometrial echo. **b** Transverse scan: left ovary 2–2.5 mL, composed largely of cystic elements; right ovary approximately 0.7 mL, less cystic. US: consistent with precocious puberty.

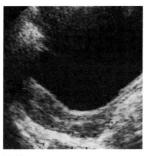 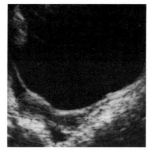 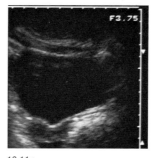

18.11a   18.11b   18.11c

18.**11   Precocious puberty** (hypothalamic cause?) in a child with retarded psychomotor development and hydrocephalus of unknown cause. Ventriculoatrial, later ventriculoperitoneal shunt. Repeated dysfunction and revision. Treatment with buserelin nasal spray (LH-RH analogue) produced gradual regression of primary and secondary sexual characteristics. Longitudinal scan **a** at 7 years, 8 months: late pubescent−type uterus, 6 cm. **b** At 8 years, 4 months: early pubescent−type uterus, 4.6 cm. **c** At 9 years, 3 months: prepubescent uterus, 3.4 cm.

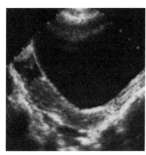 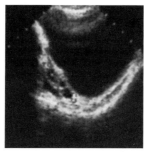 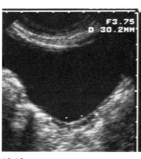 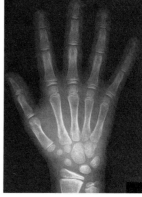

18.12a   18.12b   18.13a   18.13b

18.**12   Delayed puberty** in an 18-year-old woman. **a** Longitudinal scan: uterus thin, approximately 6 cm; fundus accentuated. Small amount of free intraperitoneal fluid, origin unclear. **b** Left longitudinal scan: ovaries 4−5 mL, each containing multiple cystic elements. Delayed puberty, presumably constitutional.

18.**13   Type I glycogen storage disease** in an 11-year-old with delayed mutaration. **a** Longitudinal scan: very narrow infantile uterus. Ovaries not visible. **b** Hand radiograph shows osseous maturity of approximately 6 years, 10 months (after Greulich and Pyle).

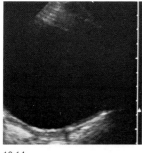 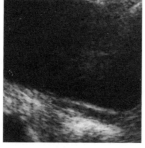 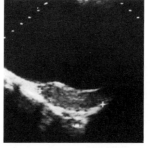 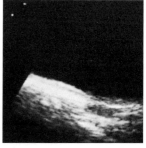

18.14   18.16   18.15a   18.15b

18.**14   Thalassemia minor** in a girl of 16 years, 2 months with gallstones and general maturation delay. Longitudinal scan: very narrow uterus approximately 4 cm long (infantile). Ovaries appear as narrow, elongated structures (not shown here).

18.**16   Hypogonadotropic hypogonadism** in a 17-year-old with x-autosomal translocation (gonadal dysgenesis, corresponding to the Turner syndrome). Longitudinal scan: uterus thin, infantile, no pubescent signs, relatively long, approximately 4.7 cm. Ovaries not demonstrable.

18.**15   Hypergonadotropic hypogonadism** (galactosemia) in a girl of 17 years, 8 months with recent menarche. US at age 14½ years showed a very narrow, infantile-type uterus and long, thin ("streak") ovaries, approximately 0.2 mL. Now: **a** Longitudinal scan: uterus approximately 6 cm, nonprominent fundus. **b** Left longitudinal scan: ovary somewhat larger than before (approximately 0.4 mL), has a similar shape.

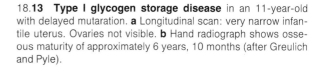

Disturbance of Menstruation

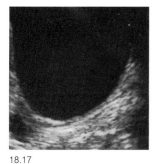 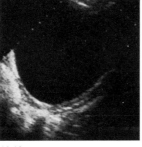

18.17 18.18

18.17 Rokitansky—Küster—Mayer syndrome in an 18-year-old with primary amenorrhea. Clinical examination: vaginal aplasia, uterus nonpalpable rectally. Longitudinal scan: no normal vaginal structure, uterus not demonstrable. Ovarian volumes approximately 10 and 7 mL, with scattered small cystic components (not shown).

18.18 Known peripheral androgen resistance in a 19-year-old with primary amenorrhea. Longitudinal scan shows normal vagina with proximal blind pouch. See also Fig. 18.**47** (same patient, with a Sertoli cell tumor).

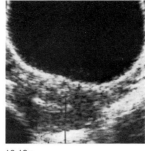 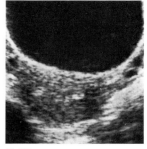

18.19a 18.19b

18.19 Menorrhagia in 13½-year-old girl. Transverse US: **a** septated uterus with one cervix, single endometrial echo in this region. **b** Double echoes in the corpus and fundal region, confirmed by longitudinal examination. Significance of findings questionable in connection with clinical presentation.

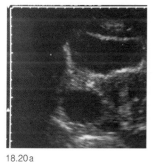 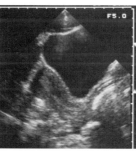

18.20a 18.20b

18.20 Suspected corpus luteum cyst in a girl of 13 years, 8 months with profuse menorrhagia. **a** Transverse scan: cystic lesion, presumably of the right ovary: approximately 30—35 mL. **b** Longitudinal scan: prominent endometrial echo. **DD:** dysfunctional (corpus luteum) cyst? malformative? neoplastic? US findings normal after a 1-month gestagen therapy; findings still normal 7 months later.

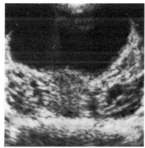 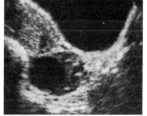

18.21a 18.21b

18.21 Suspected functional cystic ovarian change in a 13-year-old with successive episodes of polymenorrhea, dysmenorrhea, and oligomenorrhea; suspicion of "tumor" in the right adnexal region. **a** Transverse scan: relatively large ovaries (right approximately 20 mL, left approximately 12 mL) with multiple peripheral cystic components. **b** Right longitudinal scan shows a larger cystic mass: follicular cyst? Corpus luteum cyst? Normal postpubertal uterus (partially shown).

18.22 Oligomenorrhea in a 15-year-old girl with hirsutism and VATER association (spinal anomalies, anal atresia with a rectovaginal fistula, malrotation of the right kidney). **a** Right longitudinal scan: enlarged ovary, 13 mL; multiple small peripheral cysts (similar on the left). **b** Transverse scan: vaginal septum (arrow) separating two endometrial echoes in the bicornuate uterus. Stein—Leventhal syndrome unlikely (testosterone normal). No biopsy.

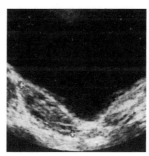 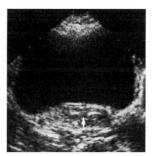

18.22a 18.22b

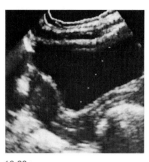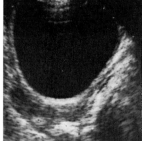

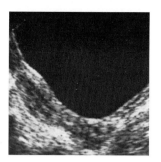

18.23a   18.23b

18.24

18.23 Primary constititional maturation delay, secondary anorexia in a 16-year-old with primary amenorrhea. Longitudinal scan: normal-appearing pubescent uterus. Presumed constitutional delay of menarche. Menarche occurred 1 month later. Normal menstruation for 3 years, then anorexia and secondary amenorrhea. **b** Scan at age 20: uterus markedly narrower and generally smaller than before menarche! Uterine atrophy (secondary).

18.24 Anorexia in a 15½-year-old with secondary amenorrhea. Longitudinal sonogram: uterus relatively long (7.5 cm) and thin: uterine atrophy.

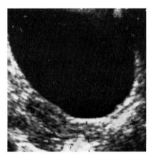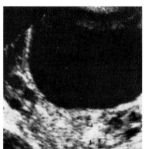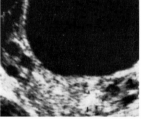

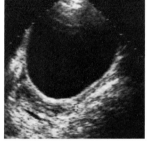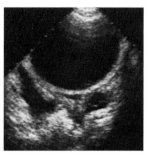

18.25a   18.25b

18.26a   18.26b

18.25 Anorexia in an 18-year-old who menstruated once 1 year before. Secondary amenorrhea. **a** Longitudinal scan: small, thin uterus, approximately 5.5 cm: uterine atrophy. **b** Transverse scan: ovaries with multiple cysts; ovarian size 6.5 and 4 mL. Normal menstruation ensued at the age of 19; uterine size adequate.

18.26 Crohn disease in an 18-year-old with secondary amenorrhea. **a** Longitudinal scan: uterus thin, approximately 6 cm. **b** Transverse scan: relatively large right-sided ovarian cyst (approximately 20 mL), smaller cyst on the left (approximately 6 mL), each with a prominent border. Note the irregular shape of the cyst on the right. A small amount of free intraperitoneal fluid. Uterine atrophy. **DD:** corpus luteum cyst(s), follicular cyst(s).

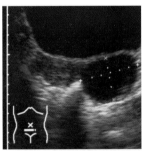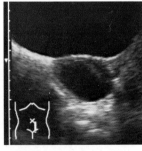

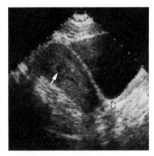

18.27a   18.27b

18.28

18.27 Juvenile dysfunctional bleeding since the age of 5 in 20-year-old female. Previous US showed intermittent small cystic ovarian components. **a, b** Transverse and sagittal scans show a larger, presumably functional cyst in the left ovarian region, approximately 75 mL. Spontaneous resolution. Partially solid at the periphery. **DD:** follicular cyst, corpus luteum cyst.

18.28 Early pregnancy in a 16-year-old with secondary amenorrhea for 7–8 weeks during a prolonged hospitalization (complex foot unjury after a jump from a window in a suicide attempt). Longitudinal scan: early pregnancy, approximately 3–4 weeks. Small cystic structure in the uterine fundus (arrow) represents the gestational sac. Prominent uterine wall.

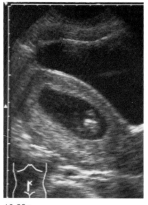
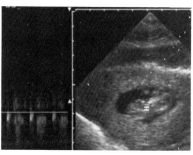

18.**29** **Pregnancy** in a 17-year-old with secondary amenorrhea. **a** Longitudinal uterine scan: embryo in transverse view (thoracic). **b** Transverse scan: embryo in longitudinal view, crown–rump lenght approximately 30 mm, consistent with an almost 10-week gestation. Normal amniotic cavity. Surrounding uterine wall more echogenic inside due to decidual structures (basal, parietal, capsular). Arterial doppler signal was presumably sampled in the aortic region.

18.29a   18.29b

Genital Anomalies

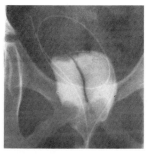
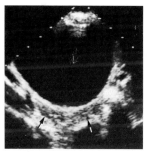

18.**30** **Duplication of the uterus and vagina** in a 7½-year-old with a history of high anal atresia and rectovaginal fistula. Fecal and urinary incontinence. **a** Vaginography: urethra opens into the anterior part of the vaginal roof (corresponds to the urogenital sinus). From there the vagina doubles; normal cervix on each side. **b** Transverse scan: complete double uterus (arrow).

18.30a   18.30b

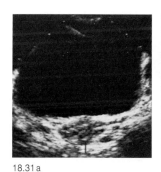
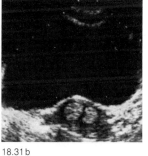
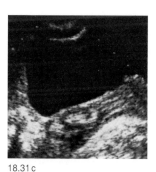

18.31a   18.31b   18.31c

18.**31** **Duplication of the uterus and vagina** in a 10-year-old with VATER association (rib anomaly, anomalous pulmonary venous drainage, anal atresia, right duplex kidney). **a** Transverse scan shows 2 vaginas, one placed obliquely above the other.

b Transverse scan shows 2 uterine cavities, each presumably containing mucus. **c** Longitudinal oblique scan: uteri and vaginas.

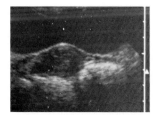
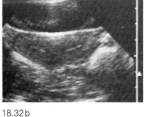
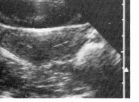
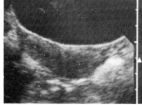

18.32a   18.32b   18.32c

18.**32** **Bicornuate uterus** in a 17-year-old with the Turner syndrome, special karyotype (45XO, 46X-isoXQ). Spontaneous

puberty. Transverse scan: **a** single cervix, **b** double endometrial echo, **c** two separate uterine fundi.

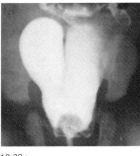 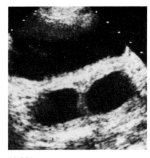 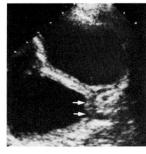 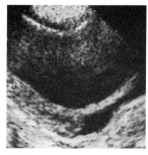

18.33a   18.33b   18.33c   18.34

18.33 Bicornuate uterus with hematometra associated with vaginal stenosis in a 16-year-old with urogenital sinus, ventralized anus, and spinal anomalies. Underwent bilateral ureteral reimplantation for reflux. Urachal remnant. Secondary urinary and fecal incontinence. Reported normal menstruation for 3 years. **a** "Vaginography" (neonatal diagnosis of a "double vagina"; in retrospect, hydrometra in a bicornuate uterus, with contrast medium in the bicornuate uterus and rectum). US at age 16: **b** transverse scan shows hematometra in the double fundus of the bicornuate uterus. **c** Longitudinal scan: cervical stenosis (arrows).

18.34 Hydrocolpus due to the hymenal membrane in a 16-month-old with an interlabial retrourethral mass. Longitudinal scan: hydrocolpos, normal uterus. Operation: hymenal incision, spontaneous drainage.

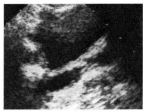 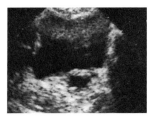

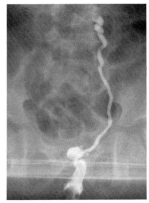

18.35a   18.35b   18.35c

18.35 Ectopic left ureteral orifice at 21 and 23 months. Clinical examination: interlabial mass, pea-size, bluish, cystic, more likely vaginal than urethral. **a** Longitudinal and **b** transverse scans: suspicion of hydrometrocolpos with uterine duplication and a solitary right kidney. Radiography: normal voiding cystogram; solitary right kidney. Operation: oblong cystic structure,

left intravaginal. **c** Retrograde contrast study: ectopic left ureteral insertion into the vagina, with rounded proximal and elongated distal ectasia. Hypoplastic left kidney. *Note:* vaginal US findings with absence of a kidney on the same side makes it tempting to presume an obstruction of the uterovaginal canal on that side (with uterine duplication).

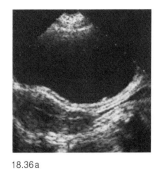 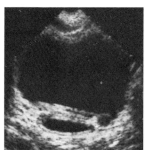

18.36a   18.36b

18.36 Vaginal urine reflux in a 14-year-old with a meningocele and neurogenic bladder, she underwent a left ureteral reimplantation for reflux. **a** Longitudinal scan: vaginal reflux of urine mimics hydrocolpos; normal postpubertal uterus. **b** Transverse scan: intravaginal urine collecton; residual distal left ureteral ectasia.

Pelvic Masses

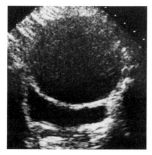 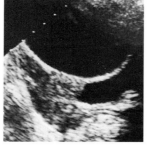 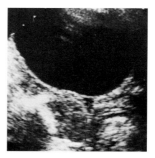

18.37a   18.37b   18.37c

18.37 Ovarian cystadenoma in a 12½-year-old with a history of colicky pain in the right hemiabdomen for several days. Pelvic mass. Ovarian cyst? **a** Transverse and **b** longitudinal scans: approximately 300 mL pre-/supravesical cyst compressing the bladder, previding. **c** Postvoiding longitudinal scan.

Laparotomy: removal of a right ovarian cyst with a twisted ovary. Histology: serous, partly papillary cystadenoma of the ovary. *Note:* voiding during US can be helpful in differentiating cyst from bladder.

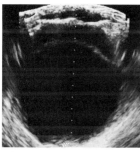 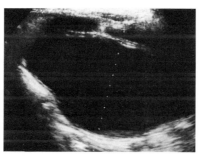

18.38a   18.38b

18.38 Hematocolpos in a 13½-year-old with primary amenorrhea, lower abdominal pain, and a soft pelvic mass. Hymenal atresia! **a** Transverse and **b** longitudinal scans:

retrovesical cystic mass, approximately 600 mL: hematometrocolpos. Evacuated through hymenotomy.

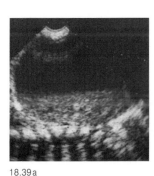 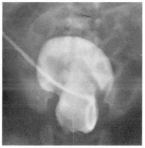 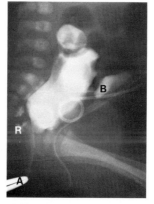

18.39a   18.39b   18.39c

18.39 Hydromucometrocolpos in a 2-day-old infant with a large, soft abdominopelvic mass. No hymenal atresia. **a** Longitudinal scan: an elliptical, thick-walled cystic structure with a layer of corpuscular sediment. Massive bilateral mechanical hydronephrosis (not shown). Pigtail catheter inserted under US guidance, yielded approximately 120 mL of opaque, pale greenish fluid (rich in squamous epithelial cells, no lymphocytes).

Contrast filling of the "cyst" **b** anteroposterior: mushroom-shaped structure; **c** lateral: "cyst" between the bladder (B) and rectum (R). Anus (A) is marked. Laparotomy at 2 months for a recurrent, unexplained reappearance of the "cyst" confirmed presumptive diagnosis of hydromucometrocolpos secondary to distal short (3−5 mm) vaginal atresia. Plastic repair, uneventful postoperative course.

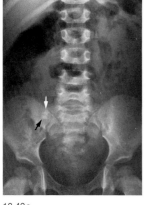

18.40a

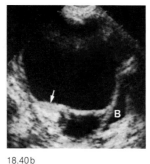

18.40b

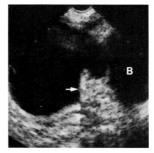

18.40c

18.**40   Cystic teratoma** in a 28-month-old infant sick for several days. Abdominal pain? Soft mass in the right lower midabdomen. **a** Radiograph: pelvic mass effect; fecolith (arrow)?

b Oblique and **c** right longitudinal scans: well-defined, thin-walled cystic lesion, volume approximately 60 mL, located above the bladder (B) and enclosing a calculus (arrow). Unusual for perityphlitic abscess. Ovarian cyst? Duplication cyst of the terminal ileum? Other malformation? Laparotomy: right ovarian cystic tumor. Histology: cystic teratoma, benign.

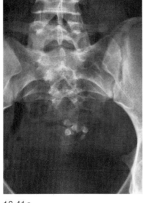

18.41a

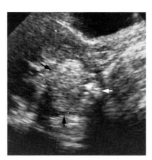

18.41b

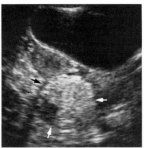

18.41c

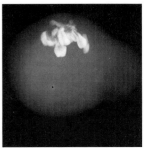

18.41d

18.**41   Differentiated teratoma** in a 16-year-old girl who developed secondary noctural enuresis at the age of 4; history of anorectal prolapse for 4 months. **a** Radiograph: toothlike calcifications on the left at the level of the coccyx. **b** Longitudinal and **c** transverse scans: rounded, well-defined, partially hyperechogenic mass (arrows) in the left retrouterine area (left

pre-/paraectal area on the radiograph, not shown). Laparotomy: removal of a left-sided ovarian tumor. Correction of a rectal prolapse. Histology: differentiated nonmalignant teratoma. **d** Surgical specimen.

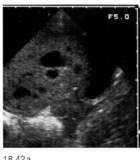

18.42a

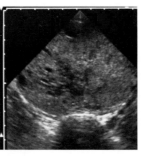

18.42b

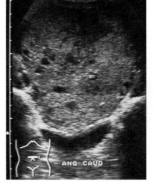

18.42c

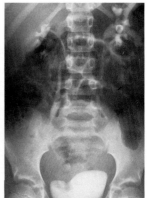

18.42d

18.**42   Yolk sac tumor** in a 7-year-old girl with pollakiruia 11 months before, vomiting and diarrhea 2 weeks before; a 1-week history of dysuria. **a** Longitudinal and **b, c** transverse sonograms: essentially a solid tumor with necrotic−hemorrhagic cavities; estimated volume 300−350 mL. **DD:** ovarian / adnexal tumor

(germ cell tumor, gonadal stromal tumor, lymphoma) or uterine tumor (rhabdomyosarcoma, lymphoma). **d** EU: supravesical mass; mild congestion; prerectal tumor (not shown). CT yielded no additional information. Laparotomy: complete removal of a left-sided ovarian tumor, weight 350 g. Histology: yolk sac tumor.

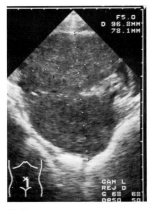
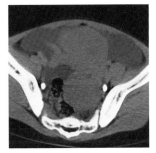
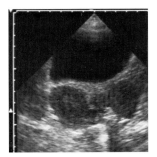

18.43a   18.43b   18.43c

18.43 Leukemia in a girl of 11 years, 10 months with a 1-week history of exertional dyspnea. Radiograph showed a massive left-sided pleural effusion. **a** Longitudinal scan: massive ascites, nephromegaly, lymphadenopathy (none shown). Two large adjacent masses in the left adnexal region (greatly enlarged ovaries).

DD: infiltrative adnexal/ovarian tumor, lymphoma, leukemia. **b** CT correlate, also showing involvement of right adnexal structures. Cytology (pleural aspirate): pre-T-cell leukemia (pre-TALL). **c** Transverse scan: ovaries in the correct location, less enlarged after 3 weeks' therapy.

18.44 Functional ovarian cyst in a 4-month-old infant born at 26 weeks, i.e., now approximately 2 weeks after term. Previous respiratory distress syndrome and staphylococcal sepsis. Very prominent genitalia with vaginal discharge; extremely high estradiol levels. Suspicion of an estrogen-producing tumor. **a** Transverse and **b** longitudinal scans: loculated cystic mass with a volume of approximately 25 mL, presumably belonging to the right ovary: hormone-producing tumor? Teratoma? Uterus 4 cm long, prominent endometrial echo. Laparotomy: removal of the right cystic ovary. Histology: benign functional ovarian cyst (effect of increased central stimulation after the loss of maternal negative feedback in the very immature preterm baby).

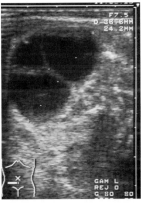
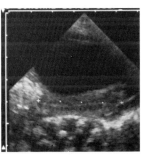

18.44a   18.44b

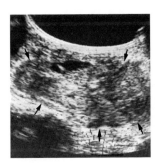
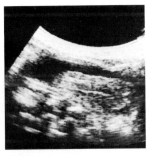
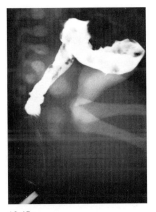

18.45a   18.45b   18.45c

18.45 Rhabdomyosarcoma in a 2-day-old infant with a soft, livid, "cystic" tumor of the left labium majus and left perineal-gluteal region. Vaginal interior could not be visualized. Anus displaced dorsally. Micturition and defecation normal. Teratoma? Rhabdomyosarcoma? Anterior longitudinal scan: **a** sharply marginated, heterogeneous, predominantly solid mass (arrows), left paramedian; **b** normal neonatal uterus, retrovesical. Rhabdomyosarcoma? **c** Radiograph: prerectal mass; clamp marks the anus. Operation: subtotal resection of a tumor arising from the left outer vaginal wall. Histology: rhabdomyosarcoma, small-cell, poorly differentiated. Unresponsive to chemotherapy. Child died 3 months later from metastasis and cachexia.

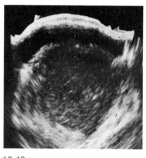 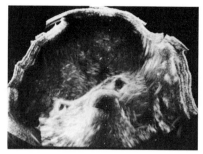 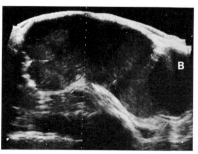

18.46a   18.46b   18.46c

18.46 Malignant teratoma in a nonmenstruating 12-year-old with rapidly progressive, painless abdominal distention over a 3-week period. Malaise. Firm visible and palpable mass in the lower midabdomen. **a, b** Transverse scans: very large, solid, homogeneous, retrovesical, subpehatic tumor. **c** Longitudinal scan: cranially lobulated tumor extending up to 8 cm above the umbilicus (cm scale) and projecting to the right (B = bladder). **DD:** arising from the uterus or an ovary? (neither structure is

defined); uterine rhabdomyosarcoma. Radiograph showed large prerectal mass with moderate mechanical obstruction of the upper urinary tract. Laparotomy: total extirpation of a solid tumor (from the right ovary); uterus clear. No metastases. Histology: malignant teratoma with seminomal and yolk-sac components. Chemotherapy: Patient doing well 6 years later; normal menstruation.

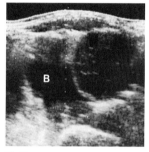 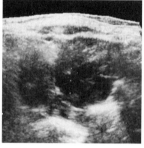

18.47a   18.47b

18.47 Sertoli cell tumor in a 21-year-old with known peripheral androgen resistance ("testicular feminization"). Transverse scans taken at clinical follow-up **a** before and **b** after micturition: rounded, hyperechogenic but solid tumor in the left paravesical area (B = bladder), volume approximately 100 mL. Painless, palpable. Suspected gonadal tumor. Laparotomy: removal of the enlarged left gonad. Histology: Sertoli cell tumor (same patient as in Fig. 18.**18**).

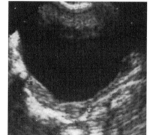 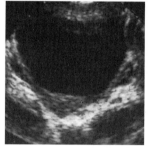

18.48a   18.48b

Vaginal Bleeding (Prepubertal)

18.48 Single episode of vaginal bleeding in a 3½-year-old with possible precocious puberty. **a** Longitudinal scan: normal infantile uterus, length 3 cm; fundus exceptionally well defined (no definite evidence of estrogen effect); no obvious endometrial echo. **b** Transverse scan: normal-size ovaries (right < 0.4 mL, left > 0.45 mL) with cystic components. True uterine bleeding doubtful. No further bleeding episodes occurred.

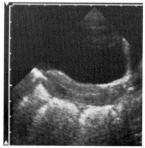 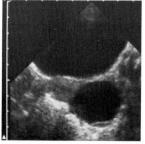 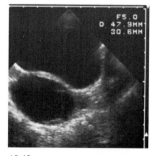

18.49a   18.49b   18.49c

18.49 Vaginal bleeding, precocious puberty in a girl of 4 years, 10 months with estrogenized genitals. **a** Longitudinal scan: pubescent uterus, 5 cm long, conspicuous endometrial echo. **b** Transverse and **c** longitudinal scans: left ovarian cyst, approximately 20 mL. **DD:** estrogen-producing cyst; teratoma of

the left ovary; higher-level stimulatory process. Cranial MRI normal. Hormonal therapy. Three weeks later, the cyst was gone (treatment response? spontaneous?). Uterus still enlarged, consistent with precocious puberty.

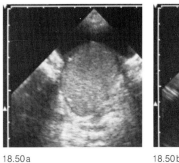 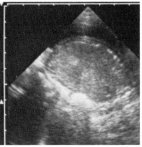

18.50a   18.50b

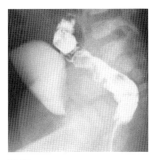

18.50c

18.50 Profuse vaginal bleeding, yolk sac tumor in an 18-month-old girl. **a** Transverse and **b** longitudinal scans: egg-shaped, solid, well-defined retrovesical mass with peripheral calcifications; may be intraperitoneal. **DD:** adnexal tumor (ovar-ian, e.g., teratoma) with invasion of the vagina; sarcomatous tumor of the uterus and/or vagina. **c** Radiograph: prerectal (exclusion of a sacrococcygeal tumor such as a neuroblastoma, etc.); normal EU. Laparotomy: removal of the tumor.

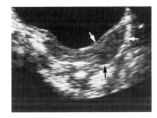 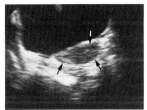

18.51a   18.51b

18.51 Vaginal bleeding, sarcoma botryoides in a 3½-year-old girl. **a** Longitudinal and **b** transverse scans: solid mass (arrows) in the proximal part of the vagina, cannot be separated from the cervix: polyp? tumor?

Abdominopelvic Pain, Pelvic Inflammatory Disease

18.52 Pain caused by cystic ovarian change? Nonmenstruating 12-year-old with two episodes of acute right lower abdominal pain, no fever. Possible torsion of an ovarian cyst. **a** Transverse and **b** longitudinal scans: elliptical cystic mass in the right adnexal region, sharply marginated, approximately 18 mL in size; suspected ovarian cyst. Laparoscopy: enlarged right ovary, no torsion; tense, livid surface. Follicular cyst? No further measures. Subsequent spontaneous resolution of the clinical symptoms and cystic structure. Assumption: follicular cyst.

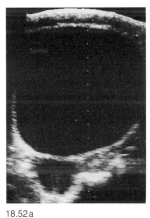 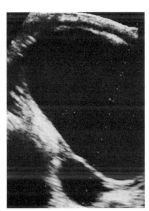

18.52a   18.52b

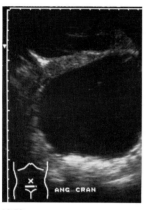 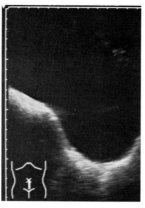 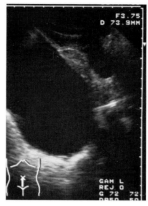 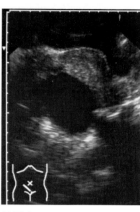

18.53a   18.53b   18.53c   18.53d

18.53 Paraovarian cyst(s) in a 15-year-old girl with a 2-week history of cramplike low abdominal pain after defecation since the onset of menses. **a** Transverse, **b, c** longitudinal, and **d** oblique scans: large retrouterine cyst, presumably of the left ovary; volume approximately 1000 mL. Laparotomy: huge left-sided paraovarian cyst ("fimbrial cyst"), aspiration yielded about 1.2 L of watery fluid. Removal. There were additionally two small, pedunculated paraovarian cysts on each side. Ovaries multifollicular. Histology: paraovarian cyst(s). *Note:* visualization of the uterus varies with the probe position. With the large cyst, neither ovary could be visualized.

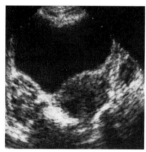 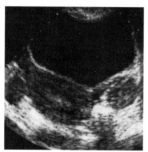 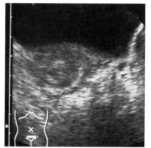 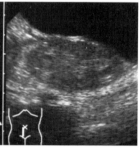

18.54a   18.54b   18.55a   18.55b

18.54 Suspected chronic ovarian torsion in a 15-year-old who has been menstruating for 2 years. Evaluated for pain in the right lower abdomen. **a, b** Transverse scan: enlarged ovaries, volume approximately 17 mL on the right, 12 mL on the left; predominantly solid, partly hyperechogenic; multiple small cystic elements. Both uterine tubes clearly visible (left shown). Laparotomy: large, firm, whitish right ovary. Ovariectomy for a suspected tumor! Left ovary was smaller and similar in appearance to the right ovary, though changes were less pronounced. The left ovary was biopsied. Uterus enlarged; "inflammatory"? Histology: no evidence of neoplasia. Torsion (recurrent) or early stage of the Stein–Leventhal syndrome? No clinical suspicion of the Stein–Leventhal syndrome.

18.55 Adnexal torsion with hemorrhagic infarction in a child of 3 years, 2 months with a 3-day history of abdominal pain. **DD:** gastroenteritis, appendicitis. Radiographs consistent with progressive bowel motility disorder. **a** Transverse and **b** longitudinal scans: solid mass with well-defined margins, volume approximately 15–20 mL, retrovesical, right paramedian or adnexal tumor. **DD:** unusual for abscess; phlegmonous process (clinical context)? Ovarian torsion with venous congestion? Laparotomy: triple twist of the right uterine tube with a hemorrhagic infarction of the adnexa including the ovary.

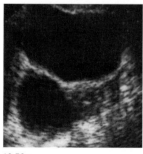 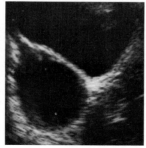 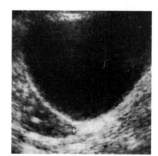

18.56a   18.56b   18.56c

18.57 Paraovarian cyst in a 15-year-old with blood-tinged vaginal discharge since the last menstruation 3 weeks before; 1-week history of right lower abdominal pain, progressive, with vomiting. **a** Transverse and **b** longitudinal scans: right paramedian retrouterine cystic mass, volume 14 mL; separate from the right ovary (arrows) **DD:** ovarian cyst, follicular cyst, hydrosalpinx, perityphlitic abscess. Laparoscopy: cyst on the right side of the cul-de-sac; fibrinous coat on the right ovary. Subsequent laparotomy: removal of the paraovarian cyst. Histology: presumably a wolffian remnant. Plausible in retrospect, considering location.

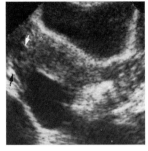 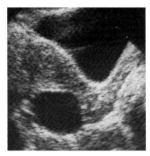

18.57a 18.57b

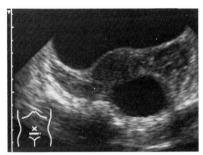 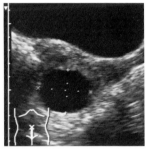

18.58a 18.58b

18.58 Fimbrial cyst in a 16-year-old with acute abdomen. **a** Transverse and **b** longitudinal scans: 20-mL retrouterine cyst, separate from both ovaries. Laparotomy performed for severe pain: torsion of the fimbrial cyst, histologically confirmed.

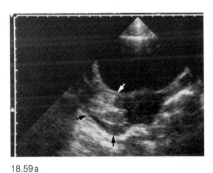 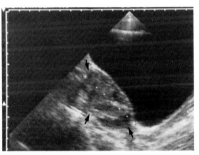 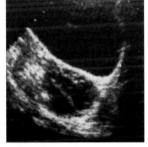

18.59a 18.59b 18.60

18.59 Hemorrhagic follicular cyst in a 16-year-old with acute right lower quadrant pain 1 day before. Pain subsided spontaneously; soft abdomen. **a** Transverse and **b** right longitudinal scans: an approximately 45-mL right ovary (arrows), heterogeneous, partly hyperechogenic. Suspicion of extensive intraovarian bleeding. Clinical suspicion of appendicitis prompted appendectomy: normal appendix. Hemorrhagic ovary; partial resection. Histology/pathology: hemorrhagic follicula cyst ("chocolate cyst").

18.60 Corpus luteum cyst in a 15-year-old regular menstrual periods for 2 years, some dysmenorrhea. History of abdominal pain "for years," persisted after appendectomy 7 months before. Right adnexal tumor? Abscess? Right longitudinal scan: approximately 80-mL elliptical lesion, presumably ovarian, echogenic cranially, predominantly cystic caudally; solid anterior border with multiple tiny cysts. **DD:** ovarian abscess, teratoma, endometriosis, postappendectomy abscess. Laparotomy: cyst in the right ovary extirpated, "leaving the ovary alone." Course: further episodes of left-sided abdominal pain! "Irritable colon?" Three follow-up US examinations: no discernible ovarian structure on the right side! Left ovary solid, volume approximately 14 mL (compensatory enlargement?).

◄ **18.56 Suspected adnexitis** in a 14-year-old, menarche 1 year before; 5-month history of menometrorrhagia with nausea, vomiting, and headache. Suspicion of acute appenditicis: appendectomy. Appendix normal; inflamed, swollen right uterine tube ("adnexitis") with serosanginous ascites. Apparently sexual contact. No bacterial growth from ascites. US 1 month later: **a** transverse and **b** longitudinal scans show a 40-mL cystic lesion in the right adnexal region. **DD:** hydrosalpinx, ovarian cyst, follicular cyst, corpus luteum cyst, abscess. Gestagen therapy. Cyst gone 3 weeks later. **c** Right longitudinal scan: normal-sized right ovary with central hyperechogenicity.

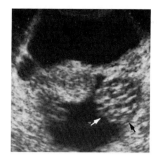

18.61

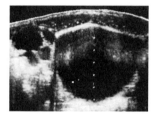

18.62 a

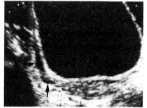

18.62 b

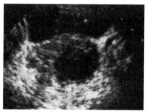

18.63 a

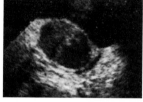

18.63 b

18.61 Lesion with abscessation? Sixteen-year-old with hemolytic/uremic syndrome in history. Renal failure; peritoneal dialysis. Recurrent peritonitis (*Staphylococcus aureus*). Severe abdominal pain. Antibiotics. Transverse scan: copious intraperitoneal fluid (dialysate). At the left posterior (belonging to ovary or adnexal structure?) is a "solid" mass, volume approximately 20 mL, with a heterogeneous echo structure (arrows): inflammatory mass? Ovary itself? Laparotomy withheld due to regression of pain. Diagnosis uncertain (may be lesion with abscess).

18.62 Suspected iatrogenic ovarian ectopy in a 13½-year-old. Puberty. Operated on as an infant for a right-sided inguinal hernia. Now evaluated for pain and a soft palpable mass in the right inguinal area. **a, b** Transverse scan: multicystic lesion directly below the abdominal wall, intraperitoneal, right paravesical, possible connection with the uterine tube (arrow). Menarche ensued within a few months. Episodic pains persisted, apparently unrelated to the menstrual cycle. Pains diminished with time, so surgery was withheld. US at the age of 14½ years: similar findings. Speculative diagnosis: right ovary fixed beneath the abdominal wall during a previous operation for inguinal hernia.

18.63 Salpingitis in a girl of 3 years, 10 months old with a 1-week history of abdominal pain, vomiting, and diarrhea. Fever of 40°C. Lower abdominal tenderness; no peritonism. **a** Transverse and **b** longitudinal scans: sharply marginated, heterogeneous left paramedian retrovesical mass, predominantly cystic, volume approximately 27 mL: abscess (postappendicitic)? Laparotomy: mass found at the expected site. Ruptured, pus evacuated. Presumptive left-sided salpingectomy. Removal of a "normal-looking" appendix. Histology: severe acute salpingitis with abscess; purulofibrinous inflammation of the parametria and of the (inadvertently) removed left ovary. "Periappendicitis."

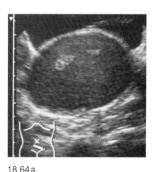

18.64 a

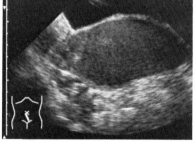

18.64 b

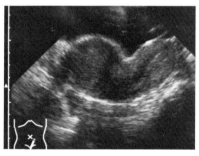

18.64 c

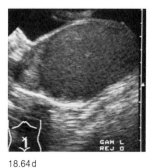

18.64 d

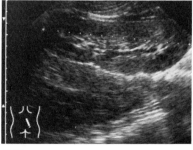

18.64 e

18.64 Left-sided hematocolpos in the double uterus of a 13-year-old with normal menses for 8 months. She presented with extremely painful dysmenorrhea. Rectal: soft anterior mass. **a–d** Hemato(metro?)colpos. **e** Solitary right kidney with compensatory enlargement, but an apparently normal uterus on the left! (One would except uterine/vaginal duplication with vaginal obstruction on the left side with an absent left kidney.) Displacement of the normal right uterus toward the left? Radiography: solitary right kidney. Gynecologic examination after massive evacuation of old blood: hemorrhagic vaginal wall. Surgical exploration: previous rupture of a left-sided hematocolpos in the double uterus with a normal uterus on both sides.

19 Testes and Thyroid

U. V. Willi

In most patients the testes and thyroid gland are easily accessible to clinical examination. Testicular lesions tend to have an acute etiology and usually are evaluated on an emergency basis.

Palpable thyroid lesions are usually followed for a longer period of time within the context of clinical findings and labortory studies. Occasionally they are investigated by ultrasound.

A common indication for sonography of the *testes* is to confirm or exclude a tumor. Clinically, a testicular hydrocele can mimic an enlarged testis or a testicular tumor. Usually the latter differentiation is easily made by ultrasound, whereas testicular enlargement, with or without a change of echo pattern, is a nonspecific finding and frequently necessitates surgical exploration. Radionuclide scanning is useful for patient selection, as acute or chronic testicular torsion and epididymitis present relatively characteristic findings.

The principal abnormalities of the *thyroid*, which often shows general or irregular enlargement, are struma, thyroiditis, hypothyroidism, hyperthyroidism, and nodular lesions. The sonographic criteria of interest are the echo characteristics (echogenicity and structure) of the gland. An (endemic) struma may be manifested by thyroid enlargement with no change in echogenicity, and morphologically it may closely resemble hypothyroidism. A struma may undergo cystic and hemorrhagic change, especially during the growth spurt, with an associated change in echo pattern. Thyroiditis is usually characterized by diffuse hypoechogenicity (chronic lymphocytic form and Graves disease), and the sonographic features are seldom distinguishable from those of hyperthyroidism. A subacute de Quervain thyroiditis exhibits locally varying, well-defined zones of reduced echogenicity (rare in children). While cystic "nodules" are generally benign, solitary solid lesions of low or mixed echogenicity are quite often malignant. Every solitary thyroid nodule, even a uniformly hyperechogenic one (often signifies a benign follicular adenoma), should be cytologically and histologically evaluated by fine-needle aspiration. Malignant nodules are generally "cold" on radionuclide scans. The examiner can usually rely on *swallowing dynamics* to distinguish an intrinsic lesion from an extrinsic lesion such as a paramedian neck cyst.

References

Dodat, H., Y. Chavrier, J. F. Dyon, R. B. Galifer, D. Aubert, J. S. Valla, G. Morisson-Lacombe: Tumeurs testiculaires primitives de l'enfant. Chir. pédiat. 27 (1986) 1–13

James, E. M., J. W. Charboneau: High-frequency (10 MHz) thyroid ultrasonography. Semin. Ultrasound 6 (1985) 294–309

Sciuk, J., O. Schober: Die Sonographie der Schilddrüse. Radiologe 29 (1989) 95–102

Testes

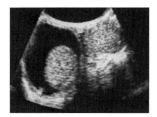
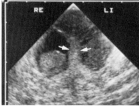
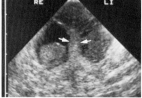
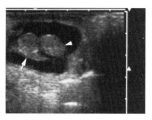

19.1   19.2

19.3

19.**1** **Testicular hydrocele** in a 5-year-old with a suspected right testicular tumor: firm, smooth on palpation. Transverse sonogram: right testicular hydrocele.

19.**2** **Testicular hydrocele** in a 2-month-old with swelling of the proximal and anteromedial thighs, scrotum, and penis. Transverse scan: testicular hydrocele, moderate on the right, mild on the left; swelling of the scrotal septum (arrows) and scrotal wall. Diagnosis uncertain (toxic?). Spontaneous remission.

19.**3** **Testicular hydrocele and epididymitis** in a boy of 4 years, 2 months with a 2-month history of left-sided scrotal pain. Acute: pain increase, swelling. Torsion? Hydatids? Left longitudinal scan: testicular hydrocele (▼); swelling of the epididymis (←): epididymitis. Operation: removal fo 2 small necrotic hydatids. Presumed diagnosis: chemical epididymitis and reactive hydrocele.

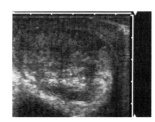
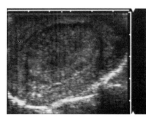
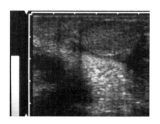

19.4a   19.4b

19.4c

19.**4** **Necrosis after torsion** in a 14-year-old with a 3-day history of increasing swelling, redness, and tenderness of the right hemiscrotum. **a, b** Longitudinal scans of the right testis: echo pattern strongly or moderately heterogeneous, depending on the plane; severe enlargement (swelling). **c** Longitudinal scan of the left testis: normal. **DD:** missed torsion, possibly with inflammatory paratesticular reaction; infection; tumor (e.g. rhabdomyosarcoma). Operation: testicular/paratesticular necrosis after torsion. Orchiectomy.

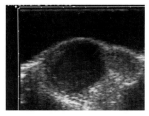
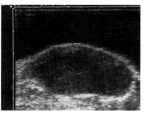
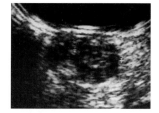
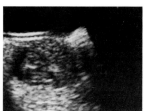

19.5a   19.5b

19.6a   19.6b

19.**5** **Rhabdomyosarcoma** in a 3½-year-old boy; bright, independent child reported the finding (enlarged testis) to his mother. Suspected tumor. **a** Transverse and **b** longitudinal scans: right testis enlarged, relatively hypoechogenic, subtle evidence of nodularity, heterogeneity. **DD:** presumed rapid growth implies malignancy: sacroma, lymphoma, leukemia. Orchiectomy. Histology: rhabdomyosarcoma.

19.**6** **Teratoma** in an 8-month-old infant. Left testis enlarged, firm. **a** Transverse an **b** longitudinal scans: enlarged left testis with a general increase in echogenicity and 2 central, very echogenic zones. **DD:** probable malignancy; germ-cell tumor (teratoma, embryonic carcinoma, seminoma, yolk sac tumor); stromal tumor (Sertoli or Leydig cell tumor); tumor derived from other tissue; infiltrative tumor (neuroblastoma, lymphoma, leukemia). Orchiectomy. Histology: teratoma with cartilaginous tissue and bony elements.

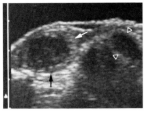 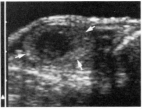

19.7a   19.7b

19.7 Suspected Leydig cell tumor in a boy of 4 years, 8 months with precocious puberty and a greatly accelerated growth rate; high testosterone level (corresponding to an adult). **DD:** adrenogenital syndrome (AGS), brain tumor **a** Transverse and **b** right longitudinal scans: normal left testis (△); greatly enlarged right testis (←); extensive, hypoechogenic center; more echogenic periphery ("egglike"). Clinical context raises the suspicion of a hormonally active testicular tumor (Leydig cell tumor). Orchiectomy. Histology: Leydig cell tumor. Testosterone level normal only 1 day after the operation, rapid return to a normal growth rate.

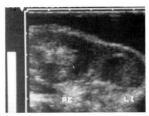 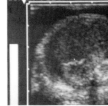

19.8a   19.8b

19.8 Inflammatory pseudotumor in a 12-year-old boy with a 1-year history of recurrent pain in the right testis. Contusional injury of the right hemiscrotum with hematoma 3 weeks before. **a** Transverse and **b** right longitudinal scans: enlargement of the testis and possibly of the epididymis. **DD:** testicular (and paratesticular?) tumor; posttraumatic/hemorrhagic lesion. Orchiectomy (see also Fig. 5.**46**).

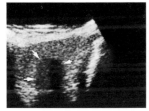 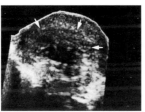

19.9   19.10

19.9 Adrenogenital syndrome (AGS) in a 15-year-old diagnosed at 6 weeks, salt loss. Testicular volume 15 mL; hard consistency; some irregularity noted on palpation. Right longitudinal scan: testicular adrenal-like tissue, hypoechogenic, well defined (arrows).

19.10 Adrenogenital syndrome (AGS) in a 17-year-old diagnosed at 3 weeks, salt loss. Testicular volume approximately 15 mL; hard consistency, palpable irregularities. Right transverse scan: testicular adrenal-like tissue, extensive; heterogeneous echo structure, less well defined (arrows).

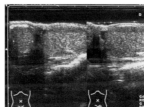 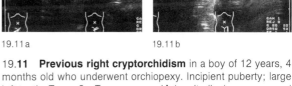

19.11a   19.11b

19.11 Previous right cryptorchidism in a boy of 12 years, 4 months old who underwent orchiopexy. Incipient puberty; large left testis. Tumor? **a** Transverse and **b** longitudinal scans: normal echo structure in both testes; right testis relatively small, left relatively large: may represent compensatory enlargement.

Thyroid

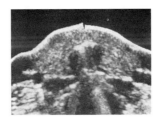

19.12

19.12 Euthyroid diffuse struma in a 15-year-old girl. Transverse scan at the level of the isthmus: normal homogeneous echo structure; possible slight accentuation of echogenicity. Organ size generally increased.

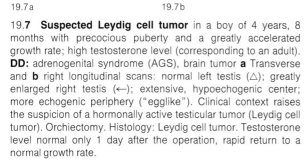
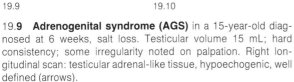

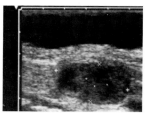 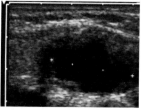

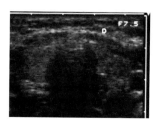

19.13a   19.13b

19.13c

19.13 Euthyroid "diffuse stroma," cystic lesion in a girl of 11 years, 8 months with painful swelling in the right suprajugular area. **a** Longitudinal scan: heterogeneous "tumor," identified dynamically (swallow) as belonging to the thyroid. Aspiration: hemosiderin-containing. Thereafter progressively cystic. **a** Lon-

gitudinal and **c** transverse scan at 12 years, 5 months: large cystic lesion in the right lower pole. Upper pole region normal on both sides. Local excision. Histology: struma nodosa colloides; chronic inflammation, local fibrosis.

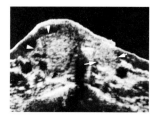 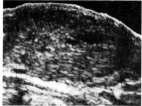

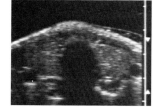 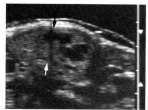

19.14a   19.14b

19.15a   19.15b

19.14 Decompensated follicular adenoma in an 11½-year-old girl with an euthyroid struma on the right side. **a** Transverse and **b** right longitudinal scans: markedly enlarged right thyroid lobe (▼); multiple moderate-sized cystic areas; small left lobe (←). (Note the marked external protuberance through the thyroid enlargement on the right.) Scintigraphy showed a "hot nodule"; decompensated follicular adenoma. Right strumectomy, leaving residual thyroid tissue. Histology: follicular, partly macropapillary adenoma; evidence of increased activity. Two years later, suspicion of a right-sided recurrence.

19.15 Pendred syndrome (labyrinthine deafness, impaired thyroxine synthesis) in an 11½-year-old girl with congenital hypothyroidism. Transverse scans through **a** the upper pole and **b** the lower pole: marked isthmic widening (arrows); enlargement of the left lower pole with cystic lesions of varying size. Resection of the left lower pole and isthmus. Histology: cystic nodular hyperplasia.

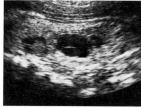 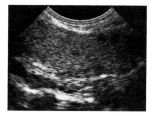

19.16a   19.16b

19.17

19.16 McCune–Albright syndrome in a girl of 13 years, 10 months. Precocious puberty: polyostotic fibrous dysplasia; narrow optic canals. Major cystic changes in both ovaries (US). **a** Left and **b** right longitudinal scans: 3 large lesions on the left with varying degrees of reduced echogenicity; multiple smaller rounded hypoechogenic areas on the right. Scintigraphy showed increased uptake in the lesions (which appeared as one "hot nodule"): compensatory autonomous adenoma.

19.17 Paramedian neck cyst in a girl of 2 years, 5 months with a cystic mass left of midline. Thyroid? Left longitudinal scan: lesion caudal to the left lower pole of the thyroid: paramedian neck cyst. Operatively removed. Diagnosis confirmed.

20 Parathyroids, Adrenals, Pancreas

U. V. Willi

The parathyroids, adrenals, and pancreas are poorly accessible to direct clinical examination. Sonography is most often indicated when there is suspicion of a functional abnormality of one of these organs or when a disorder has already been demonstrated. The goal of the examination is to identify a morphologic correlate.

Primary and secondary hyperparathyroidism are relatively uncommon in children. Hyperplasia of the *parathyroid(s)* (often involving several or all gland bodies) and adenoma (typically unifocal) are accessible to sonography, since in 85–90% of cases they are located in the expected soft-tissue structures of the neck. The value of the examination is limited by the relatively small size of the parathyroids, even when hyperplasia exists, and by the potential for ectopy. Thus, a negative examination does not necessarily rule out disease. Solitary adenoma is a common cause of primary hyperparathyroidism and is frequently associated with nephrocalcinosis or nephrolithiasis.

The principal sonographic abnormalities involving the *adrenals* are hemorrhage and neuroblastoma. Adrenal hemorrhage in newborns, unilateral or bilateral and possibly „segmental", seems largely a result of birth trauma, although rare prenatal occurrences are known. Here, as elsewhere in the body, adrenal hematoma is characterized by a relatively rapid change in echo pattern (within days) and size (within weeks). Cases of neuroblastoma are illustrated in chapter 5 (Abdominal Masses). Adrenal adenoma may be benign or malignant. Suspicion may be directed toward this lesion by the effects of its endocrine activity (virilization, precocious pseudopuberty). Adrenogenital syndrome (AGS) is theoretically associated with adrenal cortical hyperplasia, though this is not always apparent on sonograms. A case with an inflammatory adrenal mass is illustrated in Fig. 12.**12**.

Generally the *pancreas* can be satisfactorily visualized in children, but this may be difficult if there is much air in the gastrointestinal tract. Scanning on multiple planes of section is recommended:

- conventional transverse oblique scan over the liver with slight caudal angulation;
- longitudinal oblique scan from the midline, angled toward the left;
- longitudinal coronal flank scan angled anteriorly, using the spleen as an acoustic window.

Cases of pancreatic pseudocysts are illustrated in chapter 6 (Figs. 6.**14–16**). Pancreatitis (posttraumatic; chemical/toxic, e. g., opiates, L-asparaginase; associated with biliary obstruction, etc.) may be manifested solely by high amylase levels (serum, urinary) with no sonographic correlate. In other cases it may produce hypo- or hyperechogenicity, with or without swelling, or may present mixed sonographic features.

Cystic fibrosis is associated with multiple possible characteristic intra-abdominal findings. Up until about school age, it leads to a diffuse and progressive increase of pancreatic echogenicity with fibrosis (size decrease) and/or fatty infiltration of the organ.

References

Cohen, E. K., A. Daneman, D. A. Stringer, G. Soto, P. Thorner: Focal adrenal hemorrhage: a new US appearance. Radiology 161 (1986) 651–633

Daneman, A.: Adrenal neoplasms in children. Semin. Roentgenol. 23 (1988) 205–215

Siegel, M. J., K. W. Martin, J. L. Worthington: Normal and abnormal pancreas in children: US studies. Radiology 165 (1987) 15–18

Stark, D. D., G. A. W. Gooding, O. H. Clark: Noninvasive parathyroid imaging. Semin. Ultrasound 6 (1985) 310–320

Parathyroids

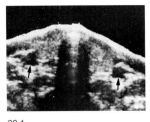 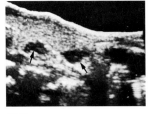 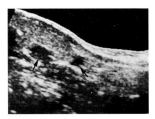 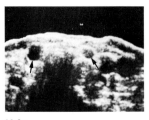

20.1   20.2a   20.2b   20.2c

20.1   End-stage renal failure, secondary hyperparathyroidism, nephronophthisis in a 16-year-old girl. Transverse cranial thyroid scan: bilateral enlargement of the upper parathyroids (arrows), each posterolateral to the thyroid lobes: hyperplasia of the parathyroids (also inferiorly; sister in Fig. 14.**40**).

20.2   End-stage renal failure and secondary hyperparathyroidism in an 18-year-old woman. **a** Right and **b** left longitudinal scans and **c** caudal transverse scan of the thyroid: all four parathyroids (arrows) are enlarged, hypoechogenic, and clearly visible at their normal locations. Parathyroid hyperplasia. Subsequent ¾ parathyroidectomy.

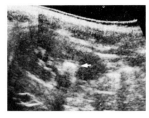 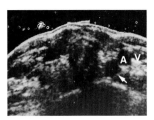

20.3a   20.3b

20.3   Parathyroid adenoma in a girl of 15 years, 5 months with recurrent urinary tract infections. **a** Right posterior longitudinal scan: renal calculus (arrow). Serum calcium and phosphorus signify primary hyperparathyroidism. **b** Caudal transverse scan of the thyroid: rounded, hypoechogenic mass (arrow) posteromedial to the carotid artery (A), approximately 0.8 cm in size (2.0 cm in the longitudinal view): suspected adenoma of the left inferior parathyroid. CT and selenium methionine scintigraphy both negative. Significant elevation of serum parathormone. Operative removal: location ectopic, corresponding to the left superior parathyroid. V = jugular vein.

Adrenals

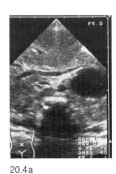 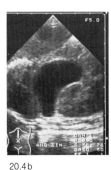 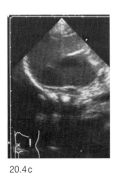 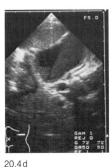 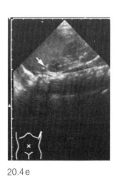

20.4a   20.4b   20.4c   20.4d   20.4e

20.4   Adrenal hemorrhage in a 3-day-old boy with a right axillary artery thrombosis and suspected left renal vein thrombosis (US). **a** Oblique transverse scan and **b** longitudinal scan angled to the left: suprarenal cystic mass, most likely adrenal hemorrhage. Four days later **c** longitudinal and **d** transverse scans of left flank: layering of corpuscular elements, corresponding change of hematoma. **e** Left flank longitudinal scan 2 months later shows small, partly calcified adrenals as residuum (arrow). *Note:* changes in the echo structure and size (reduction) of the lesion are typical of adrenal hematoma.

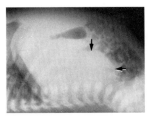 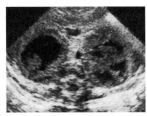 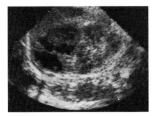

20.5a   20.5b   20.5c

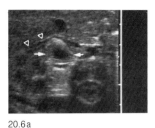
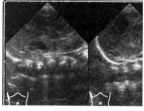
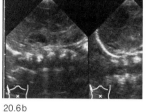

20.6a   20.6b

20.6 Segmental adrenal hemorrhage in a 2-day-old boy diagnosed 1 week prenatally with a right suprarenal cystic mass. **a** Right upper abdominal transverse scan and **b** right flank longitudinal scan: cystic, rather thick-walled lesion in the medial half of the right adrenal (→←); lateral portion appears normal (△). Left image in **b** is medial (lesion), right is lateral (normal). **DD:** segmental adrenal hemorrhage more likely than ganglioneuroma or neuroblastoma. Regressive course.

20.7a   20.7b

20.7 Adrenocortical adenoma with precocious puberty in an 11-month-old boy with penile enlargement, pubarche, weight/length > 97th percentile, but normal-sized testes. Clinical impression: adrenal virilizing tumor. **a** Left posterior longitudinal scan: relatively well-defined left-sided suprarenal mass. **b** CT with i.v. contrast: corresponds to US; high-density areas presumably represent sites of contrast enhancement (X-ray showed no calcifications). Uncomplicated operative removal. Histology: adrenal cortical adenoma, no evidence of malignancy. Growth rate normalized, pubertal signs regressed.

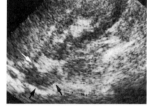

20.8

20.8 Adrenogenital syndrome (AGS) in a 36-year-old man. Left flank longitudinal scan: large adrenal (arrows): adrenal cortical hyperplasia (testicular structure normal; see also Figs. 19.**9** and 19.**10**).

Pancreas

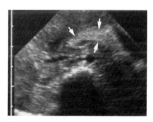
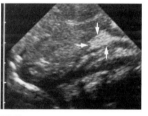
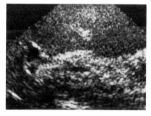

20.9a   20.9b   20.10

20.9 Insulin-dependent nonautoimmune diabetes in a 4-month-old girl with cachexia and extreme dystrophy. Radiographs showed osteoporosis. **a** Oblique transverse scan and **b** midsagittal scan show a very hyperechogenic pancreas (arrows; with moderate nephromegaly and hepatomegaly): lipoatrophic diabetes? Clinical presentation, laboratory findings, and course do not confirm the suspicion: insulin-dependent diabetes, the Fanconi syndrome, Blackfan–Diamond anemia, mitochondrial dysfunction. Transient improvement followed by deterioration and death.

20.10 Cystic fibrosis in a 6½-year-old boy. Transverse scan shows the classic pattern of diffuse increase in pancreatic echogenicity.

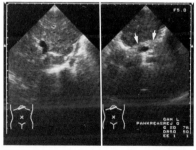

20.11a   20.11b

20.11 Cystic fibrosis in a girl of 10 years, 3 months with "congenital hepatic fibrosis." Sweat test reportedly negative. **a, b** Oblique transverse scans: pronounced increase in pancreatic echogenicity (arrows); irregular hyperechogenicity and contour of the liver (focal nodular hyperplasia?); increased periportal echoes (no visible gallbladder): findings consistent with cystic fibrosis. Repeat sweat test confirmed the diagnosis!

◀ **20.5 Bilateral adrenal hemorrhage** in a 4- and 7-day-old boy delivered by vacuum extraction. Sick neonate, vomiting, hyperexcitable. Small left intraventricular hemorrhage; abdominal mass. **a** Lateral radiograph: retroperitoneal mass (arrow). **b** Transverse and **c** longitudinal scans: bilateral adrenal hemorrhage, extensive, causing downward displacement of the kidneys. The lesions maintained a constant size for 3 weeks, showed a progressive increase of internal echoes. Ten weeks later the lesions were gone. Neurologic status normal.

21 Soft-Tissue and Joint Diseases

R. D. Schulz

Indications for sonography in these cases are:

- palpable mass,
- diffuse or localized inflammation,
- painful limitation of motion in a large joint,
- soft-tissue trauma with or without blunt thoracic or abdominal trauma,
- postoperative complications (seroma, lymphocele, abscess),
- monitoring of tumor response to therapy.

This chapter does not cover lymphadenopathy, hip dysplasia, or the thyroid and parathyroids (see Chaps. 12, 20, 22). The different echo characteristics of skin, subcutaneous tissue, fat, tendons, ligaments, muscles, cartilage, and bone permit the increasing use of ultrasound for soft-tissue imaging. Generally this is done using a 5-MHz or even a 7.5-MHz transducer. Imaging of superficial changes requires the use of a standoff pad. Problems with the application of this technique often relate to difficulties in the identification of reference structures. Scans that include images of bone, blood vessels, muscle groups and fascia, ligaments, or a joint capsule facilitate spatial orientation. When findings are equivocal, comparison of both sides is often useful for establishing an individual reference echo pattern. The manipulation of the joint by the examiner or assistant can aid in assigning echos to specific structures.

Soft-tissue ultrasound provides information on the echo pattern of a lesion: cystic, solid or complex, location, size, shape, and margination with respect to adjacent tissues: smooth, irregular, expansile, infiltrative. A specific tissue diagnosis generally cannot be made, although the clinical presentation and history often provide a basis for narrowing the differential diagnosis. Thus, for example, a superficial cyst of variable size in the popliteal fossa is most probably a Baker cyst. Foreign bodies and calcifications can also be demonstrated. Only the surface structure of bone can be imaged with ultrasound; it remains to be seen whether transmission sonography can really provide additional information on osseous changes.

From 10 to 15% of all malignant tumors in children are soft-tissue tumors. Of these, 50–60% are rhabdomyosarcomas, 10% are fibrosarcomas, and 10% are malignant synovialomas.

Even if it cannot furnish a tissue diagnosis, sonography is still a very important investigation in the general diagnostic workup. While magnetic resonance imaging is of course superior to ultrasound, it is not available everywhere. Ultrasound, moreover, can detect vascular tumors such as hemangiomas, hemangiopericytomas, lymphangiomas, tendosynovial cysts (ganglia), and tumors of the peripheral nerves like neurofibromas and schwannomas, in addition to soft-tissue metastases.

Serial follow-up examinations are both feasible and prudent for all sonographically detectable soft-tissue alterations.

When there is suspicion of a soft-tissue infection, sonography can be used about the large joints, especially the hip, to demonstrate the presence of effusion. With osteomyelitis, the hypoechogenic "cuff" on the bone surface is unlikely to escape the notice of a careful examiner. If joint effusion and osteomyelitis (scintigraphically detectable) appear unlikely on the basis of ultrasound findings, a soft-tissue abscess may perhaps be the cause of the infection.

To date there have been few reports on the sonographic diagnosis of osteomyelitis. Up to 2–3 weeks may pass before this condition produces changes on X-rays. Radionuclide bone scanning is much more sensitive, although a negative scan does not positively exclude osteomyelitis. A normal radiograph and bone scan do not exclude acute osteomyelitis in neonatal patients; a bacterial diagnosis by needle aspiration is indicated. Perhaps sonography will one day be helpful in the early phase of disease by its ability to demonstrate subperiosteal pus and/or accompanying soft-tissue edema.

Epiphyseal separation, whether due to birth trauma or occurring as a slipped capital femoral epiphysis in older children, can be diagnosed with ultrasound. The joint effusion that frequently accompanies capital femoral epiphysiolysis can also be seen. While sonography cannot reliably establish the presence of Perthes disease, it can sometimes demonstrate flattening of the epiphysis or even its fragmentation in a painful hip that is examined to exclude effusion. This study should always be followed by radiography or perhaps radionuclide scanning. Sonography has proven extremely useful in differentiating between coxitis fugax and septic arthritis. Widening of the anteromedial compartment of the hip joint combined with echo-free or hypoechogenic material within the compartment are pathognomonic for effusion; echo-free contents are more commonly seen in coxitis fugax. Synovial thickening is highly suggestive of synovitis.

Even nonneoplastic muscular disorders such as myositis and myositis ossificans can be identified. Some authors have reported sonographic changes in hereditary muscular dystrophies and the possibility of identifying conductors. However, this determination requires considerable experience and should be reserved for selected centers.

There has been little experience to date in the ultrasound evaluation of rheumatoid diseases in children. Rheumatic inflammatory nodules are demonstrable as hypoechogenic lesions.

References

Bernardino, M. E., B. Jing, J. L. Thomas, M. M. Lindell, J. Zornoza: Extremity soft tissue lesions: a comparative study of ultrasound, computed tomography and xeroradiology. Radiology 139 (1981) 53–59

Friedmann, A. P., J. O. Haller, J. D. Goodman, H. Nagar: Sonography evaluation of non-inflammatory neck masses in children. Radiology 147 (1983) 693–697

Harcke, H. T., L. E. Grissom, M. S. Finkelstein: Evaluation of the musculoskeletal system with sonography. Amer. J. Roentgenol. 150 (1988) 1253–1261

Hayden, C. K., L. E. Swischuk: Pediatric Ultrasonography. Williams & Wilkins, Baltimore 1987

Hofman, V.: Ultraschalldiagnostik in Pädiatrie und Kinderchirurgie. VEB Thieme, Leipzig 1988

v. Rohden, L., V. Steinbicker: Ultraschalltomographie. Ein Verfahren zur Differentialdiagnostik. In Lössner, J., A. Wagner: Beiträge zur klinischen Myologie. Hirzel, Leipzig 1987

Slasky, B. S., J. L. Lenkey, M. L. Sholnick, W. L. Campbell, K. L. Cover: Sonography of soft tissues of extremities and trunk. Semin. Ultrasound 3 (1982) 288–330

Yiu-Chiu, V. S., L. C. Chiu: Complementary values of ultrasound and computed tomography in the evaluation of musculosceletal masses. Radiographics 3 (1983) 46–82

Zieger, M. M., U. Dörr, R. D. Schulz: Ultrasonography of hip joint effusions. Skelet. Radiol. 16 (1987) 607–611

Hip Joint Effusion

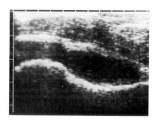
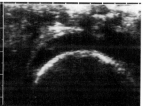
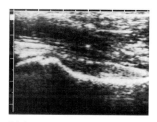

21.1a   21.1b   21.1c

21.1 Septic coxitis in a 12-year-old girl with a 2-day history of high fever and progressive, very painful limitation of hip motion. ESR 70/120. **a** Anteromedial longitudinal scan of the right hip: a wide echo-free area in the medial joint compartment with bulging of the capsule. Large hip joint effusion; in conjunction with clinical findings: septic effusion, mild synovial thickening. **b** Anterior transverse scan of the right hip: wide, crescent-shaped, echo-free band anterior to the femoral head, between the femoral head and the joint capsule. Substantial joint effusion. Effusion must be large to be seen in the transverse view. Treatment: arthrotomy for acute decompression and irrigation of the joint. The joint capsule was tense; pus spurted out when the joint was incised. **c** Anteromedial longitudinal scan of the left hip for comparison: normally hypoechogenic joint compartment of normal width; no synovial thickening.

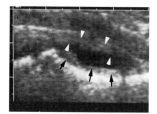
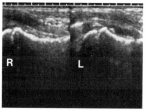
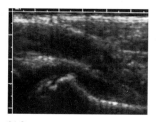
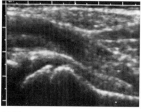

21.2a   21.2b   21.3a   21.3b

21.2 Septic coxitis with synovitis in a 4-year-old girl with a 3-day history of progressively limited motion in the left hip, a limp, and an inability to extend the left leg. Elevated temperature and ESR. **a** Anteromedial longitudinal scan of the left hip: widening of the joint compartment, synovial thickening (▼), echogenic band along the femoral neck (←), echo-free center of the compartment. Septic coxitis with synovial thickening (synovitis) and sedimentation of debris along the femoral neck. Treatment: arthrotomy. **b** Comparative anteromedial longitudinal scans of both hips: normal on the right, septic coxitis on the left. Hemorrhagic effusions or effusions associated with septic coxitis tend to be moderately echogenic rather than echo-free.

21.3 Coxitis fugax in a 6-year-old boy with a febrile infection 4 days before, now afebrile; 1-day history of left hip pain. **a** Anteromedial longitudinal scan of the left hip: expansion of the joint compartment by moderately echogenic material, bulging of the capsule: coxitis fugax. Traction and analgesic therapy relieved symptoms within 2 days. **b** Same view 7 days later: normal-appearing compartment with no effusion.

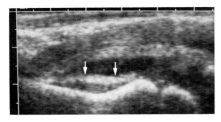

21.4

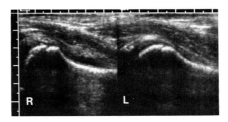

21.5

21.4 Septic coxitis, subperiosteal abscess, synovitis in a 2½-year-old boy with whooping cough, high fever, ESR 70/109, WBC 11900; 1-day history of left hip pain. Anteromedial longitudinal scan of the left hip: widening of the joint space with hypoechogenic contents, bandlike sonodensity parallel to the femoral neck (arrows) with a narrow intervening echo-free area; widening of the joint capsule: septic coxitis with subperiosteal abscess formation, synovitis. Treatment: arthrotomy, suction irrigation, then hip spica and antibiotics.

21.5 Hip joint effusion in the setting of Perthes disease in a 16-year-old boy who has had right hip pain for several months. Radiography showed Catterall stage-III Perthes disease. Comparative anteromedial longitudinal scans of the right and left hips: echo-free effusion on the right, thickening of the joint capsule, fragmentation and flattening of the femoral head: Perthes disease, chronic synovitis, joint effusion. On the left, normal findings with an intact femoral head. Diagnosis of Perthes disease established by radiography. This disease is commonly accompanied by effusion.

Inflammatory Diseases (Other than Coxitis)

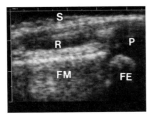

21.6

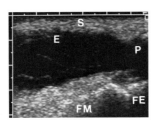

21.7

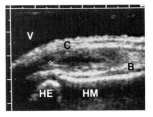

21.8   21.9

21.6 Gonitis with suprapatellar effusion in an 18-month-old boy with painful swelling of the right knee. Longitudinal scan on the extensor side of the distal right femur: FM = femoral metaphysis, FE = femoral epiphysis, P = cartilaginous patella, S = long extensor tendon, R = suprapatellar pouch. Bandlike echo-free area in the distended joint pouch: suprapatellar knee effusion in gonitis.

21.7 Gonitis with massive joint effusion in a 12-year-old boy with knee swelling, clinical suspicion of effusion, fever, pain, elevated ESR. Longitudinal scan on the extensor side of the distal left femur: S = extensor tendon, P = patella, FM = femoral metaphysis, FE = femoral epiphysis, E = effusion. Large echo-free area with septations in the suprapatellar pouch: knee effusion in gonitis.

21.8 Cellulitis in a 10-year-old boy with redness and swelling of the left thigh. Soft-tissue abscess? Longitudinal scan on the extensor side of the right midthigh: V = standoff pad (useful for imaging superficial processes), C = skin, SC = subcutaneous tissue, F = fascia, M = extensor muscles. Diffuse expansion of the subcutaneous tissue, moderately echogenic with a blurring of echo structure; well demarcated with respect to the fascia: cellulitis. **DD:** lymphangiomatosis.

21.9 Pyogenic myositis of the right proximal humerus in a 5½-year-old boy with an 8-day history of pain in the proximal right upper arm and a palpable, somewhat tender "mass" in the area of the deltoid muscle. Lateral longitudinal scan of the proximal upper arm: V = standoff pad, C = skin, B = biceps tendon, HE = humeral epiphysis, HM = humeral metaphysis. Oblong structure in the deltoid muscle with an echogenic periphery and an echo-free center. Operation: pyogenic myositis with abscessation. Antibiotic therapy.

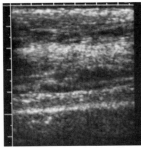

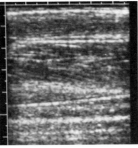

21.10a   21.10b

21.10 Myositis of the lateral right lower leg in a 4-year-old girl whose mother noted swelling on the right lower leg 4 weeks before; no fever, trauma, or signs of inflammation. Question: exclusion of soft-tissue tumor. X-ray of the right lower leg showed no osseous lesions, expansion of soft tissues on the fibular side. **a** Longitudinal scan of the lateral right lower leg: almost no normal muscle structure is apparent. Nonhomogeneous structure of mixed echogenicity. US diagnosis unclear. Operation: no tumor. Histology: myositis. **b** Comparative scan of the left lower leg at the same level: normal appearance of superficial and deep muscles with characteristic pinnation.

21.11 Osteomyelitis of the distal right tibia in a 13-year-old boy with a 6-day history of right lower leg pain, treated elsewhere as thrombophlebitis. Signs of inflammation, very high ESR. **a** Longitudinal scan of the distal right tibia: narrow, spindle-shaped, homogeneous structure over the tibial surface, with a thin anterior hypoechogenic rim: circumscribed subperiosteal abscess. **b** Transverse distal scan: narrow, uniformly echogenic crescent with an anterior hypoechogenic border directly over the tibia. Operation: subperiosteal abscess with penetration into the bone. Osteomyelitis. Radiographs initially showed no bone destruction.

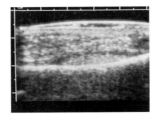 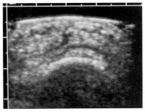

21.11a   21.11b

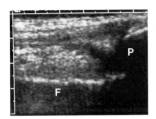 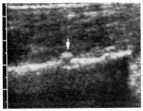   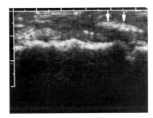 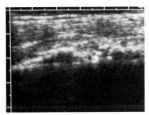

21.12a   21.12b   21.12c   21.12d

21.12 Osteomyelitis of the right distal femur in a 13-year-old boy seen for angina by the family doctor 10 days before. Six days later he felt pain in the left heel after a soccer game. X-rayed elsewhere; the foot was placed in a cast for suspected calcaneal fracture. Six days later, pain and swelling of the right knee joint and right wrist. Temperature 38°C, ESR 35/70, WBC 8000. Cast removed from the foot, X-ray of the left calcaneus showed osteolytic destruction, no fracture. Initial diagnosis wrong. **a** Anterior longitudinal scan of the right distal femur: F = femur, P = patella. Waviness and small discontinuities in the cortical contour suggest sites of bone destruction. Also, nonhomogeneous soft-tissue markings imply inflammatory changes in the surrounding soft tissues. On incision, compressed pus permeated with clots exuded from the wound: osteomyelitis. PMMA beads were inserted. Multifocal osteomyelitis progressed despite intensive antibiotic therapy, with involvement of the left knee joint, right hip joint, left elbow, right tibia, and left distal ulna. Further rise in ESR: 80/120. Repeated local surgical intervention. **b** Anterior longitudinal scan of the left distal femur 7 weeks later: irregular cortical margin with the elevation of a small bone sequestrum (arrow). Osteomyelitis of the left femur. **c** Concomitant anterior longitudinal scan of the distal right femur, 7 weeks after onset of the disease: wavy cortical contour with more pronounced discontinuities and larger sequestra in the soft tissues (arrows). **d** Medial longitudinal scan of the right mid-femur 7 weeks after onset of the disease: wide, curved area of periosteal elevation and new bone formation. Underlying cortex thinned. Intervening echo-free space represents a subperiostal abscess. **e** Radiograph of the right femur and knee joint 5 weeks after onset of the disease: bone destruction evidenced by the motheaten appearance of the distal femoral metaphysis and epiphysis and of the proximal tibial metaphysis. Sites of periosteal apposition on the femur: multifocal osteomyelitis. Numerous surgical interventions and several changes of antibiotic were necessary to bring this fulminating, multifocal infection under control.

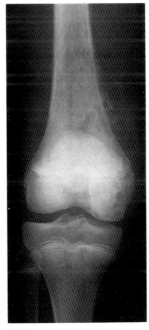

21.12e

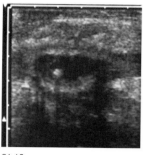
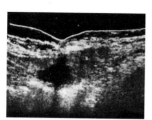
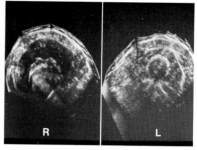

21.13   21.14   21.15a

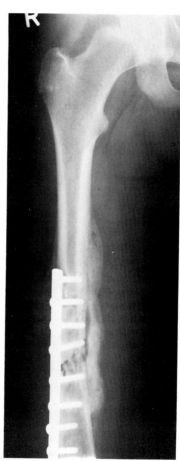

21.**13** **Inguinal scar abscess** in a 15-year-old boy who underwent bilateral orchiopexy and inguinal hernia repair 6 years before. He presented with pain in the left groin region associated with a firm egg-sized swelling in the left herniotomy scar. Oblique left inguinal scan: elongated mass, 5 cm long with a moderately echogenic border 0.5 cm wide and a central echo-free zone containing a coarse echo with an acoustic shadow. Florid abscess with a scar-tissue band. On incision, 4 ml of creamy, bloody pus was drained along with an old piece of suture. Uncomplicated course.

21.**14** **Abdominal wall abscess** in an 11½-year-old boy operated on 10 years previously for intussusception. He presented with abdominal pain and tenderness below the old scar. Parasagittal scan of the right midabdomen: dimpling of the abdominal wall in the scar area. Echo-free trapezoidal feature, tender to pressure, within the abdominal wall. Operation: one larger and three smaller abdominal-wall abscesses 10 years after laparotomy. *Note:* abdominal pain as a symptom.

21.**15** **Nonspecific inflammation of the right femur** in a 13-year-old boy with a femoral shaft fracture managed by internal fixation. He presented with pain in the midthigh region, signs of instability. **a** Transverse scans of both thighs: on the right a wide, crescent-shaped hypoechogenic area directly over the femur: inflammation associated with instability. Compare with the normal soft-tissue structure on the left. Aspiration: nonspecific inflammation with no demonstrable infectious organism. **b** Radiograph of the plated right femur: bone resorption at the upper end of the plate and about the upper screws. Fracture site not yet consolidated. Probably a mechanically induced inflammation due to unstable internal fixation.

21.15b

Trauma

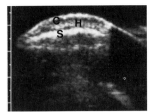

21.16

21.16 Old cephalhematoma in a 4-month-old girl with a unilateral, relatively firm paramedian swelling over the parietal skull. Parasagittal parietal scan with standoff pad: crescent-shaped, nonhomogeneous, partly hypoechogenic, partly hyperechogenic structure between the skull (S) and scalp (C): older hematoma (H) undergoing organization. Birth injury.

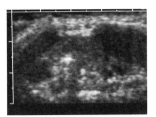

21.17

21.17 Hematoma of the sternocleidomastoid muscle in a 4-week-old girl with a marked, firm swelling of the left sterno-cleidomastoid muscle. Transverse scan of the anterior neck: marked widening and hypoechogenicity of the left sterno-cleidomastoid muscle: older hematoma. Birth injury.

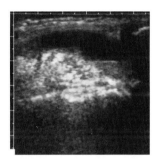

21.18

21.18 Suprapatellar hematoma in a 7-year-old boy with a comminuted fracture of the right distal femur sustained in a car accident. Longitudinal scan of the distal femur: curved, echo-free area above the patella. Contour and structure of the distal femur disrupted by the comminuted fracture. Large, fresh hematoma.

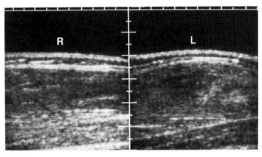

21.19

21.19 Torn muscle fibers in a 10-year-old boy who was struck on the tensed left thigh while running. Severe pain. Longitudinal scans on the extensor side of both femurs: R = normal muscle structure, L = widening of the muscle, some continuity disruption as evidenced by a thin, oblique echo band, and hypoechogenic areas consistent with hemorrhage: a partial muscular tear with a hematoma. The echo pattern of a hematoma may be anechogenic, mixed (during clot formation), or echogenic (organized hematoma) depending on the age of the collection.

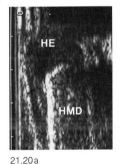 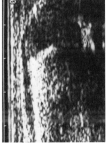 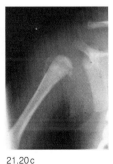

21.20a   21.20b   21.20c

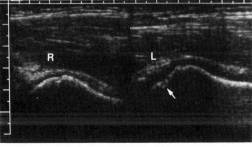

21.21

21.20 Slipped capital humeral epiphysis in a 6-day-old girl with no active left arm motion, obvious pain on passive motion. **a** Longitudinal scan of the left upper arm: hypoechogenic humeral epiphysis (HE) displaced 5 mm laterally, HMD = humeral metadiaphysis: slipped capital humeral epiphysis due to birth trauma. **b** Healthy right side for comparison: note continuity from the humeral epiphysis to the shaft. **c** Radiograph of the left arm at 12 days: classic appearance of neonatal epiphyseal separation, with periosteal callus formation on the metaphysis.

21.21 Slipped capital femoral epiphysis in a 16-year-old boy with a 3-week history of increasing left hip pain; overweight, no signs of inflammation. Anteromedial scan of the right hip joint: aside from the gap at the epiphyseal plate, a smooth transition from metaphysis to epiphysis. Scan on the left shows a conspicuous stepoff at the junction of the metaphysis and epiphysis (arrow) with epiphyseal displacement. Also, a slight expansion of the joint compartment by echo-free material: slipped capital femoral epiphysis with joint effusion.

Tumors

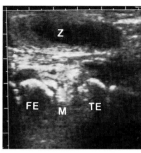 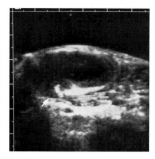

21.22a   21.22b

21.22 Baker cyst in a 6-year-old boy with tense swelling in the right popliteal fossa. **a** Longitudinal scan of the right popliteal fossa: FE = femoral epiphysis, M = meniscus, TE = tibial epiphysis, Z = superficial, echo-free, smoothly marginated soft-tissue cyst. **b** Transverse scan: Baker cyst with a hook-shaped extension to the joint space (arrow). Baker cysts can present a great variety of shapes and sizes.

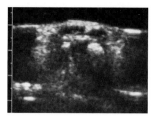 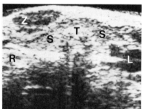

21.23   21.24

21.23 Dorsal ganglia of the hand in a 3½-year-old girl with two oblong, nontender nodules on the back of right hand; no signs of inflammation. Dorsal transverse scan of the right wrist: narrow, oval, echo-free structure over each of two carpal bones: two ganglia. Use a 5-MHz transducer and standoff pad for superficial imaging.

21.24 Paramedian neck cyst in a 7-year-old boy with palpable nodular swelling on the right side of neck, medial to the sternocleidomastoid muscle. Transverse scan through the anteroinferior neck region: S = thyroid gland, T = trachea with posterior shadowing, Z = hypoechogenic paramedian cyst.

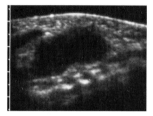 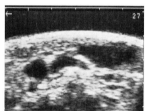

21.25   21.26

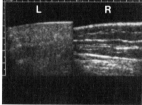 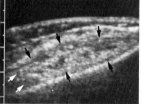

21.27   21.28

21.25 Subpectoral chest wall abscess in a 1-month-old girl with a swelling on the left side of the chest, cutaneous redness, fever. Left infra-axillary longitudinal scan: bean-shaped anechogenic lesion below the pectoralis, directly overlying the ribs. **DD:** cyst, abscess. In clinical context: abscess with liquefaction.

21.26 Cystic lymphangioma of the neck in a 3-year-old girl with a doughy swelling on the left side of neck, no apparent inflammation. Oblique scan through the left side of the neck: three intercommunicating, echo-free areas of diverse size: cystic lymphangioma. **DD:** cavernous hemangioma.

21.27 Hemangiolymphomatosis of the thigh in an 11-year-old girl with marked, painless, uniform swelling of the left thigh. Longitudinal scans of the anterior midthigh, right and left sides shown for comparison: on the left, normal soft-tissue differentiation is lost; tissues appear blurred and moderately echogenic. This pattern extends to a depth of 5 cm throughout the thigh. Contrast with normal soft-tissue differentiation on the right.

21.28 Hemangioma in a 9-year-old girl with a 2-year history of right knee problems. Radiographs normal even on repeat examination. Slight tenderness to pressure on the lateral side of the distal right thigh. Longitudinal scan of the distal right thigh: spindle-shaped, nonhomogeneous feature of mixed echogeniciy directly over the bone (arrow). Operation: deep hemangioma. Patient asymptomatic after surgery.

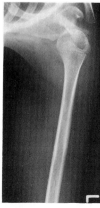 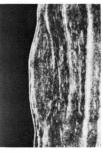

21.29a   21.29b

21.29 Lipoma of the upper arm in an 11½-year-old girl who noticed a soft, protuberant, nonpainful swelling on the inside of the right proximal upper arm. **a** Radiograph of the right upper arm: no osseous changes, but a large, well-defined egg-shaped lucency on the inside of the upper arm. **b** Longitudinal scan through the inside of the right upper arm, compound technique: subcutaneous spindle-shaped, uniformly hypoechogenic feature well delineated with respect to the muscle, indicating a solid tumor. Tumor extirpated. Histology: lipoma.

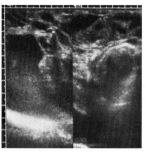
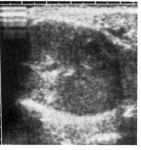

21.30   21.31

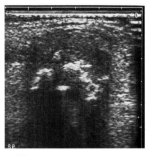
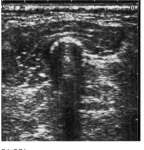

21.32a   21.32b

21.30   Thoracic cystic lymphangioma in a 1-day-old girl with a huge, spongy tumor involving the whole right side of the chest, forcing the arm into slight abduction. Longitudinal scan of the right chest wall: multilocular, intercommunicating, echo-free structures with little intervening solid tissue: giant cystic lymphangioma.

21.31   Rhabdomyosarcoma of the right pterygoid fossa in a 10-year-old boy with a firm, slightly tender swelling in the pterygoid fossa; no signs of inflammation. Oblique sonogram: nonhomogeneous, moderately echogenic mass with well-defined margins. Biopsy: rhabdomyosarcoma. Chemotherapy, radiation, then resection.

21.32   Ewing sarcoma of the right femur in a 3½-year-old boy with a radiographically and histologically established diagnosis of Ewing sarcoma. US done to check for spread into the surrounding soft tissues. **a** Anterior transverse scan of the right femur: wide, curved, hypoechogenic zone in soft tissues with scattered coarse echoes representing osseous tumor tissue. Typical crescent-shaped, echogenic shaft contour no longer visible. **b** Comparative scan through the left femur: normal soft-tissue structure of the surrounding muscles, typical echogenic crescent of long bone with a narrow, sharply defined posterior acoustic shadow. US has at most an adjunctive role in the evaluation of bone tumors.

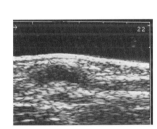
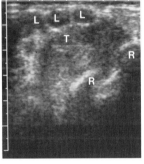

21.33   21.34

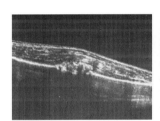

21.35   21.36

21.33   Leiomyosarcoma of the right humerus. The child's mother noticed a small, nonpainful subcutaneous swelling on the upper arm, no apparent inflammation. Longitudinal scan of the lateral upper humerus: bean-shaped, uniformly hypoechogenic feature beneath the skin in the superficial musculature. Biopsy: leiomyosarcoma.

21.34   Malignant ectomesenchymoma of the left axilla in a 14-week-old boy whose mother noticed a nodular swelling in the left axilla with an extension into the chest wall. No signs of inflammation. US scan of the left axilla and chest wall: L = three hypoechogenic superficial infiltrated lymph nodes; T = homogeneous, moderately echogenic, well-defined tumor on the chest wall; R = ribs. Biopsy: malignant tumor. Operation: tumor resection encompassing infiltrated regional nodes. Patient has been free of disease for 1½ years.

21.35   Osteogenic sarcoma of the femur in a 15-year-old boy with thigh pain and a palpable firm mass. Longitudinal midshaft scan of the femur: disruption of the cortical margin with multiple irregular echoes in the overlying soft tissues. Suspected neoplastic bone destruction. Radiograph showed typical features of osteogenic sarcoma. Chest film showed multiple pulmonary metastases. The patient underwent three operations, but did not survive.

21.36   Left supra-auricular hemangiopericytoma in a 12-year-old boy with a soft swelling above the left ear. Transverse supra-auricular scan: moderately echogenic mass, 5 × 1.8 cm in size, in contact with cranial bone, permeated by small sonolucent foci. Large, pulsating feeding vessel (arrows): highly vascular tumor, probably "microcystic" hemangioma. CT findings suggested finely structured hemangioma. Selective angiography of the external carotid artery demonstrated a heavily vascularized tumor, which was subsequently embolized with Ivalon microparticles. Swelling regressed completely; to date no recurrence.

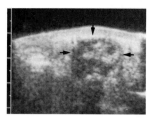
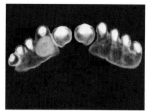

21.37a   21.37b

21.**37** **Myxolipofibroma of the foot** in a 7-year-old boy with swelling below the proximal joint of the second toe of the right foot, present for some weeks. Mass firm and slightly mobile on palpation. No signs of inflammation. Radiograph of the forefoot showed no bone destruction. **a** Transverse plantar scan over the metatarsophalangeal joints: nonhomogeneous, hazelnut-sized mass with distinct borders (arrows). **b** MRI: well-defined soft-tissue tumor of high signal intensity below the second toe of the right foot (Dr. Klott, Dr. Reichardt). Tumor extirpated. Histology: myxolipofibroma.

Other Findings

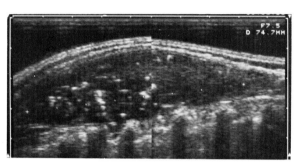

21.38a

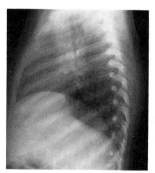
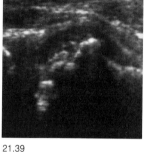

21.38b   21.39

21.**38** **Benign myofibromatosis** in a 12-year-old girl with an 8-month history of a soft mass in the right paravertebral thoracolumbar area. Mass enlarged, with a tense consistency, adherent to deeper tissues; no redness or fixation of skin. **a** Posterior longitudinal scan: spindle-shaped, nonhomogeneous, predominantly hypoechogenic mass with multiple fine to coarse echogenic foci (calcifications?). **b** Lateral chest radiograph: homogeneous soft-tissue expansion in the posterior thorax, no calcifications. **DD:** myositis ossificans, myofibromatosis, neuroblastoma, rhabdomyosarcoma. Tumor extirpated. Histology: benign myofibromatosis.

21.**39** **Perthes disease** in a 5½-year-old boy with a history of left hip pain for some weeks. No signs of inflammation. Anteromedial scan of the left hip to exclude effusion: fragmentation and flattening of the femoral epiphysis and small, echo-free effusion in the medial joint compartment. Suspected Perthes disease with effusion. Prompted pelvic survey radiograph and an axial view of the left hip: Perthes disease, Catterall stage III. US generally cannot furnish sufficient information for early diagnosis and staging.

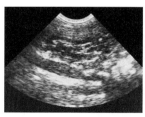
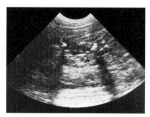

21.40a   21.40b

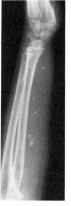
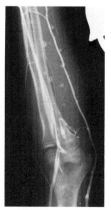

21.40c   21.40d

21.**40** **Klippel–Trenaunay syndrome** in a 10-year-old girl with swelling of the left forearm; no redness, heat, or tenderness. Longitudinal volar scan of the left forearm: **a** multiple echo-free tubular structures; **b** (slightly lateral to **a**): multiple coarse echoes with acoustic shadows in the soft tissues: calcifications. **c** Lateral radiograph of the left forearm: multiple calcifications, some lay-ered, of varying size in the swollen volar soft tissues: phleboliths. No osseous changes. Radius and ulna minimally (5 mm) longer than on the right. Venography indicated. **d** Venogram of the left arm: only the superficial forearm veins are opacified. Phleboliths outside these vessels in deep, dilated veins demonstrated by US.

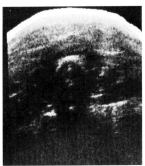

21.41

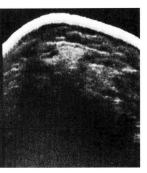

21.42

21.41 Duchenne muscular dystrophy in an 8-year-old girl. Anterior transverse compound scan of the right midthigh (7.5 MHz): uniformly echogenic musculature, fascial planes and femoral echo crescent still faintly visible, sound penetration decreased. Histology: Duchenne muscular dystrophy, Vignos stage III (Dr. v. Rohden, Dr. Wiemann).

21.42 Kugelberg—Welander type muscular atrophy in an 8-year-old girl. Anterior transverse compound scan of the right midthigh (7.5 MHz): coarse, clumped appearance of subcutaneous structures. Focally increased echogenicity in a markedly reduced muscle mass, very prominent lamellar muscular structures; femoral echo crescent. Sound attenuation by atrophic muscle accounts for the absence of acoustic shadow, i.e., echoes beyond the musculature. Histology: Kugelberg—Welander type muscular atrophy, Vignos stage IV (Dr. v. Rohden, Dr. Wiemann).

22 Neonatal and Infant Hip

R. D. Schulz

Principles of Hip Sonography and Classification of Maturity Deficits

The following indications are recognized for sonography of the neonatal and infant hip:

- suspected dislocation,
- suspected dysplasia,
- restriction of abduction,
- breech presentation,
- hypertension in pregnancy,
- family history,
- foot deformities,
- leg length discrepancy,
- oligohydramnios,
- asymmetric skin creases (?),
- general neonatal screening (?).

The early detection of hip dysplasias (maturity deficits) and especially of hip dislocation is of central concern for pediatricians and orthopedists. Radiographic examination of the neonate or small infant up to 3 months of age is controversial due to both the limited value of X-rays in this age group and the radiation risk. Preformed in cartilage, the neonatal hip is essentially nonosseous. According to the experimental and clinical studies of R. Graf, sonography provides a safe, effective technique for visualizing the osseous and nonosseous structures of the infant and neonatal hip joint. There are various sonographically reproducible dysplasias that can be accurately identified and classified according to type. This is highly advantageous both in the diagnosis of hip dysplasias and in the monitoring of therapeutic response. Real-time imaging, moreover, enables the examiner to test for excessive joint mobility. In the hands of an experienced sonographer, the method is effective and easy to use.

The structures around the infant hip joint that can be identified with ultrasound are illustrated in Figs. 22.1 and 22.2. It is vital to consider the sectional plane on which the joint is imaged. Graf defined several criteria for a reproducible and representative section through the hip joint; these are indispensable for the qualitative and quantitative interpretation of hip sonograms (see Fig. 22.2):

1. A straight, vertical (parallel to image border) iliac border above the acetabulum.
2. Visualization of the inferior border of the ileum with the acetabular fossa.
3. Visualization of the superior cartilaginous rim and bony rim of the acetabulum.
4. Visualization of the acetabular labrum.
5. Visualization of the femoral head.
6. Visualization of the femoral neck (helpful).

Hip sonograms are interpreted qualitatively and quantitatively, employing both the "standard plane" examination and the dynamic examination, in which the examiner observes spontaneous motion of the femoral head in the joint and also actively tests joint stability by pushing the femur upward against the acetabular roof (Table 22.1).

Qualitative refers to the overall visual impression: the contour of the bony acetabulum, the shape of the bony and cartilaginous rims, the echo structure of the cartilaginous rim, and the position of the labrum. The components forming the acetabular roof are subject to various changes depending on the condition that is present: delayed maturation, dysplasia, or dislocation. *Quantitative* refers to image evaluation using designated reference lines and angular parameters (Figs. 22.3 and 22.4). Based on angle measurements and

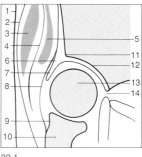 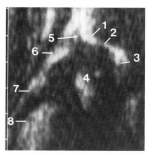

22.1   22.2

22.1 Schematic longitudinal section through the infant hip joint.
1 Skin
2 Subcutaneous tissue with the iliotibial tract
3 Gluteus medius muscle
4 Intermuscular septum
5 Gluteus minimus muscle
6 Superior cartilaginous rim of the acetabulum
7 Acetabular labrum
8 Joint capsule
9 Cartilage–bone interface in the femoral neck
10 Greater trochanter
11 Superior bony rim of the acetabulum
12 Iliac bone (acetabular roof)
13 Cartilaginous femoral head
14 Triradiate cartilage

22.2 Normal hip sonogram of a 4-month-old infant.
1 Superior bony rim of the acetabulum
2 Acetabular roof
3 Triradiate cartilage
4 Capital femoral ossification center
5 Superior cartilaginous rim of the acetabulum
6 Acetabular labrum
7 Joint capsule
8 Femoral neck

additional structural and morphologic criteria, Graf has developed a clinically proven system for the classification of hip dysplasias (Table 22.1).

The measuring technique is subject to interpersonal and intrapersonal variations relating to echo unsharpness and other factors. Angular discrepancies of ±2−5° may occur. But qualitative and quantitative image analysis combined with dynamic examination should permit the experienced examiner to achieve high accuracy. If pathologic angles are measured on a hip sonogram that presents a completely normal visual impression, either the scan plane is incorrect or the reference lines are improperly drawn (or both). The novice tends to overstate measurements due to uncertainty. Decentering of the femoral head from the acetabular floor noted in the dynamic examination is clinically significant and is known as a sonographically mobile hip. Therapeutic problems may result from neglect or delay of treatment. Mobile hips may be found in any hip type beyond type 1 and are most commonly encountered in type 3. *Caution:* the femoral head does not leave the acetabulum completely in a sonographically mobile hip; this would sigrify a dislocatable hip.

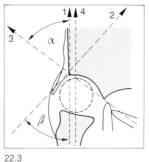 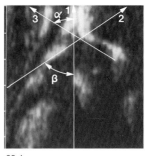

22.3   22.4

22.3 Schematic drawing of a hip sonogram showing reference lines and angular parameters. 1 = Baseline (tangent from the superior bony rim along the upper linear portion of the iliac bone), 2 = cartilage roof line (from the superior bony rim through the center of the acetabular labrum), 3 = bony roof line (from triradiate cartilage to the bony rim of acetabulum), 4 = vector line (through the center of the femoral head), α = bony roof angle, β = cartilage roof angle.

22.4 Reference lines on a hip sonogram: here line 1 corresponds to line 4 (vector line), α = bony roof angle, β = cartilage roof angle.

Table 22.1   Classification of hip types (after Graf, expanded by Schulz)

Type	Bony roof contour	Bony rim	Cartilage rim	α	β
1a Mature hip (any age)	Good	Angular	Projects far over femoral head	> 60°	< 55°
1b "Transitional form" *Physiologic delay of ossification*	Good	Usually rounded	Short, covers femoral head	> 60°	> 55°
Appropriate for age 2a (+)	Satisfactory	Round	Broad, covers femoral head	50−59°	> 55°
2a With maturity deficit 2a (−) (up to age 3 months)	Deficient	Round	Broad, covers femoral head	50−59°	> 55°
2b Delayed ossification (after age 3 months)	Deficient	Round	Broad, covers femoral head	50−59°	> 55°
2c Critical hip (any age)	Deficient	Round to flat	Broad, still covers head	43−49° Critical range	70−77°
m Mobile hip (any age) *Eccentric hips*	Deficient to poor	Round to flat	Broad or displaced	< 60°	> 55°
3a	Poor	Flat	Displaced, no structural change	< 43°	> 77°
3b	Poor	Flat	Displaced, with structural change	< 43°	> 77°
4 Dislocation	Poor	Flat	Displaced	< 43°	> 77°

If a hip joint cannot be imaged in typical fashion, as when, for example, the acetabular roof exhibits a comblike structure, then a generalized skeletal dysplasia should be suspected. A radiographic examination is essential to clarify the diagnosis in cases of this kind. We also feel that radiographs are indicated when a large discrepancy is noted between clinical and sonographic findings. At present there is diversity of opinion as to whether a pelvic survey radiograph is indicated at the termination of treatment following a dislocation or severe dysplasia.

Either a linear-array or sector scanner can be used for hip sonography. Both have advantages and disadvantages in terms of examination technique, focusing capability, and echo conditions. A 5-MHz transducer is acceptable for neonates and older infants. In pathologic hips, there is a tendency for angle measurements to come out smaller with a sector scanner than with a linear array. It is unclear whether this is due to artifacts or differences in travel times.

Sonography is excellent for monitoring therapeutic response. Follow-up scans should be scheduled at intervals of 4–5 weeks, although in dislocated hips we perform the initial follow-up at 1 week (to confirm centering or to modify treatment). In cases where treatment in an abduction splint leaves sufficient lateral access for the probe, stable centering of the femoral heads in the acetabula can be accurately confirmed, even though the strongly abducted position often does not permit imaging on the "standard plane." It is assumed that the femoral head is well centered if the greatest head diameter is seated deeply within the acetabulum.

The ossification center of the femoral head can be seen about 14–21 days earlier on sonograms than on X-rays. Some infants already have capital femoral ossification centers at birth, while 54% of infants have an ossific center by 4 months of age. Thus, the range of variation is large.

The value of sonography in the diagnosis of avascular necrosis of the femoral head remains unclear. If a comparison of both sides indicates a shortening of the distance between the femoral neck and acetabular roof, there is strong reason to suspect avascular necrosis.

If a dislocation is found, sonography can be performed after the reduction maneuver to confirm successful centering. With good ultrasound equipment, it is often possible to identify an obstacle to reduction (obstructive factor) and draw appropriate therapeutic conclusions.

Therapeutic implications for type 1a and 1b hips: no treatment. Opinions differ as to the need to treat type 2a+ or 2a− hips (abduction). An abduction pillow is indicated for type 2b hips and also for types 3a and 3b. Splinting has proved useful for type 2c and mobile hips. Management of the dislocated hip (type 4) is geared toward the age of the child following reduction or the identification of an obstructive factor. A variety of treatments are employed.

References

Graf, R.: Sonographie der Säuglingshüfte. Ein Kompendium. Bücherei der Orthopäden, Bd. 43. Enke, Stuttgart 1986

Graf, R., P. Schuler: Die Säuglingshüfte im Ultraschallbild: ein Atlas. Edition Medizin, Weinheim 1986

Schulz, R. D., et al.: Die sonographisch mobile Säuglingshüfte – Beobachtungen und klinische Relevanz. In Judmaier, G., H. Frommhold, A. Kratochwil: Ultraschalldiagnostik 1984. Drei-Länder-Treffen Innsbruck 1984. Thieme, Stuttgart 1985

Schulz, R. D., M. Zieger: Principles of ultrasonography of the hip in newborn and young infants. In Heuck, F. H. W.: Radiology Today 4. Springer, Berlin 1987

Examples of Incorrect Scan Plane Selection in the Hip of a 14-Week-Old Female Infant

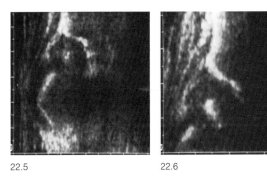

22.5

22.6

22.5 **Normal scan, type 1a hip.**

22.6 **Scan plane too far anterior,** causing lack of concavity of the acetabular roof: type 2b hip?

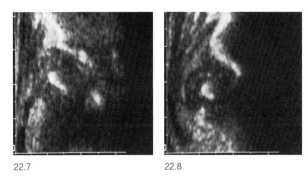

22.7

22.8

22.7 **Scan too far anterior and rotated.**

22.8 **Scan rotated anteriorly, no labrum.**

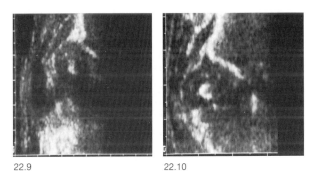

22.9

22.10

22.9 **Hip scanned from the caudal aspect.**

22.10 **Scan rotated posteriorly.**

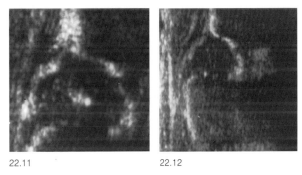

22.11

22.12

22.11 **Type 1a hip** in a 7-week-old girl with good contour of the bony and cartilaginous acetabular roof and an angular superior bony rim.

22.12 **Type 1b hip** in an 8-week-old boy with good contour of the bony and cartilaginous acetabular roof and a rounded superior bony rim: transitional form.

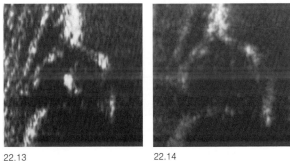

22.13

22.14

22.13 **Type 1a hip** in a 14-week-old girl with an ossified femoral head nucleus; in rare cases an ossification center may already be present at birth.

22.14 **Type 1b hip** in a 10-week-old girl with good acetabular roof contour and a rounded superior bony rim.

22.15

22.15 **Type 2a left hip** in a 4-week-old girl with restricted abduction on the left, $\alpha = 55°$, $\beta = 60°$, satisfactory roof contour, rounded bony rim.

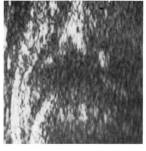
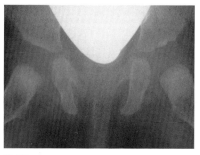
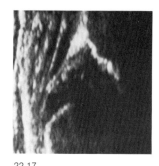

22.16a   22.16b   22.17

22.**16 a Normal findings** in a 3-month-old girl with a rounded bony rim and widened cartilaginous rim. The defect or notch in the superior rim is also visible on radiographs. **b** Pelvic radiograph of the same infant, showing symmetric notchlike defects in the superior bony rims of the acetabula.

22.**17 Type 2b** left hin in a 6-month-old girl with asymmetric skin creases and a positive family history; α = 54°, deficient acetabular roof round bony rim, centered femoral head, relatively large labrum.

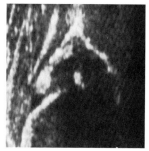
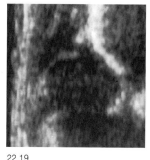
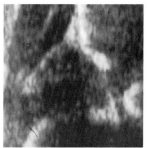
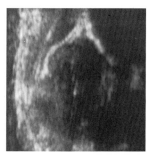

22.18   22.19   22.20   22.21

22.**18 Type 2b** right hin in a 5-month-old boy with restricted abduction on the right, deficient acetabular contour, rim defect, and centered femoral head.

22.**19 Type 2c** right hip in a 3-week-old girl with a lax hip, α = 45°, deficient acetabular contour, rim defect, flat bony rim, decentering head, displaced labrum. Treated by splinting.

22.**20 Type 2c** right hip in a 14-day-old girl, breech presentation, α = 46°, deficient acetabular development, flat bony rim, femoral head slightly eccentric. Treated by splinting.

22.**21 Type 3a** left hip in a 6-week-old girl. No clinical findings, α = 35°, deficient acetabular development, flat rim, displaced labrum, eccentric femoral head. Treated with abduction pillow.

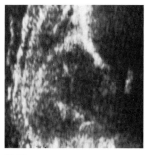
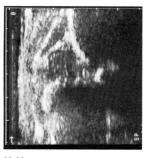
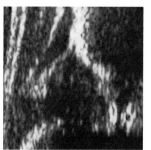
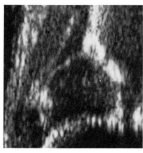

22.22   22.23   22.24a   22.24b

22.**22 Type 3b** left hip in a 6-month-old girl with a marked restriction of abduction on the left, poorly formed bony acetabulum, flat bony rim, displaced labrum, increased echogenicity of the cartilage rim, eccentric femoral head. Splinting.

22.**23 Type 3b** left hip in a 5-week-old boy, positive family history, breech presentation; α = 38°, poor bony acetabulum, flat bony rim, echogenic cartilage rim, eccentric femoral head. Splinting.

22.**24 a Type 2a** left hip in a 14-day-old boy with restricted abduction, slightly deficient bony acetabulum, α = 52°, rounded bony rim, head centered without provocative test. **b Type 2a/m** in the same patient. Femoral head decentered in dynamic testing: mobile hip, not properly classified as 2a, which would not require treatment. This case requires stabilizing treatment with an abduction pillow or splint. After 6 weeks, the head position is stable.

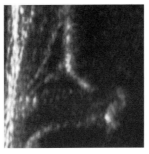
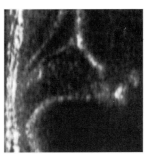

22.**25**   **a Type 2a** left hip in a 2-day-old girl with a foot deformity, unrestricted abduction, α = 52°. Somewhat deficient
acetabular development, rounded bony rim, centered femoral
head. **b Type 2a/m** left hip, same patient. Dynamic provocative
test evoked marked decentering of the femoral head: mobile hip.
Stable position after 4 weeks' treatment with a minisplint.

22.25a   22.25b

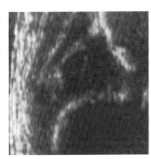
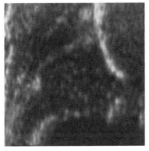
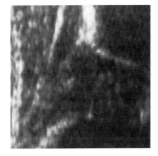

22.26a   22.26b   22.26c

22.**26**   **a Type 3a** left hip in a 10-week-old girl. Breech presentation, lax hip, α = 32°, poorly molded acetabulum, flat bony rim,
eccentric femoral head. **b Type 3a/m** left hip, same patient.
Dynamic test increased eccentricity of the femoral head, unstable position: sonographically mobile hip; treated with minisplint. **c** Same patient after application of minisplint. Head is well
centered in the acetabulum. Here the point of US is to demonstrate secure centering of the greatest femoral head diameter in
the acetabulum; the "classic" view is often unobtainable due to
the abducted limb position.

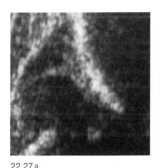
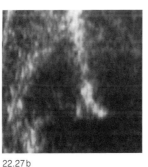
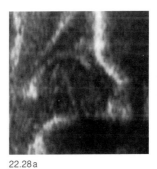
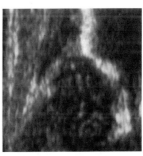

22.27a   22.27b   22.28a   22.28b

22.**27**   **Type 4 (dislocated)** right hip in a 4-day-old boy with
arthrogryposis and clubbed feet. Acetabula clinically empty.
a Acetabulum sonographically empty, acetabular contour poor,
cartilage rim everted, joint capsule tense. Femoral head is outside the acetabulum. **b** Left femoral head is also displaced
laterally upward out of the acetabulum.

22.**28**   **Type 4 (dislocated)** left hip in a 7-day-old boy with a
manually reducible and dislocatable hip. **a** Left hip, poor acetabular development, flat bony rim, displaced labrum, displaced cartilage rim. Clinically reducible, conservative treatment with minisplint. **b** Examination after reduction in abducted position: deep
centering of the femoral head.

22.**29**   **Type 4 (dislocated)** left hip in a 7-week-old girl. Family
doctor felt snap in the hip with clinical dislocation. US shows poor
acetabular development, flat bony rim, deformed labrum and
cartilage rim; femoral head has left the acetabulum. Reduction
and treatment first with flexion harness, then with splint.

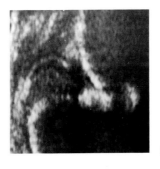

22.29

Special Problems in Hip Sonography

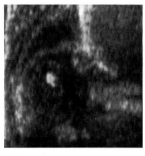 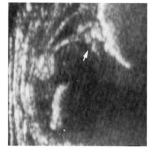

22.30   22.31

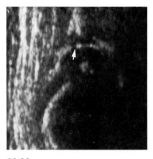

22.32

22.**30** **Type 4 hip with obstructive factor** in a 5-month-old girl. Clinical dislocation, leg length discrepancy, asymmetric skin creases. Poor acetabular configuration, flat bony rim, curved echogenic structure capping the rim. This structure consists of the ligamentum teres and the inverted labrum. Primary deep reduction not possible due to obstructing tissues. Treatment with flexion harness. Follow-up scan did not show deep centering, therefore: open reduction with resection of obstructing tissues.

22.**31** **Type 4 right hip with obstructive factor** in a 5-month-old boy with clinical dislocation. Superolateral position of the femoral head. Several small echoes (arrow) between the femoral head and bony rim: interposed labrum and ligamentum teres. Conservative treatment generally futile: surgery.

22.**32** **Pseudo-obstruction** in a 3-month-old girl with a normally developed hip joint. During examination, a crescent-shaped echogenic band was frequently noted between the acetabular roof and femoral head: vacuum phenomenon caused by traction on the leg; disappeared when traction was released.

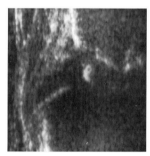 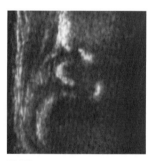

22.33 a   22.33 b

22.**33** **Avascular necrosis after dislocation** of the right hip in a 5-month-old girl treated by splinting (as a newborn) for hip dislocation. **a** US still shows poor acetabular development with rim defect and, most notably, a shortened femoral neck–acetabular distance, signifying flattening of the femoral head; small ossification center. Widened head and elongated acetabular roof. All US findings consistent with avascular necrosis. **b** Normal findings on the left side. Compare **a** with a normal femoral neck–acetabular distance, spherical femoral head, and larger ossific nucleus.

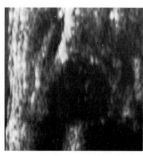 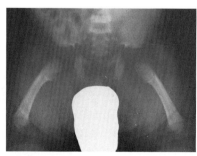

22.34 a   22.34 b

22.**34** **Achondroplastic left hip** in a 13-day-old boy. **a** US: despite patient age, the hip cannot be adequately visualized due to atypical configuration of the acetabulum; horizontal course of the acetabular roof not demonstrable. In such rare cases pelvic radiographs and clinical findings are essential for making a diagnosis. **b** Pelvic radiograph: achondroplasia (Dr. Emons, Bonn).

Monitoring Response to Treatment of Dysplasia and Dislocation

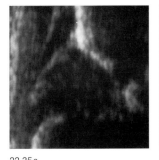 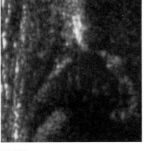 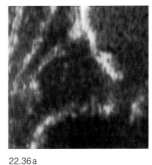 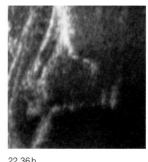

22.35a   22.35b   22.36a   22.36b

22.**35 a Type 2a** right hip in an 8-day-old girl with a positive family history, no clinical abnormalities. Abduction diapering. **b** Ten weeks later: normal findings. Normalization within 5 weeks is common in type 2a hips.

22.**36 a Type 3a** left hip in a 6-week-old girl. No clinical abnormalities. **b** After 2 months' splinting: normal findings.

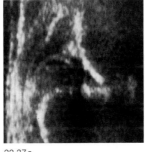 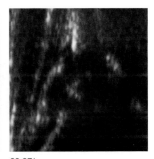

22.**37 a Type 3a/m** right hip in a 2-month-old girl with restricted abduction on the right. Several months' splinting. **b** Nine months later: normal findings with central ossification of the femoral head.

22.37a   22.37b

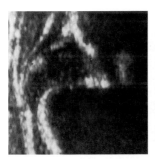 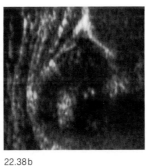 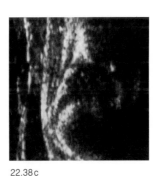

22.38a   22.38b   22.38c

22.**38 a Type 3a** left hip in a 6-week-old boy with restricted abduction on the left, clinically stable. Treated with minisplint for 4 weeks. **b** Four weeks later, improvement to type 2a. Further treatment with abduction pillow. **c** After 6 weeks in abduction pillow, type 1a.

22.**39 a Type 4 dislocation** of the right hip in a 2-week-old girl with a clinically dislocatable hip; primary reduction, retention with minisplint. **b** After 2 months' treatment, the hip is clinically and sonographically normal.

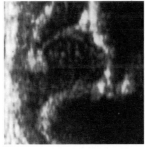 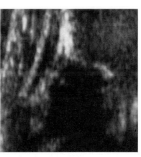

22.39a   22.39b

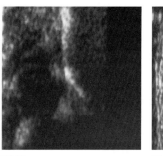

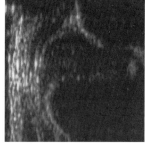

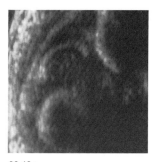

22.40a

22.40b

22.40c

22.40 a Type 4 dislocation. of the left hip in a 1-month-old girl with a clinically dislocated hip, reducible, splint therapy. **b** Ten weeks later: US progress check in splint confirms centering.

c Hip redislocated after splint removal, necessitating open reduction.

23 Transducers, Image Quality, Artifacts

K. Seitz

Transducers

Because of its superior resolution, the best overall transducer for pediatric ultrasound imaging is the 5-MHz transducer, although higher-frequency units may be appropriate for special applications. Also, it is good to have a system with both linear-array and sector-scanning options, as these transducers supplement each other (Table 23.**1**). Curved-array and trapezoid scanners represent a compromise between these two transducer types and may correspond more to a linear-array or sector scanner depending on their size.

Special applications such as hip sonography are done chiefly with linear scanners, whereas transfontanelle cranial sonography can be performed effectively only with a sector scanner or very small trapezoid scanner.

Equipment Quality

The quality of ultrasound equipment can be appraised in terms of objective and subjective parameters. The objective quality of an ultrasound image depends on physical resolution, dynamic range, and gray-scale resolution.

Physical resolution is largely a function of transducer technology. There are two components to physical resolution: axial resolution in the direction of sound propagation (x-axis) and lateral resolution, which is poorer than axial resolution by a factor of 2−3. Resolution on the z-axis is usually disregarded, since ultrasound waves are not emitted in a parallel pattern but as a lobe-shaped beam with three dimensions.

The factors critical for optimum resolution are the quality of the array technology, the number of elements and their excitation pattern, and the focusing technique. Among sector scanners, phased-array devices are not inherently superior to the mechanical types.

High resolution takes time. The best scanners at present (devices with a large aperture or annular array) give their best resolution when the frame rate is relatively low (about 8 per second). This slow image rate is not a problem in the examination of stationary organs (e. g., in transfontanelle cranial sonography), but it is quite unsatisfactory for cardiac examinations. In the abdomen, the relatively slow organ movements associated with respiration lead to significant blurriness resulting from motion.

In currently manufactured equipment, the number of gray levels (usually 64) is no longer a limiting factor in terms of resolution.

The dynamic range of the equipment determines how well echoes of similar intensities can be discriminated. Small intensity differences can determine whether a focal hepatic lesion, for example, can or cannot be detected. An adjustable dynamic range is available in higher-quality systems.

Some systems have a zoom feature that provides enhanced resolution within a designated region. Ultimately, however, resolution is limited by pixel size and monitor resolution. The latter in turn depends not just on the spacing of the screen lines but also on the transverse resolution of the CRT (cathode-ray tube).

Table 23.**1** Comparison of sector and linear-array scanners

	Advantages	Disadvantages
Sector	− small acoustic window − expanded lateral view − better, continuous visualization of canalicular structures − compression can be used to displace or bypass gas-containing bowel − better proximity (enabling use of higher-frequency scanner)	− poor near field − poor deep resolution − organ distortion from firm probe pressure − fewer landmarks for orientation
Linear-array	− good near field − uniform resolution throughout image area − little organ deformation by transducer − palpation under vision − more landmarks for orientation	− requires large acoustic window − greater disturbance from gas bubbles and rib shadows

The resolution and dynamics of a system can be objectively tested with various tissue-simulating phantoms, which ordinarily are not available to the physician. But there are also subjective criteria that can provide a very good assessment of image quality. For example, a high-resolution scanner should be able to define small-caliber blood vessels, the pancreatic duct, and the layers of the intestinal wall. The operator can quickly confirm proper imaging dynamics by differentiating the renal cortex and medullary pyramids. Near- and far-field image quality also should be checked. Abdominal wall structures, the hepatic anterior surface, and the thyroid gland occupy the near field of the transducer, while the subphrenic portions of the liver are in the far field.

Accuracy of Measurements

The accuracy of morphometric measurements on sonograms depends on the physical resolution of the equipment, but an even mor critical factor is the accuracy with which the scan plane is positioned by the examiner.

As a rule it is advantageous to perform necessary measurements along the axis of the sound beam (accuracy approximately ± 1 mm). This is not always possible, however, and the less favorable lateral resolution becomes a factor in ultrasound measurements of kidney length. This can easily result in errors of approximately 5–6 mm.

Particular difficulties are posed by the measurement of vascular diameters. High-intensity wall echoes appear larger than their true anatomic size on B-mode displays ("blooming effect"). This error is minimized by using the "inner-to-outer" measuring technique and is significant only when distances are small (< 7 mm); this technique consistently results in an overestimation of about 0.5 mm.

The greatest errors result from improper plane selection and thus are examiner-dependent.

Imaging Errors and Artifacts

Sonographic imaging is based on the pulse-echo principle and the greatly simplified assumption that ultrasound waves propagate uniformly through soft tissues. While this is not true, the slight differences in travel time generally are not significant because they are below the resolving power of the scanning equipment (exception: thickness compression artifact).

Ultrasound waves, which cannot be collimated into a truly parallel beam, are subject to reflection, refraction, scattering, absorption, and diffraction. These physical processes give rise to a variety of imaging errors and artifacts. Most artifacts are lost in the normal echo pattern due to their very low intensity.

Total Reflection and Absorption

Total reflection and absorption lead to the most familiar imaging artifact, the acoustic shadow. Large, abrupt impedance changes at interfaces between soft tissues and bone or gas lead to the production of a high-amplitude echo. On encountering such an interface, all of the ultrasound energy is reflected or reflected and absorbed. As a result, structures located behind this barrier (as seen from the transducer) are not reached by the sound. Hence they do not generate echoes, and an echo-free zone—the acoustic shadow—is seen.

On the one hand, this phenomenon can be very troublesome in examinations because it can obscure structures of interest. Yet in many cases acoustic shadowing can be utilized diagnostically as a means of identifying gallstones, renal calculi, calcifications in tissues, abnormal gas collections associated with ileus or gastrointestinal perforation, and abscesses that contain gas-forming microorganisms (Figs. 23.**1**, 23.**2**).

Not every calculus and calcification casts an acoustic shadow. This depends on the relationship between the spatial extent of the object and the transmitted ultrasound frequency. Higher-frequency ultrasound waves lead to acoustic shadowing from smaller calculi. Reflector geometry is also a factor, and more prominent acoustic shadows are seen with orthograde insonation.

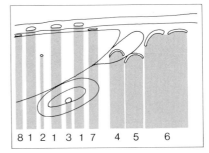

23.**1** Potentially troublesome and diagnostically helpful acoustic shadows in the right upper abdomen. 1 = Rib shadow, 2 = parenchymal calcification in the liver, 3 = kidney stone, 4 = gallstone, 5 = duodenum, 6 = colon, 7 = pleural sinus (also visible as a reverberation), 8 = free air due to gastrointestinal perforation; **DD**: the Chilaiditi syndrome (also creates reverberation).

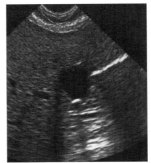 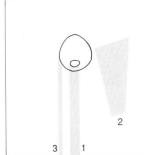

23.**2** Different types of acoustic shadow. 1 = Acoustic shadow behind a gallstone, 2 = partial shadow cast by duodenal air, 3 = edge shadowing.

Attenuation

Ultrasound energy is attenuated by absorption as it passes through tissue, and returning echoes must be amplified as a function of their travel time (time gain compensation). Increased attenuation also may signify organic changes such as hepatic fibrosis. So far, attenuation has not been quantitatively analyzed or diagnostically utilized.

Refraction and Scattering

In accordance with Snell's law of refraction, ultrasound waves deviate from a straight path when they cross an interface between dissimilar tissues. This alters both the path of the beam and the travel time of the echo. As a result, identical reflectors in soft tissue may be displayed at different coordinates in the B-mode image. The positioning error may be as large as 10–12 mm at a depth of 10 cm. This artifact can become significant in duplex and position-locating systems, especially in obese patients.

Reverberations

If echoes return to the transducer on a direct path after undergoing multiple reflections, the image spot will be displayed twice: once in its correct position, and a second time incorrectly, at twice its actual range, due to a doubling of the travel time (Fig. 23.**3**). Multiple occurrence of this phenomenon leads to reverberations, which are easily recognized by their geometric arrangement. An example is the reverberations that occur from the layers of the abdominal wall, which can obscure the superficial portions of the liver and make them difficult to evaluate (Fig. 23.**4**).

If the reflected signal returns by a different path, its positioning on the display will be altered in accordance with its travel time and the receiver position. *"Multipath"* echoes of this kind are much more difficult to assign. This artifact can cause a cyst, for example, to appear echogenic and be misinterpreted as a solid lesion (Fig. 23.**5**).

The *comet-tail* or *ring-down artifact* (Fig. 23.**6**) is a special type of reverberation occurring in closely adjacent, often plane-parallel boundary layers, especially those containing a thin fluid or gas film. It occurs at the pleural sinuses, at thin air layers (e. g., air in the bile ducts, intestinal air, free air from gastrointestinal perforation), at intrauterine devices and, to a lesser degree, in association with cholesteatosis of the gallbladder due to cholesterol deposits in the gallbladder wall. Seen consistently at the pleural sinuses, these artifacts are considered to have substantial diagnostic value.

Mirror-image artifacts occur at smooth interfaces, most notably the diaphragm (Figs. 23.**7**, 23.**8**), and can mimic a weakly echogenic effusion or pleural induration. With this and many other artifacts, confusion can often be dispelled by scanning the same region from a different acoustic window. The change in echo geometry will cause the artifact to disappear or at least alter its position.

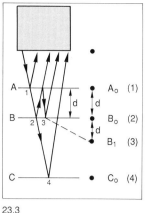
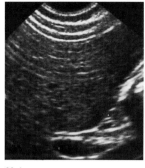

23.3

23.4

23.**3** Reverberations. The echo reflected from layer B is again partially reflected at layer A on its way to the array and undergoes a second reflection at B before returning to the source.

23.**4** Classic ripple pattern of reverberations caused by multiple relfections at the abdominal wall layers.

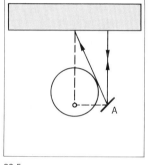
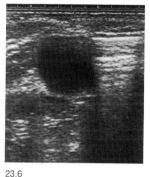

23.5

23.6

23.**5** A cystic area appears falsely echogenic when strong reflectors nearby generate "multipath" echoes.

23.**6** Ring-down artifact caused by duodenal air.

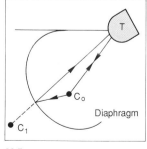
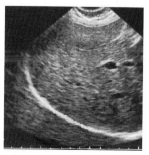

23.7

23.8

23.**7** Generation of a mirror-image artifact.

23.**8** Projection of hepatic structure onto the diaphragm due to a mirror-image artifact.

Duplication artifacts are similar to mirror-image artifacts. They result from the fact that certain anatomic structures behave as acoustic lenses.

Curvature artifacts appear when multiple elements in a transducer array receive echoes from the same reflector (Figs. 23.**9**, 23.**10**). The slight discrepancies in travel times and attenuation produce a curving effect that can be especially troublesome in the examination of fluid-filled organs and cavities. A typical example is the appearance of peripheral echoes in the gallbladder lumen due to adjacent duodenal air (Fig. 23.**11**). These echoes can easily be mistaken for small calculi, polyps, or sludge (Fig. 23.**12**).

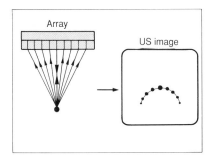

23.**9** Curvature artifact. Multiple elements in the array receive echoes from the same reflector, causing the artifactual display of a curved line.

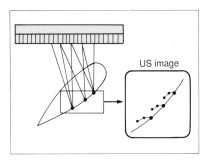

23.**10** Multiple faint curvature artifacts cause blurriness of, e. g., the gallbladder wall.

Edge Shadowing Artifact

Edge shadowing occurs when the ultrasound beam encounters the smooth, curved surface of a cystic structure. Due to the low surface roughness of the structure (e. g., a normal gallbladder wall), the reflected component is too weak to be displayed as an image spot (Figs. 23.**2**, 23.**13**, 23.**14**). The dearth of tangential echo return results in the appearance of a thin edge shadow. This artifact can be observed about all smooth-walled cysts, the gallbladder, as well as blood vessels that are cut transversely by the scan. An edge shadow from the gallbladder may be erroneously attributed to a stone.

Range artifacts occur because the propagation of ultrasound waves is not confined to the selected penetration depth. Echoes from strong reflectors deeply located may be assigned to a "wrong generation" of returning echoes and therefore incorrectly positioned on the display.

Thickness Compression Artifact

Thickness compression artifact is a travel-time artifact typically occurring when the ultrasound beam traverses the cartilage in the region of the costal arch. The velocity of sound propagation is about 1.5 to 2 times faster in the cartilage than in other soft tissues. Ultrasound waves traversing the cartilage layer at twice their usual velocity reach their receivers significantly ahead of the waves that have traversed other tissues. This results in an apparent protuberance of the

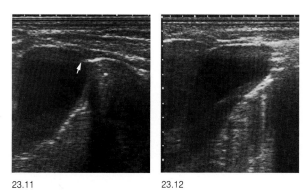

23.11   23.12

23.**11** Curvature artifact causes echoes to appear at the periphery of the gallbladder (arrow).

23.**12** Curvature artifact simulating gallbladder sludge.

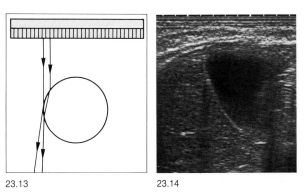

23.13   23.14

23.**13** Edge shadowing artifact. Deficient reflection as the smooth surfaces struck tangentially by the beam produces a thin acoustic shadow.

23.**14** Faint shadow at the left edge of the gallbladder accompanied by section thickness artifact at its anterior surface.

hepatic anterior surface deep to the costal cartilage. Combined with increased attenuation, this effect can cause the tissue underlying the cartilage to appear less echogenic, and it may be interpreted as a metastasis (Fig. 23.**15**). Conversely, extensive fat layers transmit ultrasound more slowly, thereby increasing the travel time and causing an apparent increase in range.

Side-lobe artifacts are rarely significant due to the very low energy content of the side lobes compared with the main lobe of the sound field. However, these artifacts may become significant when they arise from strong reflectors close to the transducer.

Section Thickness Artifact

Section thickness artifact results from the fact that the interrogating beam is not infinitely thin; the scan plane has a finite thickness of 2−4 mm depending on resolution and focusing. If an image point depicts a portion of the scan plane where there is adjacent solid and liquid material, an averaged gray level will be displayed, and the associated contour of the cyst or bladder will appear blurred (Fig. 23.**16**, see Fig. 23.**14**). The "thicker" the image slice, i. e., the poorer the physical resolution, the more pronounced the effect. These artifacts most commonly occur when the beam strikes the boundaries of a liquid structure at an oblique angle. Curvature artifacts often coexist.

Imaging Errors due to Organ Deformation

Indentation of the abdominal wall by a small transducer (sector, curved-array) can distort organ contours and alter the course of blood vessels. This is a "palpation effect" that can be utilized, for example, to evaluate the consistency of the liver (Figs. 23.**17**, 23.**18**).

Acoustic Enhancement

When ultrasound waves travel through a fluid-filled space, the absence of reflective interfaces causes less attenuation of the ultrasound compared with adjacent sound waves traversing normal soft tissues. Given equal degrees of time gain compensation, the nonattenuated waves distant from the transducer will produce echoes of relatively greater amplitude. This is not a true artifact, but the result of sound passing through a weakly attenuating structure. This effect is consistently observed behind cysts, the gallbladder, and the urinary bladder.

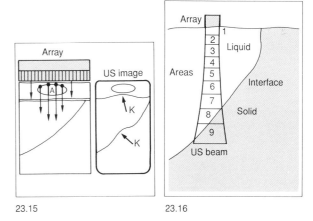

23.15   23.16

23.**15**   Thickness compression artifact causes an apparent contour distortion (K). A = region where sound propagates at twice the normal velocity.

23.**16**   Section thickness artifact. Areas 1−6 are echo-free, while areas 7−9 display an averaged gray level and so are not echo-free. A reliable cystic/solid differentiation cannot be made in this region.

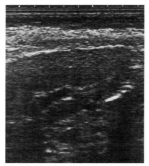 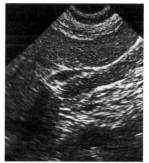

23.17   23.18

23.**17**   Biconvex liver (linear array).

23.**18**   Indentation of the anterior hepatic contour by pressure from a sector scanner (same scan plane and patient as in Fig. 23.**17**).

References

Avruch, L., P. L. Cooperberg: The ring-down artefact. J. Ultrasound Med. 4 (1985) 21

Bönhof, J. A., B. Bönhof, P. Linhart: Acoustic dispercing lenses cause artificial discontinuities in B-mode ultrasonogramms. J. Ultrasound Med. 3 (1984) 5

Bönhof, J. A., B. Bönhof, E. G. Loch: Schallkeulendimension als Artefaktursache bei der B-Bild-Sonographie. Ultraschall 5 (1984) 66

Bönhof, J. A., P. Linhart, E. G. Loch: Doppelbilder bei der B-Bild-Sonographie durch akustische Zerstreuungslinsen. Ultraschall 5 (1984) 63

Born, H. J., H. Sauer, E. Halberstadt: Mehrfachbildungsartefakte bei Linearschallköpfen. Ultraschall 5 (1984) 56

Cosgrove, D. O., P. Garbutt, C. R. Hill: Echos across the diaphragm. Ultrasound Med. Biol. 3 (1978) 385

Goldstein, A., B. L. Madrazo: Slice-thickness artifacts in gray-scale ultrasound. J. clin. Ultrasound 9 (1981) 365

Müller, N., P. L. Cooperberg, V. A. Rowly, J. Mayo, B. Ho, D. K. B. Li: Ultrasound refraction by the rectus abdominis muscles, the double image artifact. J. Ultrasound Med. 3 (1984) 515

Powis, L. R., W. J. Powis: A Thinkers Guide to Ultrasonic Imaging. Urban & Schwarzenberg, München 1984

Ziskin, M. C., D. I. Thickman, N. J. Goldenberg, M. S. Lapayowker, J. M. Becker: The comet-tail artifact J. Ultrasound Med. 1 (1982) 1

Index